Surgical Advances in Gynecology

Surgical Advances in Gynecology

Editor: Florence McClure

AMERICAN
MEDICAL PUBLISHERS
www.americanmedicalpublishers.com

AMERICAN
MEDICAL PUBLISHERS
www.americanmedicalpublishers.com

Cataloging-in-Publication Data

Surgical advances in gynecology / edited by Florence McClure.
p. cm.
Includes bibliographical references and index.
ISBN 978-1-63927-500-7
1. Generative organs, Female--Surgery. 2. Gynecology. 3. Surgery. I. McClure, Florence.
RG104 .S87 2022
618.105 9--dc23

American Medical Publishers,
41 Flatbush Avenue,
1st Floor, New York,
NY 11217, USA

ISBN 978-1-63927-500-7 (Hardback)

Contents

Preface

The world is advancing at a fast pace like never before. Therefore, the need is to keep up with the latest developments. This book was an idea that came to fruition when the specialists in the area realized the need to coordinate together and document essential themes in the subject. That's when I was requested to be the editor. Editing this book has been an honour as it brings together diverse authors researching on different streams of the field. The book collates essential materials contributed by veterans in the area which can be utilized by students and researchers alike.

Gynecological surgery is performed on the female reproductive system for the treatment of benign conditions, incontinence, infertility and cancer. It may also be performed for cosmetic and elective purposes. Some of the procedures included in the scope of gynecological surgery include appendectomy, dilation and curettage, tubal ligation, oophorectomy, hysteroscopy, etc. The techniques of exploratory laparotomy are used for the investigation of the progression of benign or malignant disease, or for the assessment and repair of the damage to the pelvic organs. Laparoscopy has clinical applications such as in the diagnosis and treatment of abdominal and pelvic pain. Minimally invasive gynecologic surgery is used for the treatment and evaluation of noncancerous gynecological conditions including irregular menstrual periods, heavy menstrual periods, ovarian cysts, pelvic pain and endometriosis. This book discusses the fundamentals as well as modern approaches of gynecology. It unfolds the innovative aspects of gynecology and women's health which will be crucial for the progress of this field in the future. The extensive content of this book provides the readers with a thorough understanding of the subject.

Each chapter is a sole-standing publication that reflects each author´s interpretation. Thus, the book displays a multi-facetted picture of our current understanding of application, resources and aspects of the field. I would like to thank the contributors of this book and my family for their endless support.

Editor

1

Combining NovaSure® endometrial ablation and Essure® hysteroscopic sterilization: a feasibility study to evaluate the confirmation tests

R. J. Detollenaere · M. P. H. Vleugels · H. W. F. van Eijndhoven

Abstract Since NovaSure® endometrial ablation (GEA) is not reliable as contraception, a reliable permanent contraceptive method which can be offered during the same operative session is often preferred by patients. We present a series of 24 patients treated by NovaSure® GEA followed by Essure® hysteroscopic sterilization at the same session. Bilateral placement of the micro-inserts after GEA was successful in all 24 patients. Confirmation by ultrasound and plain X-ray of the pelvis indicated a correct position in all 48 tubes. Routine follow-up by hysterosalpingography (HSG) to document bilateral tubal occlusion was only possible in 17/23 (74%) patients; these 34 tubes were blocked. In 6/23 (26%) patients, tubal occlusion could not be determined by HSG because of minimal filling of the uterine cavity with contrast medium. The latter was caused by severe uterine synechiae. All patients were satisfied with the result of GEA at 3 months; 19 women (83%) reported amenorrhea and the others, a strong reduction in menstrual blood loss. The combination of Essure® hysteroscopic sterilization and NovaSure® GEA is feasible and safe. However, after this combined approach the HSG as confirmation test is not always useful because of severe synechiae.

Keywords Endometrial ablation · NovaSure® · Hysteroscopic sterilization · Essure® · Hysterosalpingography

R. J. Detollenaere · H. W. F. van Eijndhoven (✉)
Isala klinieken,
P.O. Box 10400, 8000 GK Zwolle,
The Netherlands
e-mail: h.w.f.van.eijndhoven@isala.nl

M. P. H. Vleugels
Rivierenland hospital,
Tiel, The Netherlands

Introduction

NovaSure® bipolar impedance-controlled GEA (Cytyc/Hologic, Palo Alto, CA, USA) is a safe and effective method to resolve heavy menstrual bleeding [1]. Radiofrequency energy destroys the regenerative ability of the endometrium and creates an iatrogenic Asherman's syndrome [2]. Patients treated with GEA tend to develop an amenorrheic state in 48–75%, which is persistent even 5 years after the operation [3, 4].

Though risk of pregnancy is low, endometrial ablation cannot be regarded as an anticonceptive method [5]. In case of pregnancy after GEA, the risk of miscarriage, preterm delivery, and abnormal placental attachment is increased [6, 7]. Because contraception after GEA is necessary, patients may prefer a permanent form of birth control.

Essure® sterilization (Conceptus, Inc, San Carlos, CA, USA) is a minimally invasive hysteroscopic technique for permanent tubal occlusion. This procedure can be performed without anesthesia [8]. The inserts in the fallopian tubes induce an inflammatory response, causing occlusion of the intramural part of the fallopian tubes 3 months after placement. Advantages of this method compared to laparoscopic sterilization are obvious because it is less invasive with lower cost and shorter recovery time and hospitalization [9–11].

Recently, two studies presenting data of the combined approach of Essure® hysteroscopic sterilization and NovaSure® endometrial ablation were published [12, 13]. It was recommended to perform the hysteroscopic sterilization after GEA because the Essure® micro-inserts could potentially conduct the radiofrequency energy thereby damaging the surrounding tissue. Although GEA is known for its capacity to create Asherman's syndrome follow-up by HSG showed only mild synechiae in 24% of the patients and subtle filling defects in 33% of the cases [12]. The HSG as confirmation test was not impaired by the adhesions. Follow-up by 3D ultrasound was also described and considered to be reliable [13].

After an uneventful Essure®-only procedure, it is common in the Netherlands to confirm correct placement by transvaginal ultrasound 3 months after the procedure under the strict condition that a validated protocol is followed to recognize improper placements [14]. In this Dutch protocol follow-up by HSG after 3 months is only required in case of unsatisfactory placement.

The objective of this study was to evaluate the feasibility and results of Essure® hysteroscopic sterilization combined with NovaSure® endometrial ablation as well as to determine the effectiveness of transvaginal 2D ultrasound and hysterosalpingography in documenting proper localization of the micro-inserts and tubal occlusion.

Material and methods

In the period of April 2007 to July 2009 24 patients with menorraghia and the desire for permanent contraception underwent GEA followed by hysteroscopic Essure® sterilization. Pre-operatively, all patients underwent transvaginal ultrasound and endometrial sampling when indicated. Patients were excluded for the following conditions: suspected endometrial carcinoma, submucous myomas, polyps larger than 2 cm, abnormal uterine sounding length, and active pelvic inflammatory disease or hydrosalpinx. All procedures were performed under general anesthesia. To decrease the amount of post-ablation debris, they were timed in the early follicular phase of the menstrual cycle. The endometrium was not routinely pretreated with progesterone. The combination of any GEA and placement of a foreign body can increase the risk of chronic infection [15]. Therefore all patients received a prophylactic dose of antibiotics (Cefazolin/Metronidazole). Before GEA, a standard hysteroscopy, using a 4.3- or 4.9-mm CF hysteroscope (Karl Storz, Germany), was performed to identify the tubal ostia and to confirm the absence of intracavitary abnormalities. After GEA, the hysteroscope was reinserted and the tubal ostia were visualized. The Essure® micro-inserts were placed according to manufacturer's instructions. Procedure time (minutes) was registered as the time between the insertion of the hysteroscope before the GEA till the moment that the scope was withdrawn from the vagina after the sterilization. All procedures in our hospital were performed by the same gynecologist who was experienced and skilled to perform GEA, hysteroscopic Essure® sterilization, and transvaginal ultrasound detection of the micro-inserts. He also reviewed the HSG images together with a member of the radiology department. Until Essure® sterilization was proven to be successful, all patients were advised to use alternative contraception.

The choice of the confirmation test was based on the standard protocol used in the Netherlands for the Essure®-only procedure. In this protocol the confirmation test is limited to ultrasound after 3 months in uncomplicated procedures. Whether or not placement of the Essure® micro-inserts is considered as complicated depends on the number of coils in the uterine cavity, procedure time, and resistance during the insertion. In case of unsatisfactory placement ultrasound is performed after 1 month and HSG after 3 months. This protocol is validated [14] and the choice for ultrasound after 1 month inspired by the idea that it is not rational to wait for 3 months when ultrasound already demonstrates abnormal placement. For safety reasons, we considered the combined GEA and Essure procedure as "complicated" and performed a transvaginal ultrasound after 1 month. Placement was considered to be successful in case the reflections of the micro-insert crossed the outer line of the uterine wall and the proximal ends of both devices were visualized inside the outer line or in the region of the endometrial cavity [14]. The HSG after 3 months was done in an outpatient setting by the same gynecologist who performed the operative procedure. We started the HSG with a plain pelvic X-ray and used lipiodol as contrast medium. Most important objective of a HSG is to evaluate the relationship of the proximal end of the inner coil of the micro-insert to the uterine cornua. Only when maximal distension of the cornua is achieved and contrast meets or obscures the proximal portions of the Essure® micro-insert, a HSG can be used to evaluate tubal occlusion [16]. HSG was thought to be satisfactory when (1) both micro-inserts were visible with <50% of the length of the inner coil trailing into the cavity, (2) the proximal ends of the inner coils appear to be <30 mm into the tube from where the contrast fills the uterine cornua, and (3) no contrast visible in the tubes beyond micro-inserts or in the peritoneal cavity [16]. At the follow-up visit after 3 months rate of satisfaction with the outcome of the procedure was evaluated using a three point scale: very satisfied, satisfied, and unsatisfied. Monthly blood loss was recorded as: amenorrhea, bleeding less than before treatment, bleeding same as before treatment, and bleeding more than before treatment. Amenorrhoea was defined as cessation of bleeding immediately after ablation until the control visit at least 3 months after the procedure.

Results

The mean age of the 24 patients was 39 years (32–46) and mean parity 2.1 (range 0–5). Eighteen women had previously received medical therapy for their bleeding disorder: oral contraceptives (22%) or a levonorgestrel IUD (72%). The procedure time ranged between 5 min and 25 min (mean 10.6 min±5), including hysteroscopy before GEA. Bilateral placement of the micro-inserts after GEA was successful on the initial attempt in all 24 patients. All tubal ostia could be identified with one to six expanded Essure® coils visible trailing in the uterine cavity after placement. No complications occurred per- or postoperatively and all patients were discharged the same day (Fig. 1).

It was possible to identify all micro-inserts with transvaginal ultrasound in all women 4 weeks after the procedure. All micro-inserts appeared to be in good position. After this initial ultrasound examination at 4 weeks, one patient was lost for follow-up, so 23 patients received a pelvic X-ray and HSG 3 months after the procedure. The plain pelvic X-ray documented appropriate placement of both micro-inserts in all 23 patients. The HSG could be done properly in 17 patients (74%) and documented bilateral tubal occlusion in all these 17 patients (Fig. 2a). In these patients, no patent tubes or spill of contrast in the peritoneal cavity was found. In the other six patients (26%), HSG demonstrated minimal contrast medium in the uterine cavity probably caused by severe uterine synechiae. Tubal occlusion could not be determined by HSG in these patients (Fig. 2b, c).

No pregnancies were reported during follow-up. All patients were satisfied with the result of the GEA 3 months after procedure; 83% of the women reported amenorrhea, while 17% had a strong reduction in menstrual blood loss (bleeding less than before treatment). One patient returned after 10 months because of dysmenorrhea, which already existed before the procedure. Although she had significantly reduced loss of blood each month, this patient underwent a vaginal hysterectomy. Histological examination of the uterus revealed the presence of severe adenomyosis. In a second patient, a diagnostic hysteroscopy was performed 14 months after the combined procedure for reason of pain. The uterine cavity was not accessible due to an Asherman's syndrome. This finding was compatible with her amenorrhea and her complaints resolved spontaneously after a while. The third patient came back after 7 months with complaints of cyclic abdominal pain. In this patient the 3-month follow-up HSG failed because of synechiae. Transvaginal ultrasound showed hematometra due to Asherman's syndrome. The uterus was drained of 200 ml blood after which treatment the complaints resolved completely.

Discussion

NovaSure® endometrial ablation is a safe and effective alternative to hysterectomy for women with menorraghia when treatment with oral medication or levonorgestrel IUD fails [3, 4]. Because pregnancy is still possible after GEA, with higher risk of complications, supplementary contraception is necessary. Advantage of Essure® hysteroscopic sterilization is the transcervical approach with its minimal invasive properties.

This study demonstrates that combination of Essure® hysteroscopic sterilization and NovaSure® GEA is easy to perform and safe for women with persistent menorraghia and

Fig. 1 Study design

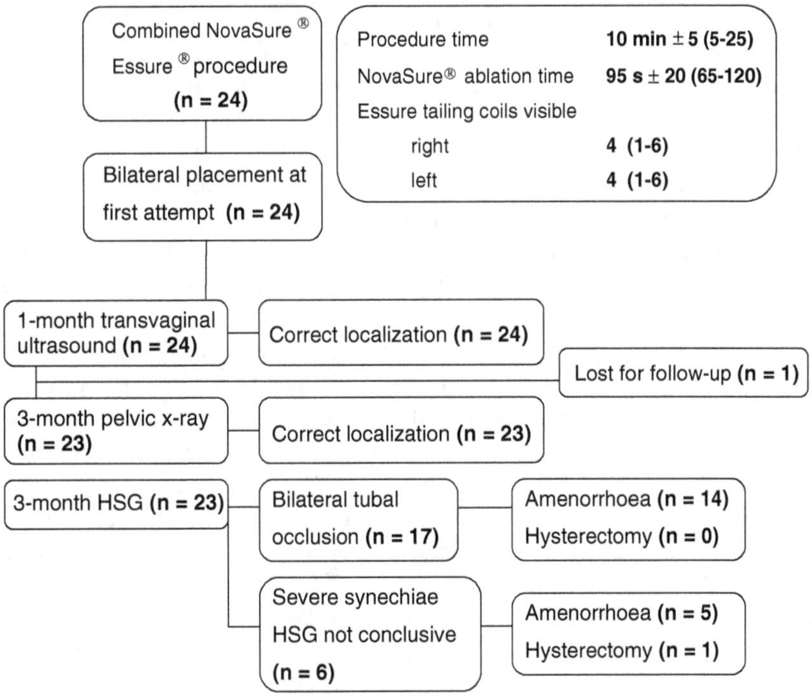

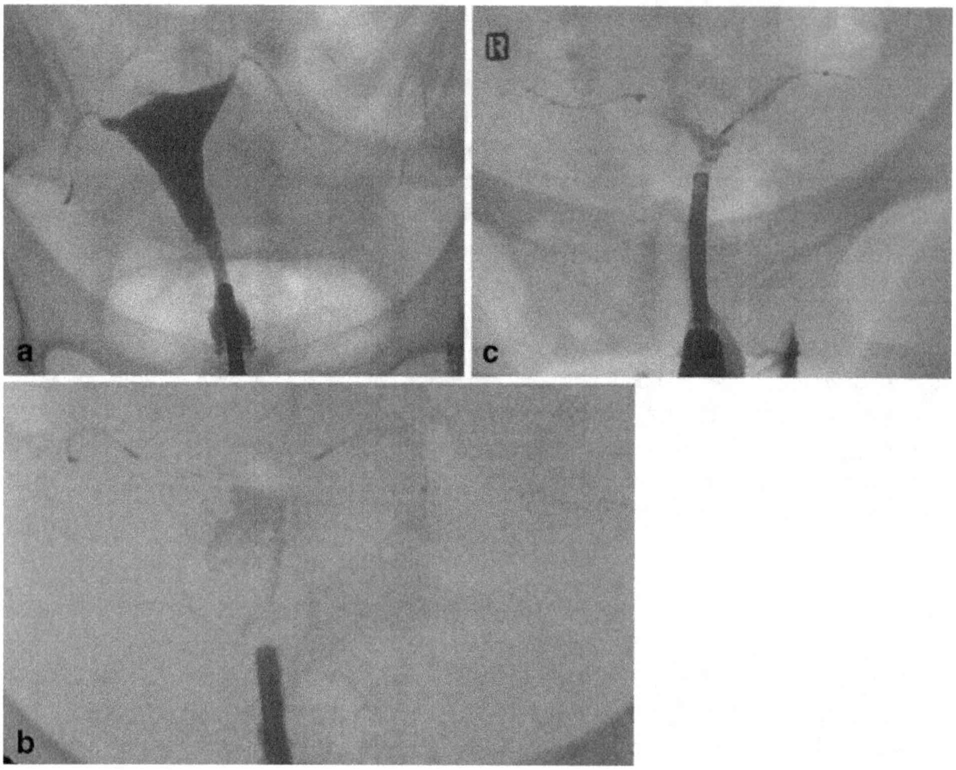

Fig. 2 HSG image after combined NovaSure® / Essure® procedure. **a** HSG showing proper localization of both micro-inserts, good filling of the uterine cavity, and no contrast visible in the tubes beyond micro-inserts or in the peritoneal cavity. **b** HSG performed at 3 months follow-up after an uncomplicated combined procedure. Normal visualization and location of Essure® inserts. Almost no distension of the uterine cavity by the contrast medium. **c** HSG 3 months after the combined procedure with almost no filling of the uterine cavity

wish for permanent contraception. No complications occurred and mean procedure time was short. All patients were (very) satisfied at 3 months follow-up and a high amenorrhea rate was reported. In our study, one adverse event (hematometra) was reported. A recent Cochrane review concluded that women undergoing newer ablative procedures are less likely to have fluid overload, uterine perforation, cervical lacerations and hematometra than women undergoing the more traditional procedures [17]. Although the risk for an adverse outcome is low for NovaSure® GEA, it is possible that a combined procedure may increase the risk for hematometra and eventually hysterectomy.

Transvaginal ultrasound and pelvic X-ray revealed a proper placement of all micro-inserts. However, these techniques are not yet validated as confirmation test for the combined procedure. On the other hand, the HSG as confirmation test was not conclusive in 26% of the women. Severe uterine synechiae hampered a sufficient filling with contrast medium of the uterine cavity. It was therefore impossible to determine both the proper placement of the micro-inserts and the occlusion of the fallopian tubes.

Only one other study has been published with a comparable number of patients with the GEA followed by Essure® sterilization [12]. In that study successful Essure® sterilization after GEA was achieved in all 25 patients. In contrast to our data, the authors reported only mild synechiae not interfering with the ability to document proper placement of the micro-inserts. They were able to assess tubal blockage by HSG in 90% of cases and tubal patency in 10%.

The advantages of the transvaginal ultrasound compared to pelvic X-ray and HSG are no radiation exposure, more comfortable examination, and lower costs. Ultrasound has the ability to locate the device and visualize its relationship with surrounding tissue. Contrast infusion sonography (CIS) is another technique to assess micro-insert placement in the post-Essure® setting. In a pilot study with a small sample, the authors concluded that CIS has comparable accuracy to HSG [18]. Although pelvic X-ray and transvaginal ultrasound can demonstrate proper placement of the micro-inserts, tubal occlusion can only be determined by HSG.

In the Dutch protocol follow-up by HSG after 3 months is only required in case of unsatisfactory placement [14]. Follow-up according to this protocol after a combined procedure will reduce the number of useless HSG's by synechiae as confirmation test. However, in case of unsatisfactory placement HSG remains the gold standard for determination of tubal occlusion. In this perspective, we have to consider a different sequence of procedures. That is to say, to start with the hysteroscopic sterilization and in case of an uneventful placement as defined in this protocol, continue immediately with the GEA, followed by ultrasound after 3 months. In case an HSG is needed according to the criteria of the Dutch protocol, GEA could be postponed until after the 3-month HSG. Performing GEA after Essure® sterilization implicates a theoretical risk of thermal injury of the tubes or intraperitoneal organs by the energy conductance over the micro-inserts. However, there is growing evidence that this risk is negligible. In a series of 77 patients GEA after hysteroscopic Essure®

sterilization turned out to be safe and well tolerated [19]. In a perihysterectomy safety study, GEA after Essure® sterilization was found to cause no thermal serosal injury. The rise in serosal temperature during GEA was similar in the tubes with and without an Essure micro-insert [20].

Whether the above-mentioned Dutch protocol is applicable for the group of patients described in this feasibility study has to be evaluated. In this evaluation study, the Essure® sterilization is done first after which the type of confirmation test needed according the Dutch protocol decides whether the GEA is performed in the same session or after the 3-month HSG.

Today, all combined procedures in our hospital are performed under general anesthesia thereby adding costs and risks to the treatment. Recent studies demonstrated that Essure® hysteroscopic sterilization was feasible and safe in the outpatient setting [8, 9, 21, 22]. NovaSure® GEA can also be performed without problems in an office setting [23]. Therefore, it is interesting to conduct a randomized controlled trial comparing pain and acceptance of the combined approach in the inpatient and outpatient setting.

In conclusion, NovaSure® endometrial ablation followed by Essure hysteroscopic sterilization is feasible and safe. Transvaginal ultrasound and pelvic radiography are effective methods to confirm proper localization of bilateral micro-inserts after combined procedure. Proper follow-up by HSG is not always possible because of impairment by synechiae. Whether or not the sequence of both treatments can be changed to bypass the difficulty in performing and evaluating the HSG remains to be validated.

Declaration of interest R.J. Detollenaere reports no conflicts of interest. M.P.H. Vleugels is a trainer for Essure sterilization method. With regard to H.W.F. van Eijndhoven, the institution received payments for training courses in Essure sterilization for Dutch Gynecologists (entity: Sigma Medical Netherlands). The authors alone are responsible for the content and writing of the paper.

References

1. Sharp HT (2006) Assessment of new technology in the treatment of idiopathic menorrhagia and uterine leiomyomata. Obstet Gynecol 108:990–1003
2. McGurgan P, O'Donovan P (2007) Second-generation endometrial ablation—an overview. Best Pract Res Clin Obstet Gynaecol 21:931–945
3. Gallinat A (2007) An impedance-controlled system for endometrial ablation: five-year follow-up of 107 patients. J Reprod Med 52:467–472
4. Kleijn JH, Engels R, Bourdrez P, Mol BW, Bongers MY (2008) Five-year follow up of a randomised controlled trial comparing NovaSure and ThermaChoice endometrial ablation. BJOG 115:193–198
5. Gervaise A, de Tarac R, Fernandez H (2005) Contraceptive information after endometrial ablation. Fertil Steril 84:1746–1747
6. Mukul LV, Linn JG (2005) Pregnancy complicated by uterine synechiae after endometrial ablation. Obstet Gynecol 105:1179–1182
7. Lo JS, Pickersgill A (2006) Pregnancy after endometrial ablation: English literature review and case report. J Minim Invasive Gynecol 2006:88–91
8. Vleugels MPH, Veersema S (2005) Hysteroscopic sterilisation in the outpatient department without anaesthesia. Gyn Surgery. doi:10.1007/s10397-005-0118-4
9. Sinha D, Kalathy V, Gupta JK, Clark TJ (2007) The feasibility, success and patient satisfaction associated with outpatient hysteroscopic sterilisation. BJOG 114:676–683
10. Hopkins MR, Creedon DJ, Wagie AE, Williams AR, Famuyide AO (2007) Retrospective cost analysis comparing Essure hysteroscopic sterilization and laparoscopic bilateral tubal coagulation. J Minim Invasive Gynecol 14:97–102
11. Duffy S, Marsh F, Rogerson L, Hudson H, Cooper K, Jack S, Hunter D, Philips G (2005) Female sterilisation: a cohort controlled comparative study of Essure versus laparoscopic sterilisation. BJOG 112:1522–1528
12. Hopkins MR, Creedon DJ, El-Nashar SA, Brown DL, Good AE, Famuyide AO (2007) Radiofrequency global endometrial ablation followed by hysteroscopic sterilization. J Minim Invasive Gynecol 14:494–501
13. Donnadieu AC, Deffieux X, Gervaise A, Faivre E, Frydman R, Fernandez H (2007) Essure sterilization associated with endometrial ablation. Int J Gynaecol Obstet 97:139–142
14. Veersema S, Vleugels MPH, Timmermans A, Brolmann HAM (2005) Follow-up of successful bilateral placement of Essure® microinserts with ultrasound. Fertil Steril 84:1733–1736
15. Jansen NE, Vleugels MPH, Kluivers K, Vierhout ME (2007) Bilateral cornual abscess after endometrial ablation following Essure sterilization. J Minim Invasive Gynecol 14:509–511
16. Conceptus. Physician training manual. San Carlos, CA: Conceptus, 2003.
17. Lethaby A, Hickey M, Garry R, Penninx J (2009) Endometrial resection/ablation techniques for heavy menstrual bleeding. Cochrane Database Syst Rev 7: CD001501
18. Connor V (2008) Contrast infusion sonography in the in the post-Essure setting. J Minim Invasive Gynecol 15:56–61
19. Basinski CM, Price P (2009) Essure® tubal sterilization combined with subsequent NovaSure® endometrial ablation: a retrospective analysis. J Minim Invasive Gynecol 16:S62
20. Garza-Leal J, Castillo L, Hernandez I, Livengood R, Price P, Coad J (2008) Essure® transcervical sterilization combined with the Hydro Thermablator® system for endometrial ablation: a perihysterectomy safety study. J Minim Invasive Gynecol 15:1S
21. Levie MD, Chudnoff SG (2006) Prospective analysis of office-based hysteroscopic sterilization. J Minim Invasive Gynecol 13:98–101
22. Arjona JE, Miño M, Cordón J, Povedano B, Pelegrin B, Castelo-Branco C (2008) Satisfaction and tolerance with office hysteroscopic tubal sterilization. Fertil Steril 90:1182–1186
23. Samuel NC, Karragianniadou E, Clark TJ (2009) Outpatient versus day-case endometrial ablation using the NovaSure® impedance-controlled ablative system. Gyn Surgery. doi:10.1007/s10397-008-0394-x

2

Endometriosis in the African American woman—racially, a different entity?

George H. Shade · Mieke Lane · Michael P. Diamond

Abstract Endometriosis has been identified in up to 10% of women in some reports; however, few studies have evaluated African American women. The purpose of this study was to localize the implantation sites of endometriosis in urban Detroit female patients. This study was a retrospective chart analysis of patients with laparoscopes for endometriosis at St. John Detroit Riverview Hospital in Detroit, Michigan. All women had concomitant disease involving the uterus and multiple genital structures. In total, 93% had uterine implants, 62% had ovarian implants, 51% had posterior cul-de-sac disease, and 44% had fallopian tube involvement. Forty-five percent had abdominal wall spread, 8% with large bowel implants, and 13% with small bowel involvement. Fifty percent had uterosacral implants, 2% had bladder involvement, 2% had perihepatic involvement, and 4% had omental implants. African American women appear to have a predilection for uterine implants of endometriosis, which may be due to genetic, environmental, or previously presented theories. Further study of urban African American females is necessary to investigate the departure from typical sites of endometriotic implant localization.

G. H. Shade · M. P. Diamond (✉)
Department of Obstetrics and Gynecology, Wayne State University/Detroit Medical Center,
60 West Hancock Street,
Detroit, MI 48201, USA
e-mail: mdiamond@med.wayne.edu

M. Lane
Cascadia Women's Clinic,
Vancouver, WA, USA

Keywords African American · Endometriosis · Implantation · Uterus

Background

Endometriosis, which is the pathologic localization of endometrial glands and stroma at non-endometrial and myometrial locations, will forever be linked to Dr. Sampson and his well-known theory of retrograde menses as its etiology in 1921. Since then, the study of endometriosis has evolved immensely. However, one area where research of endometriosis still needs to improve is in the study of this disease process in the urban African American female.

In reviewing the current literature, there are only two articles that are devoted to endometriosis and the African American woman. Both of those articles were written by Dr. Donald Chatman in 1975 and 1976. His focus was to prove the chief complaint of abdominal pain in the African American female was not typically pelvic inflammatory disease, as was so often labeled in the Emergency Departments, but was indeed endometriosis [1, 2]. A recent report however showed that among women presenting for infertility care, African American women were significantly more likely to have salpingitis than non-African Americans; however, in this report, endometriosis was only identified in 2.6% of 77 African American women [3].

In Chatman's papers, he states that the implants he found were visualized in the typical locations including the uterosacral ligaments, cul-de-sac, and ovarian surfaces. We propose that although African American women have typical implantation sites, they may have a higher preponderance of atypical sites including the uterus. This may be explained by genetic factors, environmental influences, or previous presented theories.

Materials and methods

This retrospective chart review was conducted at St. John Detroit Riverview Hospital in Detroit, MI. The study was approved by the Institutional Review Board of St. John Detroit Riverview. The target population included African American women with a known diagnosis of endometriosis who had a laparoscopy performed by one of us (GS) over the time period of 1995–2002. These included women undergoing surgery indicated because of pelvic pain, masses, and/or infertility. This represents all women whose charts were able to be located from an archival storage facility. The basis for the diagnosis of endometriosis was laparoscopic pictures, which were available for review in 56% of the charts, while in the remaining patients, the locations of the endometriotic implants were taken directly from the chart. Histologic confirmation was not required.

The study parameters included were age, parity, age of menarche, age of diagnosis of severe pain, number of emergency room visits, race, surgical history, treatment history, and pelvic adhesions. There were 44 patients identified who met these criteria.

Findings

Among the population group of African American women, the age range for the participants was 17–57, with a mean age of 38.9 years. The mean age of menarche was 11.9 years in the 31 women with a documented age for menarche. The mean age of severe pain was 31 years of age. The average gravida and para were G2.4 and P 1.9. CA-125 was obtained in ten of the patients; two were found to be elevated. As far as prior therapies, 8 had previously received Provera, 17 had received Lupron, 5 had received oral contraceptives, and 1 patient had received Danocrine. Three women had documented cases of pelvic inflammatory disease.

Regarding the surgical management history, these women had a variety of procedures. Twenty-one patients had a total of 32 laparoscopies. Eighteen had undergone hysterectomies, five had myomectomies, and three had prior adnexal surgery. Additionally, one woman underwent an endometrial ablation procedure, while another had undergone hysteroscopy.

The proportion of patients found to have uterine implants was overwhelming, occurring in 93% of subjects. The women who were found to have uterine implants also had adhesions that affected other pelvic organs. It was found that 39% of patients had posterior uterine implants only, 2% had anterior implants only, 20% had both anterior and posterior uterine implants, and 32% had uterine implants that were not designated as anterior or posterior. Thus, a total of 93% had uterine endometriotic implants. Additionally, there were 62% of patients with ovarian implants, 51% with posterior cul-de-sac disease implants, and 44% with fallopian tube involvement. Forty-five percent had abdominal wall spread, 8% with large bowel implants, and 13% with small bowel involvement. Fifty percent had uterosacral implants, 2% with bladder involvement, 2% with perihepatic involvement, and 4% with omental implants. There was one patient with a prior history of endometriosis that had no endometriotic lesions identified at the time of her laparoscopy.

Discussion

In this retrospective study, the objective goal was to examine the sites involved with endometriosis. Traditionally, the most typical site for implantation of endometriosis has been the dependent portions of the pelvis, including the uterosacral ligaments, posterior cul-de-sac, and ovaries. While these sites were frequently involved in this study population, it was overwhelmingly found that the most common site for implants was the uterus. There was a greater predilection of the implants to attach to the posterior uterus vs. the anterior uterus. This suggestion of a possible racial difference in characteristics of endometriosis is consistent with a prior report of an increased incidence in Asian women as compared to Caucasian women [4], as well as the more recent report of endometriosis in 17 African American women in whom the rate of diagnosis was 40% lower than Caucasian women [5].

Establishing this pattern of occurrence raises the question as to why this may occur. There may be a variety of reasons why, but first, it is important to review the history of implantation theories. The embryonic rest theory developed by Von Recklinghausen and Russell in 1890 proposed that a nonspecific stimulus activated cells of mullerian origin at rest to differentiate into endometrium. In 1919, Meyer postulated that endometriosis develops from metaplasia of coelomic epithelium, from which the mullerian duct is derived in embryonic development. Sampson in 1921 further attempted to explain the genesis of endometriosis by proposing the theory of retrograde menstruation. It is well accepted today that an amalgamation of these, and other theories, represents the multiple origins of endometriosis.

Although the origin of endometriosis in African American women may be the same, there are multiple possible reasons for this discrepancy. First would be genetic-based variation, although candidate genes responsible for the difference are not identified or readily apparent. The dominant site of implantation in our population was not. One possibility could be hypothesized as an immunologic difference. For example, women with endometriosis have been documented to have increased number of peritoneal leukocytes. These leukocytes secrete growth factors and cytokines that promote proliferation of endometriosis. Natural killer cells (NKC) have also been intensely studied as a part of this immune deregulation in women with endometriosis [6]. It has been shown that NKCs are suppressed in women with endometriosis, which would affect the body's ability to adequately remove ectopic endometrium. The two main areas that may influence the African American female disease state are environment and immunology.

Alternatively, differences seen may not represent a genetic variation but rather be a function of socioeconomic or environmental issues of Detroit. In major metropolitan areas such as Detroit, African Americans predominately live in an urban setting rather than a rural environment. Living primarily in an urban setting presents its own unique social issues that reflected in the environment. Issues such as clean water, availability of adequate nutrition, and accessibility to health care are all of concern.

The impact of adequate nutrition is a significant one in Detroit. It was recently named one of the most overweight cities in the USA. To be classified as obese, the body mass index (BMI) must be greater than 30; in this study, 36% were obese.

Women with higher BMIs tend to have higher levels of estrogen, as a function of aromatization of androgens into estrogens in adipose tissue. One hypothesis is that there may be a correlation with uterine endometriotic implants and African American with obesity secondary to the estrogen receptors in the uterine tissue [7]. The higher the BMI, the more estrogen.

However, obesity does not explain all of the cases of endometriosis in this population. Another possible issue would include the exposure to environmental toxicants. One of the major environmental toxins that have been studied is 2,3,7,8-tetrachlorodibenzo-p-dioxin, otherwise known as dioxin. Dioxins are a part of the polychlorinated diaromatic hydrocarbons, which are unwanted by-product of many industrial and combustion processes. This toxin degrades slowly, builds up in the food chain, and is ingested by humans. It is known that dioxin can inhibit ovarian progesterone synthesis and can have antiestrogenic effects.

A study by Bois et al. [8] reviewed residents in a town in Italy who were exposed to a chemical plant explosion that involved dioxin. His study was conducted in response to a study by Rier et al. [9] that looked at dioxin exposure in monkeys, and found that monkeys exposed to high levels of dioxin were prone to develop endometriosis. Bois et al. [9] revealed that dioxin is stored in adipose tissue and concluded that this particular Italian community had an increased risk of developing endometriosis. Thus, in general, humans may develop endometriosis based on the level of exposure to dioxin, or perhaps other organochlorine compounds. However, the relationship of dioxin to endometriosis remains controversial, as exemplified by the recent report of Guo et al. [10], questioning the existence of significant evidence supporting such a link.

Detroit is known as the motor city secondary to its vast industry of auto production. There are also a multitude of other industries present in the Detroit area. In our study based on African American population, there is potential exposure to dioxins or other agents. Exposure may be via ingestion of contaminated water, air, and/or food supply. Since dioxin is indeed stored in fat, the hypothesis for uterine implants may be the same as above for obesity.

Environmental factors may also influence the immunological system. Dysregulation within the immune system may promote the growth of endometriosis. Halme et al. [11] showed that women with endometriosis have an increased number of macrophages, which could have altered responses to retrograde construction products, although the specific mechanism for promotion of endometriotic lesions is unclear.

Gazvani et al. [12] discussed a strong role for the system's immune cells and mediators in the pathogenesis of endometriosis. Our population may have an altered immune system secondary to the urban environment in which they were raised in and/or currently live. The resulting deregulated immune system may contribute to the higher propensity of uterine implants in this group of women [3].

We acknowledge the limitations of this study include the limited number of participants that comprised the population [13], the lack of histological confirmation to make the diagnosis of endometriosis, the lack of a comparable Detroit Metropolitan population of non-African American women, and the non-controlled factor of incomplete ability to obtain charts from an archival storage facility. Nonetheless, we believe the observation of an apparent difference in the location of endometriotic implants in African American women, as compared to previously described populations, warrants future systematic examination.

Conclusion

In the end, these African American women appear to have a higher predisposition to uterine endometriotic implants. Reasons may include environmental, lifestyle, and/or immunological factors or a combination of the various factors. This study reveals the need to have further investigation into this important subject.

Statement of Responsibility George H. Shade, M.D. provided clinical care for these patients and contributed to the initial concept of the study, data analysis, interpretation, writing and critical review of the manuscript.

Mieke Lane, D.O. conducted the chart review and contributed to the initial concept of the study, data analysis, interpretation, writing and critical review of the manuscript.

Michael P. Diamond, M.D. contributed to the initial concept of the study, data analysis, interpretation, writing and critical review of the manuscript.

Declaration of interest The authors report no conflicts of interest. The authors alone are responsible for the content and writing of the paper.

References

1. Chatman DL (1976) Endometriosis and the black woman. J Reprod Med 16(6):303–306
2. Chatman DL (1976) Endometriosis in the black woman. Am J Obstet Gynecol 125(7):987–989
3. Green JA, Robins JC, Scheiber M, Awadalla S, Thomas MA (2001) Racial and economic demographics of couples seeking infertility treatment. Am J Obstet Gynecol 184(6):1080–1082
4. Arumugam K, Templeton AA (1992) Endometriosis and race. Aust N Z J Obstet Gynaecol 32(2):164–165
5. Missmer SA, Hankinson SE, Spiegelman D, Barbieri RL, Marshall LM, Hunter DJ (2004) Incidence of laparoscopically confirmed endometriosis by demographic, anthropometric, and lifestyle factors. Am J Epidemiol 160(8):784–796
6. Garzetti GG, Ciavattini A, Provinciali M, Fabris N, Cignitti M, Romanini C (1993) Natural killer cell activity in endometriosis: correlation between serum estradiol levels and cytotoxicity. Obstet Gynecol 81(5 (Pt 1)):665–668
7. McCann SE, Freudenheim JL, Darrow SL, Batt RE, Zielezny MA (1993) Endometriosis and body fat distribution. Obstet Gynecol 82(4 Pt 1):545–549
8. Bois FY, Eskenazi B (1994) Possible risk of endometriosis for Seveso, Italy, residents: an assessment of exposure to dioxin. Env Health Perspect 102(5):476–477
9. Rier SE, Martin DC, Bowman RE, Dmowski WP, Becker JL (1993) Endometriosis in rhesus monkeys (*Macaca mulatta*) following chronic exposure to 2,3,7,8-tetrachlorodibenzo-p-dioxin. Fundam Appl Toxicol 21(4):433–441
10. Guo SW, Simsa P, Kyama CM, Mihályi A, Fülöp V, Othman EE et al (2009) Reassessing the evidence for the link between dioxin and endometriosis: from molecular biology to clinical epidemiology. Mol Hum Reprod 15(10):609–624
11. Halme J, Becker S, Haskill S (1987) Altered maturation and function of peritoneal macrophages: possible role in pathogenesis of endometriosis. Am J Obstet Gynecol 156(4):783–789
12. Gazvani R, Templeton A (2002) Peritoneal environment, cytokines and angiogenesis in the pathophysiology of endometriosis. Reproduction 123(2):217–226
13. Kyama MC, D'Hooghe TM, Debrock S, Machoki J, Chai DC, Mwenda JM (2004) The prevalence of endometriosis among African-American and African-indigenous women. Gynecol Obstet Invest 57(1):40–42

3

Clinical outcome after laparoscopic and open abdominal myomectomy

Guri Baardstu Majak · Marit Lieng · Erik Qvigstad

Abstract This paper details a retrospective study evaluating long-term outcomes after laparoscopic and abdominal myomectomy, including improvement of abnormal vaginal bleeding, periodic blood loss, pelvic pain, and fertility. This is a retrospective study based on a postal questionnaire and the women's medical journal. A total of 233 women were identified as having had a myomectomy during the period 2003–2006 and were sent a postal questionnaire. The response rate was 70%. After surgery, pain score was significantly reduced. The number of days with bleeding and the degree of discomfort due to bleeding was also reduced after the surgery. Among 31% of the women who stated infertility as a reason for the myomectomy, 52% became pregnant during the observational period of 4.5 years on average. Few studies report long-term outcomes after laparoscopic and abdominal myomectomy. Despite the limitations of this retrospective study, the results imply improvements regarding periodic pain, number of days with bleeding and discomfort due to bleeding after myomectomy.

Keywords Endoscopic surgery · Myoma · Pain · Infertility · Patient satisfaction

G. B. Majak (✉) · M. Lieng · E. Qvigstad
Department of Gynecology, Oslo University Hospital—Ullevål, Kirkeveien 166,
0407 Oslo, Norway
e-mail: majg@uus.no

E. Qvigstad
University of Oslo, Norway,
Oslo, Norway

Background

Myomas are the most common benign tumor in women, with a reported incidence as high as 70–80% [1]. They are shown to be clinically apparent in up to 25% of all women, increasing to 30–40% of women over 40 years of age [2]. Myomas present with a variety of symptoms. In addition to abnormal vaginal bleeding, pelvic pain, and pressure-related symptoms, the reproductive function may also be compromised, leading to subfertility and early pregnancy loss [3].

The treatment options and modalities for myomas are increasing, but the outcome after different interventions have not been fully evaluated [4]. As yet, the treatment is mainly surgical including myomectomy or hysterectomy.

The impact of myomectomy on fertility is debated, and there is no consensus whether myomas cause infertility or if they simply are an association [5]. Studies including women undergoing assisted reproduction treatment, however, give strong evidence that submucous and intramural fibroids distorting the uterine cavity impair fertility and that removal improves the outcome in terms of pregnancies [6–8].

A study from 2003 performed by Seracchioli et al. [9] reports improvement in symptoms after myomectomy, but few studies have focused on relief of symptoms such as heavy bleeding and pelvic pain. Thus, the aim of this retrospective study was to analyze the clinical outcome after myomectomy, performed by laparotomy or laparoscopy, in terms of improvement in abnormal vaginal bleeding, periodic blood loss, pelvic pain, and fertility.

Method

Following an ethical approval in March 2009 (Regional Committee for Medical Research Ethics in Eastern Norway,

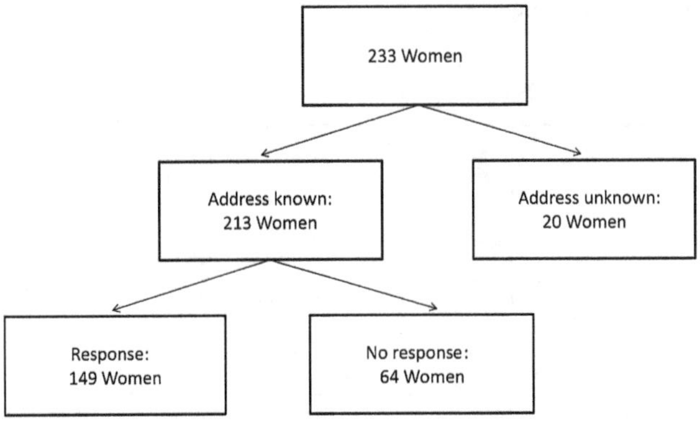

Fig. 1 Flow chart of study population

Ref: S-09128, 2009/2128), all women who were treated by myomectomy at the Department of Gynecology, Oslo University Hospital Ullevål from 2003 till 2006 were sent a questionnaire ("Electronic supplementary material"). A 4-year inclusion period was chosen in order to achieve a relatively large sample size. We consider the years before 2003 as being too long ago to ask women regarding their preoperative symptoms. The last years were omitted to ensure an acceptably long follow-up. Questions related to vaginal bleeding, pelvic pain, and fertility were raised for the preoperative period and the first two postoperative years, respectively. Standard 10-point visual analogue scales (VAS) were used to measure pain intensity and the extent to which bleeding gave discomfort. In addition, information about concomitant surgical procedures and postoperative complications were collected from the women's medical records.

Data were analyzed using SPSS for Windows (SPSS 17.0; SPSS, Inc. Chicago, IL, USA). All statistical tests were performed two-sided, with 5% significance level. Normally distributed continuous data were analyzed using a two-sided independent samples Student's t test and, when paired, the paired samples t test. Categorical data were analyzed using Pearson's chi-square test.

Findings

A total of 233 women were sent the questionnaire. The 233 procedures were equally divided between the four inclusive years. Myomectomy was performed by laparoscopy in 161 women (69%) and by laparotomy in 72 women (31%). The mean age at time of surgery was 36.8 years. We were unable to reach 20 women due to unknown adresses. A total of 149 women returned the questionnaire, providing a response rate of 70% (Fig. 1).

The dominating indications stated for the myomectomy was pain (43%), abnormal uterine bleeding (36%), and infertility (31%). A total of 18 women (12%) stated other reasons, mostly pressure symptoms and/or that the procedure was recommended by a medical practitioner. There were 88 women (59%) who stated two or more indications for having the myomectomy.

A total of 122 women (82%) reported to have suffered from periodic pain before the myomectomy, with a mean score of 5.0 (SD 2.9) on a ten-point VAS. After myomectomy, the overall mean pain score was reduced to 3.0 (SD 2.8), giving a statistically significant mean pain reduction of 2.0 (SD 2.2; 95% CI, 1.5, 2.5; $p<0.001$) (Table 1). Women who stated pain as an indication for myomectomy (64 women) had a higher mean pain reduction than women not stating pain as indication (Table 1). In addition, 52 (35%) of the women stating pain as indication for myomectomy reported to be completely pain-free after the myomectomy. A total of 45 women reported absence from work due to menstrual pain before the myomectomy, which was reduced to 19 women after the myomectomy.

Self-reported preoperative menstrual data were available for all 149 women who returned the questionnaire. Mean days with bleeding were reduced for all women after the myomectomy, with the highest reduction for women with bleeding as indication for the myomectomy (Table 2).

In all 149 women, the mean degree of discomfort caused by vaginal bleeding, scored on a ten-point VAS, was significantly reduced after the myomectomy. The highest reduction was seen in women stating bleeding as indication for the myomectomy (Table 2).

During the follow-up period, 58 out of the 149 responders conceived and 51 women gave birth. A total of 29 women delivered by cesarean section. Ten women reported that complications occurred during their pregnancy and/or delivery, but except for one pre-labor rupture of the uterus, no complications seemed related to the previous myomectomy.

Table 1 Intensity of pelvic pain before and after the myomectomy as measured by a standard ten-point visual analogue scale

	VAS pain score before myomectomy, mean (SD)	VAS pain score after myomectomy, mean (SD)	Difference pain score, mean (SD); 95% CI	p-value
Overall pain intensity (n=122)	5.0 (2.9)	3.0 (2.8)	2.0 (3.0); 1.5, 2.5	<0.001
Pain intensity in women with pain as indication for myomectomy (n=64)	5.9 (2.9)	3.5 (3.0)	2.4 (3.7); 1.5, 3.3	<0.001
Pain intensity in women without pain as indication (n=58)	4.2 (2.7)	2.6 (2.5)	1.6 (2.2); 1.1, 2.1	<0.001

Table 2 Days of bleeding and degree of discomfort due to bleeding before and after the myomectomy

	Before myomectomy, mean (SD)	After myomectomy, mean (SD)	Difference, mean (SD); 95% CI	p-value
Overall days of bleeding (n=149)	5.9 (2.2)	4.9 (1.8)	1.0 (2.2); 0.7, 1.5	<0.001
Days of bleeding in women with bleeding as indication (n=54)	7.4 (2.6)	5.1 (2.3)	2.3 (2.7); 1.5, 3.2	<0.001
Degree of discomfort due to bleeding (n=149)	5.3 (2.6)	3.3 (2.6)	1.9 (3.2); 1.3, 2.5	<0.001
Degree of discomfort due to bleeding in women with bleeding as indication (n=54)	8.3 (1.7)	3.6 (2.9)	4.6 (3.4); 3.6, 5.7	<0.001

Out of the responders, 46 (31%) reported infertility as indication for the myomectomy. The mean age for these women was 36.0 years at the time of surgery and the median observational time was 4.5 years (range 2.0–6.0 years). Out of these 46 women, 24 conceived and 20 gave birth, resulting in a pregnancy rate of 52% and a live birth rate of 45%, respectively.

A high proportion of the included women (n=122, 82%) reported being satisfied or very satisfied with the myomectomy. There was no difference in satisfaction related to the indication for myomectomy or the surgical approach (Fig. 2).

Immediate postoperative complications occurred in 11 out of the 149 responders (7%). The complication rate was 9% in laparoscopic procedures and 7% in open procedures, respectively. The complications were as follows: accidental morcellation of the bowel in one woman, peroperative bleeding requiring blood transfusion in three women, postoperative abdominal infection/intraabdominal abscess in five women and urinary tract infection in two women. In addition, one woman reported uterine rupture which may represent a late complication to the surgery.

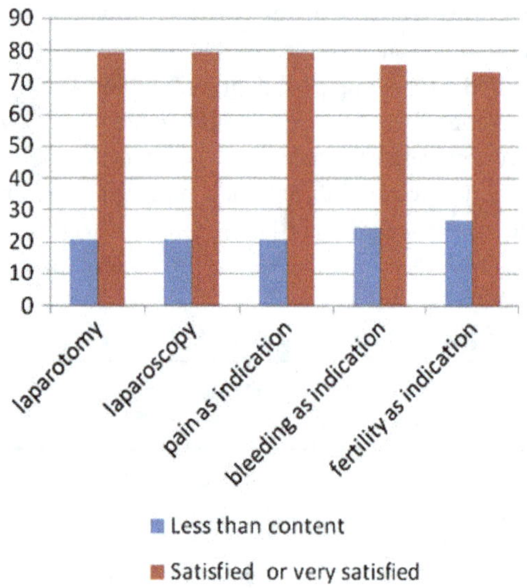

Fig. 2 Satisfaction related to surgical procedure and stated indication

Conclusions

The results of our study indicate that the women who underwent myomectomy experienced significantly reduced periodic pelvic pain after the procedure. They also reported reduced number of days with vaginal bleeding and significantly reduced discomfort due to bleeding. The overall patient satisfaction was very high after the procedure, with 82% reporting to be very satisfied or satisfied postoperatively.

Although all women reported significantly reduced periodic pain after myomectomy, the largest reduction of pain score was observed in women who reported pain as indication for the myomectomy. Eighty-eight women stated two or more indications for having the myomectomy, and the combination of abnormal uterine bleeding and pain was the most common. This supports a previous theory suggesting that increased blood flow may be associated with dysmenorrhea, especially if there is passage of blood clots [10]. Myomas are also associated with adenomyosis, which again is associated with menstruational pain [10]. There is reason to believe that most of the women treated by laparoscopic or abdominal myomectomy suffered from intramural or subserosal myomas since submucosal myomas are preferably treated surgically by hysteroscopic resection. Wegienka et al. have shown that intramural and subserosal myomas had the same tendency to cause menorrhagia as the submucosal ones [11].

The exact mechanism by which myomas may cause excessive bleeding is unknown, though abnormal vaginal bleeding, and usually menorrhagia, is stated as the most common symptom reported by women with myomas [12]. The relation between increased periodic blood loss and myomas may be caused by factors such as increased endometrial surface area, increased vascularity of the uterus, interference with the normal uterine contractility and pressure, and impingement on the uterine venous system causing the dilatation of venules within the myometrium and endometrium [13–15]. Furthermore, dysregulation of local vasoactive growth factors is thought to promote vasodilatation [16]. When enlarged venules are disrupted during the periodical bleeding, the bleeding from dilated venules may exceed the usual hemostatic mechanisms [17]. Our findings of reduction of periodic blood loss after myomectomy substantiate such theories, and our results indicate that myomectomy shortened the menstrual period and significantly reduced discomfort related to periodic bleeding.

When all other causes of infertility are excluded, it is generally thought that myomas may be responsible for infertility in only 2–3% of infertility cases [17]. In our study, the women reporting infertility as indication for the myomectomy had a postoperative pregnancy rate of 52%. The 5-year review by Olufowobi et al. after myomectomy reported that the spontaneous pregnancy group had a pregnancy rate of 46%, which is approximately the same as the findings in our study [12]. Literature reviews imply that submucosal myomas have a strong association with lower ongoing pregnancy rates and decreased implantation, while women with intramural myomas experience more miscarriages. Data from women undergoing assisted reproduction technology (ART) suggest that removal of submucosal myomas and intramural myomas that distort the uterine cavity improves the fertility outcome, but the cause–effect relationship is poorly understood [18]. A limitation in our study is the lack of information regarding ART in the reported pregnancies.

The strength of our study is its originality, reporting the beneficial outcome of relatively commonly performed procedures, which previously were scarcely evaluated. Furthermore, the sample size is relatively large. The major limitation of the study is that we have no information about the size, site, and number of myomas removed in each patient. Prospective, randomized studies are needed to assess the impact of these factors regarding the effect of myomectomy.

Another limitation is the retrospective nature of this study. However, while women may not have been able to recall their preoperative symptoms with great precision, we believe that they were able to present a reasonably accurate view of the whole experience from the pre- to postoperative period, and therefore the change in symptoms is likely to reflect improvements or deteriorations. The response rate was 70%, and we were not able to reach 20 patients because of unknown address. The reported treatment efficacy could therefore be considered as overestimated. The information from the womens medical journals and the questionnaire implies that this is a heterogeneous group, and the reported improvements are significant.

In conclusion, this retrospective study indicates improvements regarding periodic pain, number of days with bleeding, and discomfort due to bleeding after myomectomy. Despite the limitations described, we believe that the significant benefits observed after myomectomy are promising and should be proven in future prospective studies.

Conflicts of interest The authors report no conflicts of interest. The authors alone are responsible for the content and writing of the paper.

References

1. Baird DB, Dunson DB, Hill MC, Cousins D, Scechtman JM (2003) High cumulative incidence of uterine leiomyoma in black and white women: ultrasound evidence. Am J Obstet Gynecol 188 (1):100–107
2. Buttram VC Jr (1986) Uterine leiomyomata—aetiology, symptomatology and management. Prog Clin Biol Res 225:275–296
3. Stewart EA (2001) Uterine fibroids. Lancet 357:293–298
4. Istre O (2008) Management of symptomatic fibroids: conservative surgical treatment modalities other than abdominal and laparoscopic myomectomy. In: Arulkumaran S, Manyonda IT (eds) Best practice and research, vol 22, 4. Elsevier, New York, pp 735–747
5. Khaund A, Lumsden M (2008) Impact of fibroids on reproductive function. In: Arulkumaran S, Manyonda IT (eds) Best practice and research, vol 22, 4. Elsevier, New York, pp 749–760
6. Keltz M, Varasteh N, Levin B, Neuwirth R (1998) Pregnancy rates following hysteroscopic polypectomy, myomectomy and a normal cavity in infertile patients. Prim Care Update Ob Gyns 5(4):168
7. Connolly G, Doyle M, Barrett T, Byrne P, De Mello M, Harrison RF (2000) Fertility after abdominal myomectomy. J Obstet Gynaecol 20:418–420
8. Campo S, Campo V, Gambadauro P (2003) Reproductive outcome before and after laparoscopic or abdominal myomectomy for subserous or intramural myomas. Eur J Obstet Gynecol Reprod Biol 110:215–219
9. Seracchioli R, Colombo FM, Bagnoli A, Govoni F, Missiroli S, Venturoli S (2003) Laparoscopic myomectomy for fibroids penetrating the uterine cavity: is it a safe procedure? BJOG 110 (3):236–240
10. Lippman SA, Warner M, Samules S, Olive D, Vercellini P, Eskenazi B (2003) Uterine fibroids and gynaecologic pain symptoms in a population based study. Fertil Steril 80:1488–1494
11. Wegienka G, Baird DD, Hertz-Picciotto I, Harlow SD, Steege JF, Hill MC et al (2003) Self-reported heavy bleeding associated with uterine leiomyomata. Obstet Gynecol 101:431–437
12. Olufowobi O, Sharif K, Papaionnou S, Neelakantan D, Mohammed H, Afnan M (2004) Are the anticipated benefits of myomectomy achieved in women in reproductive age? A 5-year review of the results at a UK tertiary hospital. J Obstet Gynecol 24:434–440
13. Sehgal N, Haskins AL (1960) The mechanism of uterine bleeding in the presence of fibromyomas. Am Surg 26:21–33
14. Farrer-Brown G, Beilby JO, Tarbit MH (1970) The vascular pattern in myomatous uteri. J Obstet Gynecol Br Commonw 77:967–975
15. Farrer-Brown G, Beilby JO, Tarbit MH (1971) Venous changes in endometrium of myomatous uteri. Obstet Gynecol 38:743–751
16. Stewart EA, Nowak RA (1996) Leiomyoma-related bleeding: a classic hypothesis updated for the molecular era. Hum Reprod Update 2:295–306
17. Buttram VC Jr, Reiter RC (1981) Uterine leiomyomata: etiology, symptomatology and management. Fertil Steril 36:433–445
18. Klatsky PC, Tran ND, Caughey AB, Fujimoto VY (2008) Fibroids and reproductive outcomes: a systematic literature review from conception to delivery. Am J Obst Gyn 198(4):357–366

4

Parallel hysteroscopic and laparoscopic myomectomy in infertile patients

Béla G. Molnár · Zsolt Kormányos · Virág Márton · Luka Anðelic · Andor Góli

Abstract The past decades have brought about numerous new methods in the treatment of the most frequent benign gynaecological tumour, the myoma, while at the same time, the indications of traditional surgical treatment have also been reassessed. The constant procrastination of pregnancy to older and older age, the frequency of myoma growing by age and the wider application of assisted reproduction techniques have created new conditions for the treatment of myoma. In our research, we analysed the data of 30 infertile patients out of a group of 99 who had hysteroscopic and laparoscopic myomectomy carried out in one session. In the course of 2 years, nine women got pregnant. Besides two miscarriages, the others could carry their pregnancy for at least 34 weeks. Out of the seven deliveries, five (71%) ended with caesarean section, for obstetrical reasons in all cases. In case of uterus with multiplex myoma, hysteroscopy and laparoscopy can safely be applied in parallel and it does not necessarily imply the termination of the occurring pregnancy by caesarean section.

Keywords Fibroid · Infertility · Hysteroscopy · Laparoscopy

Background

Among infertile patients, the frequency of occurrence of myoma is 2–22%. Although it may seem evident that especially submucous myomas may be responsible for infertility, the significance of myomas in infertility is still questioned by many. Undoubtedly in numerous cases, patients with myoma become pregnant spontaneously and carry their pregnancy up to their terminus. However, it unfortunately occurs rarely that one single node deforms the uterus; we are much likely to face uterus with multiplex myoma. In such cases, the elimination of submucous and intramural or subserous nodes in different sessions would result in a loss of time (repeated scheduling, waiting lists) for the infertile patients. Moreover, the patients would be exposed to the risks of anaesthesia and occurrence neopathy for two times. Apparently, in the case of patients suffering from the parallel presence of submucous myoma and intramural or subserous myoma, the elimination of all fibroids is to be realised in one session.

Methods

In the past 5 years, we have carried out 663 myomectomies, of which 453 were laparotomies, while 163 were hysteroscopic and 161 were laparoscopic eliminations of the fibroid. In 99 cases, the hysteroscopic and laparoscopic enucleation of the myoma node was realised in the course of one single surgical intervention. We hereby disregard the cases in which the intervention had to be transferred into laparotomy. We included those 30 infertile patients in our analysis who, in the course of gynaecological examination, were diagnosed with myoma as well and who underwent parallel hysteroscopic and laparoscopic surgical interventions aiming at eliminating the fibroids. At four of these patients, the lead symptom besides sterility was metrorrhagia. The examination and the surgical treatment of the

B. G. Molnár (✉) · Z. Kormányos · V. Márton
Obstetrics and Gynaecology, University of Szeged,
Szeged, Hungary
e-mail: molnargb@gmail.com

L. Anðelic · A. Góli
Obstetrics and Gynaecology, Opšta Bolnica Subotica,
Subotica, Serbia

patients at the two institutions were based on identical principles. In order to identify the precise position of the myoma, we used TVS. Of the 30 patients, 15 had already undergone IVF-ET treatment. Twenty-six patients had never been pregnant; one woman had been pregnant once but lost the pregnancy. Abortion occurred in one case among the anamnestic data. Two members of the group had already had deliveries. We had not used hormonal treatment to decrease the size of the myoma, not even in cases where it was larger than 4 cm. We strived for scheduling the interventions for the proliferative period but, due to the waiting lists, operation may have taken place in the secretion phase.

Submucous myomas were eliminated by a monopolar myoma resectoscope (STORZ GmbH, Tuttlingen, Germany and Wisap, Sauerlach, Germany). The splitting of the operation into two sections did not become necessary in either of the cases. When there was a type II fibroid, we applied 5 NE Oxytocin intravenously in order to support the removal of the node, when the resection of the fibroid had already been started.

In the course of the resection of intramural and subserous myomas, we used three (Szeged) and two (Subotica) assistant trocars, respectively. We did not apply vasopressin or hydropreparation during resection. We used monopolar needle only to incise the capsule of the fibroid; the enucleation of the myoma was carried out partly mechanically and, to treat the vessels leading to the lump, partly by a bipolator. The myoma bed was treated, in most of the cases, by serosa–serosa type interrupted stitches (Fig. 1). We had the chance to try the Bearded stitch sewing material as well with which we could sew the myoma bed positioned on the anterior wall, on the bladder base. Should the myoma be of a diameter larger than 4 cm and of totally intramural position, its bed was sewed in two layers. The enucleated fibroid was eliminated by an electric morcellator (STORZ GmbH, Tuttlingen, Germany and Wisap, Sauerlach, Germany) and was sent for histological examination.

Findings

The average age of patients was 34.8 years (min., 24 years; max., 42 years). Parallel hysteroscopic and laparoscopic myomectomy was carried out on 30 patients. For 13 patients one myoma was removed by hysteroscopy and one by laparoscopy. For the other 17 patients, more than one myomas were removed either through hysteroscopy or laparoscopy. An overall number of 78 myomas were removed from the 30 patients. Four was the largest number of fibroids removed from one single patient. The average size of submucous myomas was 26 mm (min., 10 mm; max., 50 mm); the average size of intramural nodes was 38 mm (min., 10 mm; max., 100 mm); the average size of subserosal fibroids was 35 mm (min., 10 mm; max., 50 mm). In the course of hysteroscopic myomectomies, the absorption of irrigation fluid remained below 1,500 ml in all of the cases. The average fluid absorption was 350 ml (min., 100 ml; max., 1,500 ml). The average operation time was 99 min (min., 40 min; max., 210 min). Of the whole operation time, hysteroscopy accounted for 25% and laparoscopy for 75%. Twenty-five patients left the inpatient institution within 24 h and five patients left on the second day after the operation.

In the course of hysteroscopic interventions, perforation or fluid overload did not occur in either of the cases. In the course of laparoscopic myomectomies, the cave did not open once. Within 1 year, nine women became pregnant. Outside two miscarriages, the others were able to carry their pregnancy for at least 34 weeks. Of the seven deliveries, five (71%) ended with caesarean section. The reason for caesarean section was obstetrical in all of the cases. During the caesarean sections, we did not meet significant adhesions.

Discussion

When hysteroscopic and laparoscopic interventions are carried out in one session, we should start with the

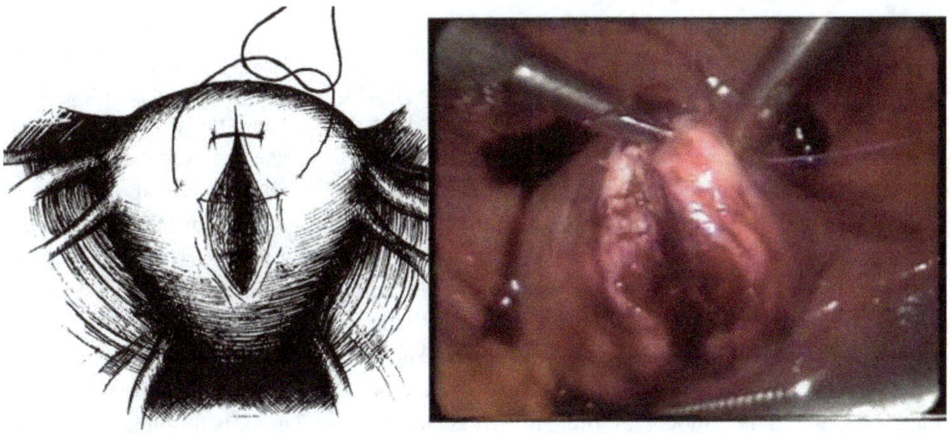

Fig. 1 Serosa–serosa type stitches to close the nest fibroid

hysteroscopic intervention for practical reasons: this way the justification of diagnosis of perforation, its treatment, the suction of the distending fluid from the abdominal cavity and the impediment of its absorption from the peritoneum become possible. In the case of infertile patients, the diameter of the resectoscope should be the smallest possible [1], in order to minimise the dilatation of the cervix, by which the risk of cervix incompetence at future possible pregnancy is also minimised.

At pregnancies proceeding expanded myomectomies, the question whether the woman can be led into vaginal delivery is always raised. According to our experience, as long as no perforation occurred in the course of the hysteroscopic intervention and the uterine cavity did not open during laparoscopic myoma enucleation, that is, the patient suffered no injury affecting the wall of the uterus in the whole of its thickness; caesarean section is not to be applied as a routine. Unharmed myometrium provides sufficient flexibility and resistance in the course of advancing pregnancy. In the first and second stage of labour, intensified monitoring and the frequent control of the sensitivity of the uterine scar is necessary. Should the uterus become increasingly sensitive to pressure, caesarean section is to be applied. Although theoretically not justified, we do not apply Oxytocin infusion at deliveries following myomectomy for generating or intensifying contractions, similarly to our practice pursued at preceding caesarean sections.

In line with the findings of other work teams [2–4], we did not experience uterus rupture in our patient sample. There have been publications on uterus rupture following myomectomy, but in all of these cases, forced intensification of contractions appeared in the anamnesis [5].

If the myomas are found on the same side, e.g. on the anterior wall of the uterus, the risk of perforation of the uterine wall arises at parallel elimination. The theoretical possibility for this advancement does exist but we have not met any such case in our practice. The perforation of the uterus is rare in the course of hysteroscopic myomectomies; its possibility based on literature findings is ca. 1–2% [6]. Regarding laparoscopic myomectomies, the opening of the uterine cavity is experienced more often. If we strictly constrain ourselves to stay within the so-called “fake skin” of the myoma while enucleating it, the risk of the opening of the cavity can practically be reduced to zero. Should the cave open even so, it is advisable to close the myoma bed in two layers and provide antibiotic treatment in the post-operative period. This circumstance does not affect the time of hospitalisation [7].

There is no consensus on when a woman may become pregnant after myomectomy [8]. As for us, we share the view that at least 3 months (that is, at least two terminated menstrual cycle) should pass before starting the aspiration for pregnancy. This amount of time is sufficient for the endometrium to regenerate so that, even if conception takes place immediately, there are no more obstacles in front of the fertilised ovum to imbed. Expectation time is not affected by the size of the eliminated myoma; it is rather the size of the wound created during elimination that may act as an influencing factor. Consequently, in cases of hysteroscopic eliminations of large size type I and type II myomas and, for laparoscopic myomectomies, after eliminating myomas positioned mainly intramurally, longer recovery period is expected. In such cases we recommend to wait for 6 months. On the other hand, in our patient sample, one woman became pregnant 3 months after the enucleation of a 4-cm submucous and a 6-cm subserosal–intramural myoma and delivery occurred by a caesarean section on the 38th week. One year after delivery, she repeatedly became pregnant spontaneously; at present she is in the 30th week of her pregnancy.

Proceeding endoscopic myomectomies, provided that neither perforation (hysteroscopy), nor the opening of the uterine cavity (laparoscopy) occurred, there is no obstacle in front of vaginal delivery. However, the majority of these pregnancies are terminated by a caesarean section [9]. Besides obstetrical reasons, the indication for caesarean section is underpinned by previous operation on the active section of the uterus, the striving for safety and the fact that these patients tend to arrive at delivery following a multiannual infertility treatment so they are regarded as high-risk patients. It is important to highlight the difference between the uterus of patients with preceding caesarean section and those undergone myomectomy. In the course of caesarean section, we incise the uterus on the passive part which does not get under tension before, at the end of the next pregnancy, labour begins and contractions become regular. On the contrary, following myomectomy, the uterine wound is practically constantly under tension as pregnancy advances. That is why, in the latter case, increased awareness in pregnancy attendance is by all means justified and, at delivery, the sensitivity of the scar or the explicit extenuation of the scar implies caesarean section [10].

In the course of deliveries led by caesarean section, we did not find significant adhesions due to previous myomectomies. We claim that this circumstance is deducible to the fact that, in the course of laparoscopic myomectomy, we used a sewing technique (serosa–serosa type stitches) which, after application, results in the full covering of the wound by the uterine serosa and only minimal sewing substance runs on the surface of the uterus. This observation is underpinned by the fact that, following our 161 laparoscopic myomectomies, we have not found expressive adhesion formation at those, originally not infertile patients either who later underwent laparotomy due to other reasons (e.g. new myoma formation, ovarian tumour). On the other hand, in the course of myomectomies carried out through laparotomy, expressive adhesions had occurred with higher frequency. Therefore, based on our positive experience gained in respect of serosa–serosa type stitches, we have lately turned to applying this sewing technique in laparotomy as well. In order to explain whether less frequent adhesion formation is deducible to laparoscopic intervention or the application of serosa–serosa type stitches, we need to conclude further examinations. Other studies have also come to the conclusion that de novo adhesion formation is deducible to surgery duration, blood loss, number and size of incisions, suturing and number of knots [11].

It may occur that, in the course of caesarean section, we still find myoma on the uterine wall which brings up a further problem of how the myoma should be treated during the intervention. A widely accepted view implies that, during caesarean section, only pedunculated myomas are allowed to be removed as the resection of intramural myomas may result in profuse bleeding and, eventually, in losing the uterus [12]. However, there are tracks of successful myomectomies carried out during caesarean section where the myoma bed was secured by a previously inlaid purse string stitch [13]. Another solution of ligating the uterine arteries parallel to caesarean section in order to decrease post-operative bleeding has also been published [14]. As for ourselves, we pursue the practice of not eliminating the myomas during caesarean section, provided their position does not disturb the sewing of the uterine wound, but we recommend eliminating them in another session, should they cause complains or symptoms.

The deformation of the uterine cave following the hysteroscopic elimination of submucous myomas or the formed scar tissue following the elimination of type II fibroids may become an impediment to the realisation or carriage of planned pregnancy [15]. Proceeding interventions affecting the uterine cave, we provide oestrogen for a month which, by the rapid thickening of the endometrium, decreases the risk of adhesion formation. The placement of mechanical instrument (Folley-catheter, IUD) after intervention may, according to our experience, lead to adhesion formation so it rather worsens than improves the status of the uterine cave.

Conclusion

In the case of multiplex myomas causing infertility, the parallel hysteroscopic and laparoscopic elimination of myomas is technically possible and does not necessarily imply that future pregnancy can only be terminated by caesarean section. However, taking into consideration that, in this patient group, persistent infertility or previous unsuccessful pregnancies are often included among anamnestic data, the majority of deliveries are carried out through caesarean section.

Acknowledgements The analysis (including the purchase of a few equipment) was carried out in the framework of the project No. HUSRB/0901/214/082 co-financed by the European Union under the Hungary–Serbia IPA Cross-Border Cooperation Programme 2007–2013. The drawing part of the figure was made by Dr. József Imre.

Conflicts of interests The authors report no conflicts of interest. The authors alone are responsible for the content and writing of the paper.

References

1. Papalampros P, Gambadauro P, Papadopoulos N, Polyzos D, Chapman L, Magos A (2009) The mini-resectoscope: a new instrument for office hysteroscopic surgery. Acta Obstet Gynecol Scand 88(2):227–230
2. Campo S, Campo V, Gambadauro P (2003) Reproductive outcome after laparoscopic or abdominal myomectomy. Eur J Obstet Gynecol Reprod Biol 110:215–219
3. Soriano D, Dessolle L, Poncelet C, Benifla JL, Madelenat P, Darai E (2003) Pregnancy outcome after laparoscopic and laparoconverted myomectomy. Eur J Obstet Gynecol Reprod Biol 108:194–198
4. Landi S, Fiaccavento A, Zaccoletti R, Barbieri F, Syed R, Minelli L (2003) Pregnancy outcomes and deliveries after laparoscopic myomectomy. J Am Assoc Gynecol Laparosc 10(2):177–181
5. Lieng M, Istre O, Langebrekke A (2004) Uterine rupture after laparoscopic myomectomy. J Am Assoc Gynecol Laparosc 11 (1):92–93
6. Mettler L, Wendland EM, Patel P, Caballero R, Schollmeyer T (2002) Hysteroscopy: an analysis of 2-years' experience. JSLS 6 (3):195–197
7. Seracchioli R, Colombo FM, Bagnoli A, Govoni F, Missiroli S, Venturoli S (2003) Laparoscopic myomectomy for fibroids penetrating the uterine cavity: is it a safe procedure? BJOG 110 (3):236–240
8. Kucera E, Mandys F, Drahonovský J, Martin D, Procházka B (2009) Reproductive outcome after laparoscopic myomectomy—retrospective analysis 1994–2007. Ceska Gynekol 74(6):431–436
9. Seracchioli R, Manuzzi L, Vianello F, Gualerzi B, Savelli L, Paradisi R, Venturoli S (2006) Obstetric and delivery outcome of pregnancies achieved after laparoscopic myomectomy. Fertil Steril 86(1):159–165
10. Cheng YW, Eden KB, Marshall N, Pereira L, Caughey AB, Guise JM (2011) Delivery after prior caesarean: maternal morbidity and mortality. Clin Perinatol 38(2):297–309
11. Trew G, Pistofidis G, Pados G, Lower A, Mettler L, Wallwiener D et al (2011) Gynaecological endoscopic evaluation of 4% icodextrin solution: a European, multicentre, double-blind, randomized study of the efficacy and safety in the reduction of de novo adhesions after laparoscopic gynaecological surgery. Hum Reprod 26(8):2015–2027
12. Roman AS, Tabsh KM (2004) Myomectomy at time of cesarean delivery: a retrospective cohort study. BMC Pregnancy Childbirth 4(1):14
13. Lee JH, Cho DH (2011) Myomectomy using purse-string suture during cesarean section. Arch Gynecol Obstet Suppl 1:35–37
14. Liu WM, Wang PH, Tang WL, Wang IT, Tzeng CR (2006) Uterine artery ligation for treatment of pregnant women with uterine leiomyomas who are undergoing cesarean section. Fertil Steril 86(2):423–428
15. Deans R, Abbott J (2010) Review of intrauterine adhesions. J Minim Invasive Gynecol 17(5):555–569

5

Feasibility and long-term efficacy of hysteroscopic myomectomy for myomas with intramural development by the use of non-electrical "cold" loops

Francesco Paolo Giuseppe Leone • Stefania Calabrese • Carmelo Marciante • Irene Cetin • Enrico Ferrazzi

Abstract This study aimed to assess the feasibility and the short- and long-term efficacy of hysteroscopic myomectomy for submucous myomas with intramural development [grade 1 (G1) and grade 2 (G2)] by using non-electrical "cold" loops and to verify the role of preoperative variables on surgical outcomes. Symptomatic (bleeding and infertility) premenopausal patients with the diagnosis of submucous myoma at transvaginal sonography, and with G1 and G2 grading at sonohysterography, were included in this prospective study. Hysteroscopic myomectomy was performed by the combined monopolar electrical slicing and traction-and-leverage manoeuvres by non-electrical "cold" loops. One hundred fifty-nine patients were recruited, and 169 procedures were performed. Operating time, fluid deficit, complications and complete resection at first procedure (perioperative outcomes) and persisting symptoms and additional surgery for persisting symptoms (long-term outcomes) were not significantly different for G1 vs. G2 myomas. Perioperative outcomes were significantly different when comparing myoma mean diameter <3.0 vs. ≥3.0 cm (75th percentile). Multivariate analysis and multiple regression analysis proved that myoma mean diameter was the only significant variable for surgical outcomes. Hysteroscopic myomectomy by non-electrical "cold" loops is an effective and efficient treatment for submucous myomas with intramural development. Myoma mean diameter is the only significant preoperative variable for perioperative outcome, while myoma grading loses its role as a prognostic factor.

Keywords Hysteroscopic myomectomy · Non-electrical "cold" loops · Submucous myoma · Long-term follow-up · Hysteroscopic complications

Background

Hysteroscopic myomectomy is an efficient and effective technique and is considered the standard of care for conservative surgical removal of symptomatic (bleeding and infertility) submucous myomas [1–3]. The size and the different grading (G) of intramural extension of submucous myomas determine the chance of a complete resection and are strictly related to the risk of intraoperative complications (haemorrhage, perforation and fluid overload) [4–8].

Resectoscopic myomectomy is usually performed by the slicing technique with electrical loops. This technique is optimal for intracavitary myomas (G0) but may lead to partial section of the myometrial fibres on the uterine wall when myomas have a partial (G1) or prevalent (G2) intramural development. Moreover, thermal injury by mono- or bipolar unmodulated pure cutting electrosurgery might extend to more than 1.0 mm [9, 10], with additional damage to the myometrium and to the endometrial cavity. This might lead to late fertility complications, such as intrauterine synechiae [11].

In mid-1990s, non-electrical loops ("cold loops") were introduced as an additional tool for hysteroscopic myomectomy [12]. The use of cold loops to enucleate the intramural

F. P. G. Leone (✉) · S. Calabrese · C. Marciante · I. Cetin
Department of Obstetrics and Gynecology,
Clinical Sciences Institute L. Sacco, University of Milan,
Via G.B. Grassi 74,
20157 Milan, Italy
e-mail: leone.francesco@hsacco.it

E. Ferrazzi
Childrens' Hospital Buzzi, University of Milan,
Milan, Italy

portion of submucous myomas might avoid the unnecessary extensive electrical cut of surrounding myometrial fibres and the thermal injury of the adiacent myometrium. This "mechanical" approach minimises direct myometrial damage and unnecessary fibrosis in the area of surgical intervention. Recently, this pioneering technique has proved to be effective in a small series of large submucous myomas (≥5 cm) [13]; however, it has never been scrutinized in large and long-term prospective studies. The aim of this study was to assess the feasibility and the short- and long-term efficacy of the combined use of non-electrical "cold" loops and monopolar electrical loops for resectoscopic removal of G1 and G2 submucous myomas in a prospective series of symptomatic (bleeding and infertility) premenopausal patients.

Methods

Patients Premenopausal patients complaining abnormal uterine bleeding and/or infertility with G1 and G2 myomas were consecutively recruited between January 2000 and December 2009. Relevant demographic data were recorded. The study design was approved by the institutional review board.

Sonographic assessment Number, site and size of myomas, the myometrial free margin and endometrial thickness and pattern were assessed by high-quality transvaginal sonography and saline contrast sonohysterography (SCSH). SCSH was always performed according to previously published 2D and 3D imaging criteria in order to preoperatively classify myoma grading [14, 15]. Grade 1 (G1) was defined as a sessile fibroid, with the endocavitary part protruding into the cavity dilated by saline solution ≥50%, and grade 2 (G2) with the endocavitary part <50% and prevalent intramural development. The myometrial free margin was considered the shortest distance between the outer margin of the myoma and the perimetrium as assessed by SCSH. Inclusion criteria were: number ≤3 and size ≤5 cm of submucous myomas and myometrial free margin ≥3 mm. The mean diameter of myomas was calculated from the three diameters: $(d1+d2+d3)/3$.

Medical preoperative treatment GnRH analogue triptorelin or leuprorelin were prescribed for 2–3 months to patients with myomas >3 cm, in order to reduce myoma volume, to induce endometrial hypotrophy, and/or for patients suffering from secondary anaemia.

Hysteroscopic removal When no preoperative medication was prescribed, all patients underwent surgery in the early proliferative phase of the cycle. Resectoscopic procedures were performed using a rigid 8-mm (27 Fr) continous-flow resectoscope for intrauterine high-frequency electrosurgery with rotatable inner tube and a 12° fore-oblique telescope (Karl Storz GmbH & Co., Germany). The uterine cavity was distended and irrigated with a nonconductive, hypo-osmolar solution of 2.7% sorbitol and 0.54% mannitol, instilled under manometric control by a hysteroscopic pump. The basic fluid setting was: intrauterine pressure 50 mmHg (never exceeding 120 mmHg during surgery), inflow 150 ml/min, aspiration pressure 0.2 bar. The lowest pressure compatible with a clear vision was used during the procedure by "tailoring" opening and closure of inflow and outflow stopcocks.

The combined procedure consisted of a sequence of three different operating steps. At first, traditional slicing of the protruding intracavitary portion of the myoma is carried out by repeated and progressive passages of the semicircular monopolar cutting electrotome, with pure cutting current at 90 W. This action stopped at the level of the plane of the endometrial surface so that the passage between the myoma and the adjacent myometrium was clearly identified (pseudocapule, i.e. cleavage plane). Secondly, cold enucleation of the intramural portion of the myoma was achieved by traction-and-leverage manoeuvres with rectangular and hooked non-electrical "cold" loops. Once the intracavitary portion was resected, the usual cutting loop was substituted on the same resectoscope by a suitable blunt dissection cold loop. By gentle traction on the myoma, the pseudocapsule was clearly identified and the cold loops were then inserted in this avascular space between the whitish and compact surface of the myoma and the pinkish and smooth adjacent myometrium. These loops were then progressively used in a mechanical way by hooking and lacerating the connective bridges joining the myoma to normal tissue (see video). Finally, the removal of the enucleated intramural portion was completed by progressive slicing, being now completely dislocated and therefore safely treatable as a lesion with a total intracavitary development and/or by using the rake cold loop (Mazzon Non-Electrical Loops, Karl Storz GmbH & Co., Germany) (Fig. 1). All resected specimens were sent for histologic analysis.

Operating time was considered as the time between initial insertion and final removal of the resectoscope. Fluid deficit was calculated as the difference between the total amount of instilled solution into the uterus and the amount of fluid recovered from the suction bottle and the plastic draping that funnelled escaping fluid through the cervix into a calibrated pouch. According to the AAGL guidelines [16], a strict fluid monitoring was assessed every 10–15 min. In cases exceeding 60 min of intervention and/or a fluid deficit >1,000 ml, intra-operative sonography was used to decide if the remaining part of the lesion might be removed in few additional minutes or if stopping the procedure.

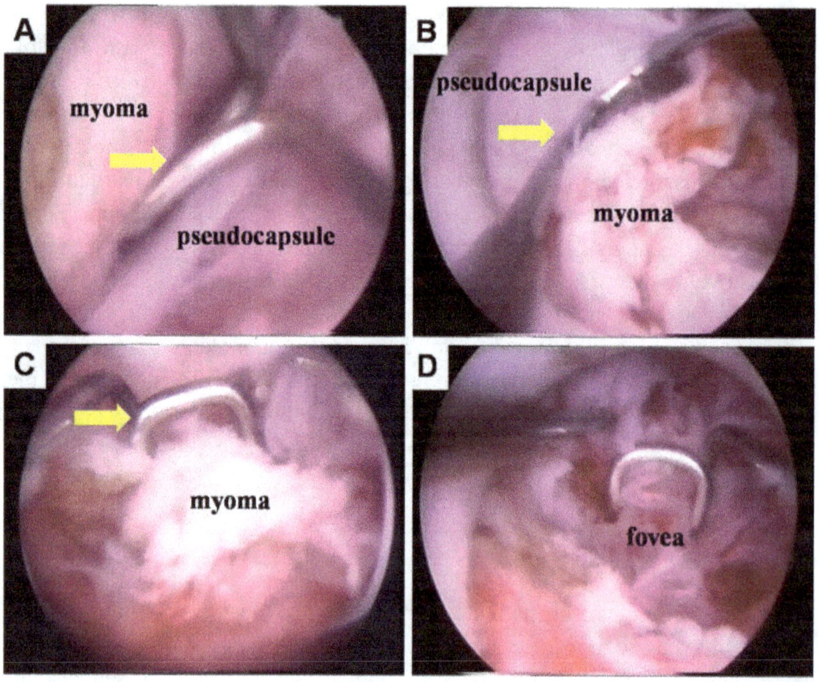

Fig. 1 **a** Myoma enucleation by pointed hooked knife-shaped loop (*arrow*), used to hook and lacerate the connective bridges which join the myoma to the adjacent myometrium. **b** Myoma enucleation by rectangular loop (*arrow*), used to identify the cleavage plane between the myoma and myometrium. **c** Myoma removal by rake loop (*arrow*), used to remove the residual deep portion of the myoma once enucleated. **d** Residual myometrial fovea after myoma removal by non-electrical loops

A short-term preoperative antimicrobial prophylaxis with cephalosporins was administered to all patients (cefazolin 1 g i.v.). All the surgical procedures were performed by one senior hysteroscopist (F.P.G.L.) in a day-surgery regimen. Within 2 months after the procedure, a SCSH was scheduled to evaluate disease persistence and to exclude uterine cavity lesions.

Intra-operative surgical outcomes were considered as follows: operating time, fluid deficit, surgical complications and complete resection at first procedure. Fluid deficit >1,500 ml, perioperative haemorrhage and uterine perforation were considered as complications. Intrauterine lesions (synechiae) at follow-up and surgical and/or medical treatment for persisting uterine bleeding were considered as unfavourable long-term outcomes.

A telephone or direct interview follow-up after 6 and every 12 months was scheduled to assess menstrual pattern, pregnancy occurrence and outcome. All patients had at least a 1-year follow-up.

Analysis Demographic and baseline characteristics were analyzed by parametric and nonparametric descriptive statistics where appropriate. Continuous and dichotomous variables before and after surgery were compared using *t* test, nonparametric test and the Fisher's exact test, respectively.

The 75th percentile of mean myoma diameters was used to define the categorical variable small/large myoma. A multivariate logistic analysis was performed to identify variables independently and significantly associated to surgical outcomes. Similarly, a multiple regression analysis was performed using myoma mean diameter and submucous myoma grading as continuous variables. Probability values less than 5% were considered significant. The time to event (abnormal uterine bleeding) analysis for all the patients was performed by the Kaplan–Meyer curve.

Findings

One hundred fifty-nine patients were recruited. Of these, 139 complained abnormal uterine bleeding, 6 were infertile and 14 had both symptoms. Median age (interquartile range) was 44 years (IR 35–48). Mean body mass index (±SD) was 24±5 kg/m^2. Mean parity (±SD) was 1±1. The median mean myoma diameter was 2.1 cm (IR 1.6–3.0). Seventy-seven patients had additional intramural and/or subserous myomas and/or adenomyosis. Eighty-one patients (51%) received preoperative medical treatment with GnRH analogue.

One hundred sixty-nine resectoscopic procedures were performed. Overall, 196 G1–G2 myomas were removed. In the 20 patients with multiple submucous myomas, the worst grading degree was considered for data analysis. Seventy-three myomas were classified as G1 (46%) and 86 as G2 (54%). No women required perioperative blood transfusion. The histological report confirmed the diagnosis of leiomyoma in the vast majority of patients; only three cases of adenomyoma were reported. In 20 patients (13%), concomitant simple endometrial hyperplasia was reported.

The multivariate logistic regression analysis of surgical results defined as perioperative outcomes (operating time

>50 min—75th percentile, fluid deficit >500 ml—75th percentile, incomplete resection, complications such as haemorrhage and uterine perforations), and as long-term outcomes (additional surgery and/or uterine cavity lesions), showed that myoma mean diameter ≥3 cm (75th percentile) was the only significant independent variable associated to abnormal perioperative outcomes (Table 1). None of the considered variables were significantly associated with abnormal long-term surgical outcome. The mean (±SD) myoma diameter of patients with perioperative unfavorable outcome (at least one abnormal outcome parameter) was 3.3 cm (±1.0 cm), significantly different to the 2.2 cm (±0.9 cm) myoma mean diameter of patients with favourable outcome ($p \leq 0.001$).

In order to strengthen the above results, a multiple regression analysis was performed. Myoma mean diameter and submucous myoma grading were considered as continuous variables in relation to both operating time and fluid deficit. By a 1-cm increase of the myoma mean diameter, a significant mean operating time increase of 9.6 min was observed ($p \leq 0.0001$); conversely, a submucous myoma G2 required a not significant operative time increase of 4.4 min compared to a G1 ($p=0.25$). Similarly, by a 1-cm increase of the myoma mean diameter, a significant mean fluid deficit increase of 190 ml was observed ($p<0.001$); conversely, a G2 required a not significant fluid deficit increase of 100 ml compared to a G1 ($p=0.06$).

Table 2 reports surgical outcome of the whole study group and distinguished in details according to myoma grading and mean diameter. The prevalence of myomas ≥3 cm (75th percentile) was not significantly different between G1 and G2 myomas (19% vs. 27%; p=n.s.). One case of uterine perforation occurred by the non-electrical "cold" loop. In the absence of unpredictable thermal damage, this lesion was conservatively managed by transvaginal sonographic monitoring, sulprostone i.v. and prolonged antibiotic therapy.

We compared the first 50 consecutive procedures (learning curve period) with the remaining 119. Perioperative results in the learning period and at steady state were not significantly different both for G1 and G2 myomas and for myomas smaller and larger than 3 cm.

Ten patients (6%) were lost at follow-up.

Irregular bleeding persisted in 23/143 patients (16%), successfully controlled with medical therapy in 13 cases. Figure 2 shows the 7 years (75th percentile of follow-up) of cumulative proportion of women with recurrence of abnormal uterine bleeding. No significant differences were found in the surgery-free survival curve considering grading groups (G1 vs. G2) or myoma mean diameter groups (<3 vs. ≥3.0 cm).

At a median follow-up period of 63 months (IR 36–85), five patients required myomectomy and five hysterectomy for persisting symptoms. Intrauterine adhesions occurred in four of 156 patients (2.6%), which were successfully removed by office hysteroscopy. One patient showed at SCSH a myometrial defect due to electrical damage.

Nine of the 20 infertile patients conceived. Three patients delivered vaginally at term; three patients delivered by caesarean section for breech presentation, foetal macrosomia and foetal distress during labour. One twin pregnancy and one singleton complicated by pre-eclampsia were delivered preterm by caesarean section. One patient had a first trimester miscarriage.

Conclusions

In this prospective study of 159 premenopausal patients with G1 and G2 submucous myomas, we report the combined use of electrical (slicing) and non-electrical loops (enucleation) to respect myometrial fibres functional anatomy and to reduce intravasation and bleeding. We obtained excellent surgical results with a high rate of single step complete resection (88%) with minimal myometrial thermal injury with a negligible number of synechiae (2.6%) and myometrial lesions (0.6%). This compares well to the best

Table 1 Multivariate logistic regression analysis of perioperative and long-term surgical outcomes

	Perioperative surgical outcomes (#159)			Long-term surgical outcomes (#153)		
	Odds ratio	95% CI	p>Chi^2	Odds ratio	95% CI	p>Chi^2
Age (>35 years)	1.03	0.98–1.08	0.29	0.99	0.91–1.08	0.83
Myoma pre-surgical mean diameter (≥3.0 cm)	8.2	1.13–21.0	0.001	1.37	0.23–8.24	0.73
Grading (G2)	1.05	0.48–2.32	0.90	0.61	0.16–2.32	0.47
Number of submucous myomas (>#1)	2.4	0.86–6.85	0.09	3.98	0.79–20.0	0.09
Preoperative GnRH analogue (yes)	1.08	0.45–2.55	0.87	0.72	0.14–3.68	0.69
Coexisting uterine lesions (yes)[a]	0.96	0.46–2.0	0.90	0.32	0.08–1.3	0.11

GnRH gonadotropin-releasing hormone

[a] Intramural myomas, adenomyosis and endometrial hyperplasia

Table 2 Surgical outcomes of the whole study group (159 patients) and related to submucous myomas grading (G) and to myoma mean diameter (*d*)

	Study group	G1	G2	*p*	*d*<3.0 cm	*d*≥3.0 cm	*p*
Patients, no.	159	73	86	–	119	40	–
Procedures, no.	169	76	93	–	123	46	–
Operating time (min) (median–IR)	35 (20–50)	30 (20–50)	45 (25–50)	0.19	30 (20–50)	50 (37–85)	0.0001
Fluid deficit (ml) (median–IR)	150 (90–500)	120 (70–400)	200 (100–570)	0.06	100 (80–300)	400 (225–700)	0.0001
Complications, no. (%)	10 (6)	3 (4)[a]	7 (8)[b]	0.3	4 (3)[c]	6 (15)[d]	0.008
Complete resection at first procedure, no. (%)	140 (88)	67 (92)	73 (85)	0.18	116 (96)	24 (60)	0.0001

IR interquartile range, *G1* grade 1, *G2* grade 2

[a] Two fluid deficit >1,500 ml, one perioperative haemorrhage

[b] Three perioperative haemorrhage, one uterine perforation, three fluid deficit >1,500 ml

[c] Two fluid deficit >1,500 ml, one uterine perforation, one perioperative haemorrhage

[d] Three perioperative haemorrhage, three fluid deficit >1,500 ml

reported results (1–12%) and to unpublished data by Mazzon [3, 11, 17].

In particular, the complete removal for G1 and G2 submucous myomas was 92% and 85%, respectively, not significantly different. This result was in line with the best results of previous studies reporting a complete removal by traditional monopolar slicing of 73–93% for G1 and 50–85% for G2, respectively [4, 6, 7, 18–21].

By means of cold loops traction-and-leverage technique itself, combined with a basic low intrauterine pressure setting (50 mmHg), complete resections were more easily achieved also in large myomas, with a limited number of complications. In fact, the maintenance of the integrity of myometrial fibres, particularly the function of archimetrial layer [22], and of myoma pseudocapsule permitted to avoid deep and larger myometrial vessels damage and to obtain adequate haemostatic myometrial contractions. This reduced the risk of fluid overload, achieving a median fluid deficit significantly lower than in previous studies [5, 7] and similar to those reported more recently [21] which might have adopted similar low intrauterine fluid pressure.

The need of repetitive changing of electrical and non-electrical "cold" loops during the same procedure might appear to be time-consuming. However, as well as in Formula 1 races, where the changing of tires at pit stop improves the car's performance, by this technique, the complete dislocation of the intramural portion of the myoma into the uterine cavity leads to a faster and safer complete removal.

To our surprise, myoma grading was not significantly associated with any of the adverse perioperative and long-term outcome. Beyond fluid deficit, which was nearly similar in G1 and G2, all other surgical outcomes were not affected by grading in this cohort in which myomas were enucleated by cold loops and not by electrosurgical slicing. The 75th percentile of myoma mean diameter of this cohort was 3 cm. This occurred to be equal to the dimension cut-off value adopted by previous authors to differentiate small and large myomas [6, 21, 23]. This myoma mean diameter proved to be the only independent significant determinant correlated to perioperative surgical outcomes (operating time >50 min, fluid deficit ≥500 ml, surgical complications and incomplete resection at first procedure). These relevant data were strictly confirmed by the multiple regression analysis. Long-term outcomes (persisting symptoms and additional surgery for persisting symptoms) were not significantly different neither for the severity of grading

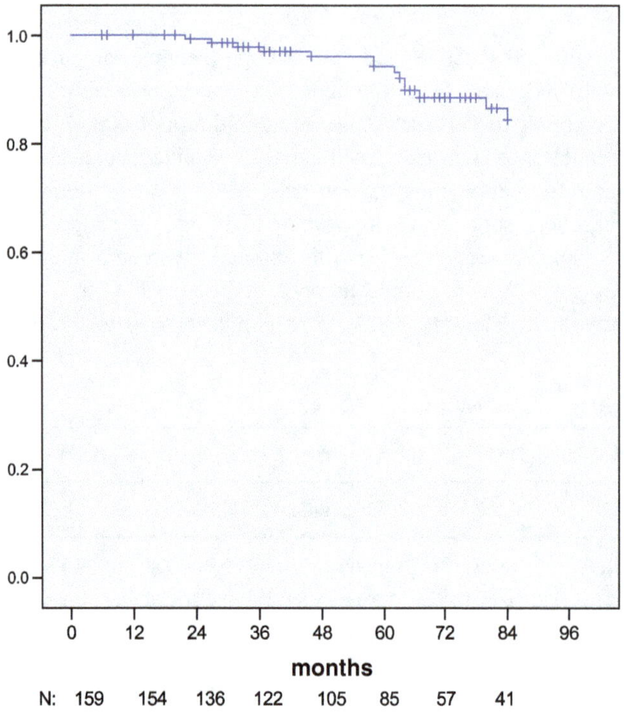

Fig. 2 Kaplan–Mayer curve of overall surgery-free survival. The percentage of patients free of surgery at 3 years was 97% (95% CI, 94–99.9), 94% (95% CI, 90–98) at 5 years and 87% (95% CI, 83–91) at 7 years

nor for the myoma mean diameter and were comparable to those previously reported with a 7-year surgery-free rate of 87% [18, 24].

Operation time, fluid decifit and complete resection at first procedure were highly significantly correlated to myoma dimension >3 cm. The importance of myomas size underlines the debatable role of pre-surgical medical treatment with the aim to reduce large submucous myomas [25, 26]. GnRH analogues are significantly more efficacious on submucous when compared to the effect on intramural or subserosal myomas [27]. However, its use in this series was not significant (Table 1), probably due to the higher technical difficulties arising in the removal of the myoma from the pseudocapsule.

Perioperative complications (fluid deficit >1,500 ml, uterine perforation and perioperative haemorrhage) occurred in ten cases (6%). These data were comparable to reported rates in series considering advanced hysteroscopic procedures, i.e. involving the myometrium [3, 19, 20].

The only uterine perforation occurred in a case with a coexisting intramural myoma adjacent to the submucous which prevented myometrial progressive thickening during enucleation as observed at sonography by Yang [28] and Casadio [29]. This perforation occurred by using cold loops avoiding further thermal damage on surrounding organs.

The negligible number of synechiae (2.6%) and myometrial lesions (0.6%) are strictly correlated with the surgical technique, clearly demonstrating that no thermal damage by monopolar current into the myometrium is an important factor for the adhesion formation, significantly lower than the reported variable incidence of 7.5–45.5% [11, 17, 30]. These results, added to the high rate of G2 and >3 cm submucous myomas one-step complete resection (85% and 60%, respectively) and the low rate of intra-operative complications, clearly evidenced the proven practical advantages derived by the use of this combined electrical and non-electrical "cold" technique. Obstetric outcomes in infertile patients were satisfactory, with a pregnancy rate of 45%, similar to previously published data (36–45%) [31, 32].

Surgeon skills might be a remarkable bias in this series, being all procedures performed by an experienced hysteroscopist [3, 13, 23]. However, the learning curve analysis by comparing the first 50 procedures with the following did not detect any significant worse outcomes in the learning phase.

Although the study group was limited for the evaluation of short- and long-term complications, the population was very well defined and the surgical conditions were also well standardized (one technique, one operator and one centre).

In conclusion, hysteroscopic myomectomy by cold loops revealed to be an effective (low complication rate and high single-step complete resection) and efficient (day-surgery procedure and low long-term failure rate) surgical approach to the removal of submucous myoma with intramural development. Furthermore, by using this technique, myoma mean diameter proved to be the only prognostic factor of perioperative outcomes.

Conflicts of interest The authors report no conflicts of interest. The authors alone are responsible for the content and writing of the paper.

References

1. Hidlebaugh DA (2001) Relative costs of gynecologic endoscopy vs traditional surgery for treatment of abnormal uterine bleeding. Am J Manag Care 7:SP31–SP37
2. Brumsted JR, Blackman JA, Badger GJ, Riddick DH (1996) Hysteroscopy versus hysterectomy for the treatment of abnormal uterine bleeding: a comparison of cost. Fertil Steril 65(2):310–316
3. Di Spiezio SA, Mazzon I, Bramante S, Bettocchi S, Bifulco G, Guida M et al (2008) Hysteroscopic myomectomy: a comprehensive review of surgical techniques. Hum Reprod Update 14 (2):101–119
4. Wamsteker K, Emanuel MH, de Kruif JH (1993) Transcervical hysteroscopic resection of submucous fibroids for abnormal uterine bleeding: results regarding the degree of intramural extension. Obstet Gynecol 82(5):736–740
5. Emanuel MH, Hart A, Wamsteker K, Lammes F (1997) An analysis of fluid loss during transcervical resection of submucous myomas. Fertil Steril 68(5):881–886
6. Hart R, Molnar BG, Magos A (1999) Long term follow up of hysteroscopic myomectomy assessed by survival analysis. Br J Obstet Gynaecol 106(7):700–705
7. Vercellini P, Zaina B, Yaylayan L, Pisacreta A, De Giorgi O, Crosignani PG (1999) Hysteroscopic myomectomy: long-term effects on menstrual pattern and fertility. Obstet Gynecol 94 (3):341–347
8. Darwish A, Zareh HZ (2002) Haemodynamic, biochemical and haematological changes during hysteroscopic myomectomy. Gynecol Endosc 11:349–355
9. Baggish MS, Tucker RD (1995) Tissue actions of bipolar scissors compared with monopolar devices. Fertil Steril 63(2):422–426
10. Munro MG, Fu YS (1995) Loop electrosurgical excision with a laparoscopic electrode and carbon dioxide laser vaporization: comparison of thermal injury characteristics in the rat uterine horn. Am J Obstet Gynecol 172(4 Pt 1):1257–1262
11. Yang JH, Chen MJ, Wu MY, Chao KH, Ho HN, Yang YS (2008) Office hysteroscopic early lysis of intrauterine adhesion after transcervical resection of multiple apposing submucous myomas. Fertil Steril 89(5):1254–1259
12. Mazzon I (1995) Nuova tecnica per la miomectomia isteroscopica: enucleazione con ansa fredda.In Testo-Atlante di Chirurgia Endoscopica Ginecologica. Edited by E Cittadini, A Perino, M Angiolillo, et al. Palermo, Italy, Cofese Ed.
13. Camanni M, Bonino L, Delpiano EM, Ferrero B, Migliaretti G, Deltetto F (2010) Hysteroscopic management of large symptomatic submucous uterine myomas. J Minim Invasive Gynecol 17 (1):59–65
14. Leone FP, Lanzani C, Ferrazzi E (2003) Use of strict sonohysterographic methods for preoperative assessment of submucous myomas. Fertil Steril 79(4):998–1002
15. Leone FP, Bignardi T, Marciante C, Ferrazzi E (2007) Sonohysterography in the preoperative grading of submucous fibroids:

considerations on three-dimensional methodology. Ultrasound Obstet Gynecol 29:717–718
16. Loffer FD, Bradley LD, Brill AI, Brooks PG, Cooper JM (2000) Hysteroscopic fluid monitoring guidelines. J Am Assoc Gynecol Laparosc 7(1):167–168
17. Touboul C, Fernandez H, Deffieux X et al (2009) Uterine synechiae after bipolar hysteroscopic resection of submucosal myomas in patients with infertility. Fertil Steril 92:1690
18. Emanuel MH, Wamsteker K, Hart AA, Metz G, Lammes FB (1999) Long-term results of hysteroscopic myomectomy for abnormal uterine bleeding. Obstet Gynecol 93(5 Pt 1):743–748
19. Cravello L, Agostini A, Beerli M, Roger V, Bretelle F, Blanc B (2004) Results of hysteroscopic myomectomy. Gynecol Obstet Fertil 32(9):825–828
20. Polena V, Mergui JL, Perrot N, Poncelet C, Barranger E, Uzan S (2007) Long-term results of hysteroscopic myomectomy in 235 patients. Eur J Obstet Gynecol Reprod Biol 130(2):232–237
21. Lasmar RB, Xinmei Z, Indman PD, Celeste RK, Di Spiezio SA (2011) Feasibility of a new system of classification of submucous myomas: a multicenter study. Fertil Steril 95(6):2073–2077
22. de Ziegler D, Bulletti C, Fanchin R, Epiney M, Brioschi PA (2001) Contractility of the nonpregnant uterus: the follicular phase. Ann N Y Acad Sci 943:172–184
23. Donnez J, Polet R, Smets M, Bassil S, Nisolle M (1995) Hysteroscopic myomectomy. Curr Opin Obstet Gyencol 7:311–316
24. Cravello L, Farnarier J, Roger V, D'Ercole C, Blanc B (1998) Hysteroscopic myomectomy. Functional results with an average follow-up of 6 years. J Gynecol Obstet Biol Reprod (Paris) 27 (6):593–597
25. Muzii L, Boni T, Bellati F, Marana R, Ruggiero A, Zullo MA et al (2010) GnRH analogue treatment before hysteroscopic resection of submucous myomas: a prospective, randomized, multicenter study. Fertil Steril 94(4):1496–1499
26. Mavrelos D, Ben-Nagi J, Davies A, Lee C, Salim R, Jurkovic D (2010) The value of pre-operative treatment with GnRH analogues in women with submucous fibroids: a double-blind, placebo-controlled randomized trial. Hum Reprod 25(9):2264–2269
27. Brosens J, Campo R, Gordts S, Brosens I (2003) Submucous and outer myometrium leiomyomas are two distinct clinical entities. Fertil Steril 79(6):1452–1454
28. Yang JH, Lin BL (2001) Changes in myometrial thickness during hysteroscopic resection of deeply invasive submucous myomas. J Am Assoc Gynecol Laparosc 8(4):501–505
29. Casadio P, Youssef AM, Spagnolo E, Rizzo MA, Talamo MR, De Angelis D et al (2011) Should the myometrial free margin still be considered a limiting factor for hysteroscopic resection of submucous fibroids? A possible answer to an old question. Fertil Steril 95(5):1764–1768
30. Taskin O, Sadik S, Onoglu A, Gokdeniz R, Erturan E, Burak F, Wheeler JM (2000) Role of endometrial suppression on the frequency of intrauterine adhesions after resectoscopic surgery. J Am Assoc Gynecol Laparosc 7(3):351–354
31. Somigliana E, Vercellini P, Daguati R, Pasin R, De Giorgi O, Crosignani PG (2007) Fibroids and female reproduction: a critical analysis of the evidence. Hum Reprod Update 13:465–476
32. Shokeir T, El-Shafei M, Yousef H, Allam AF, Sadek E (2010) Submucous myomas and their implications in the pregnancy rates of patients with otherwise unexplained primary infertility undergoing hysteroscopic myomectomy: a randomized matched control study. Fertil Steril 94(2):724–729

6

Handheld articulating laparoscopic instruments driven by robotic technology: First clinical experience in gynecological surgery

A. Hackethal • M. Koppan • K. Eskef • H.-R. Tinneberg

Abstract Kymerax, a new robotic-driven, handheld articulating laparoscopic device, that provides improved triangulation while preserving precise motions, has just recently been introduced to the European market. The KYMERAX System consists of a generator, handles, and interchangeable instruments. We describe a case in which KYMERAX was successfully used during a total laparoscopic hysterectomy. A 42-year-old patient (IIG/IIP) presented with a history of hypermenorrhagia and dysmenorrhagia. Because of a prior cesarean section and to rule out further pathologies possibly associated to dysmenorrhagia, the patient was prepared for a total laparoscopic hysterectomy in our department. The world's first human use of the KYMERAX System was discussed in details with the patient prior to the procedure. The first clinical use in gynecologic laparoscopy proved to be feasible with the new robotic-driven, articulating, handheld surgical system. KYMERAX may offer benefits in advanced laparoscopy, NOTES, and single-port surgery.

Keywords Motor-driven · Triangulation · Total laparoscopic hysterectomy · KYMERAX · Robotic

A. Hackethal (✉) · K. Eskef · H.-R. Tinneberg
Department of Obstetrics and Gynaecology,
Justus-Liebig-University of Giessen,
Klinikstr. 33,
35385 Giessen, Germany
e-mail: andreas.hackethal@gyn.med.uni-giessen.de

M. Koppan
Department of Obstetrics and Gynecology, Health Science Center,
University of Pécs,
17 Édesanyák Street,
7624 Pécs, Hungary

Background

Laparoscopic surgeons have evolved to operate without the flexibility of wrist movements. Compared to daily human manual activities, the conventional laparoscopic instrument, which has an approximate length of 35 cm, offers an active instrument tip for grasping, cutting, dissecting, coagulating tissue, and similar activities which frequently require rotation. However, triangulation or articulation of instrument tips, just as the wrists, was exclusively offered in the overly expensive laparoscopic robotic system, called Da Vinci [1].

A new motor-driven, handheld system that offers precision-driven, articulating instruments, called KYMERAX (Terumo, Japan) has recently been introduced to the medical market in Europe.

The KYMERAX System is comprised of a console, handles, and interchangeable instruments. Up to two handles can be connected to the console, which provides power to the motors located within the handle component of the system. These motors are activated by the user through the manipulation of the buttons and controls of the handle interface, and allows for rotation and yawing motions of the instrument tips (Figs. 1, 2). The motors for the instruments rotation and yawing speed can be adjusted from 1 to 5 (slow to fast) within the console.

The four available instruments attach to the handle component, are 8.8 mm in diameter and include a Monopolar scissors, Maryland dissector, needle driver, and monopolar L-hook.

The Department of Gynecology and Obstetrics at the University Clinic of Giessen, Germany was the second facility to use the KYMERAX System clinically, after the Urology Department at the University of Salzburg, Austria, and was the first facility worldwide to perform a gynecologic case, a total laparoscopic hysterectomy. First clinical

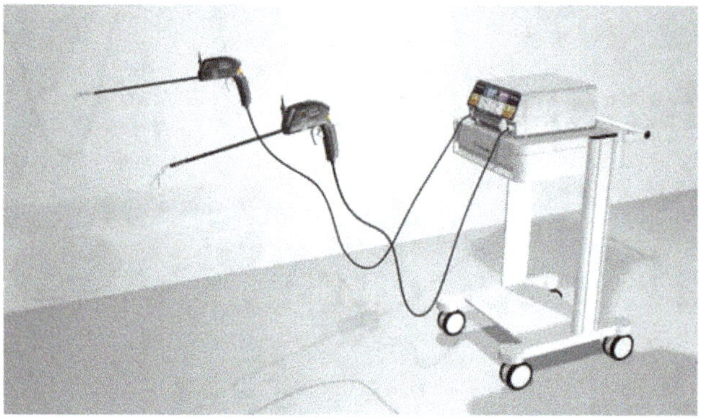

Fig. 1 The KYMERAX System is comprised of a console, handles, and interchangeable instruments

experiences and a guide for familiarization with the new motor-driven, articulating instrument system are discussed.

Method

A 46-year-old patient (IIG/IIP) with known uterine myomas presented with hypermenorrhagia and dysmenorrhagia. Earlier dilatation and curettage revealed no pathologies and hysterectomy was discussed with the patient for treatment. Because of a previous cesarean section, and to rule out further pathologies possibly associated to dysmenorrhagia, the patient was prepared for a total laparoscopic hysterectomy in our department.

Before the procedure, adequate explanation was given to the patient about the KYMERAX System and its first time use in gynecologic laparoscopy. On the 13th of May, 2011, a total laparoscopic hysterectomy (TLH) was performed at the Department of Gynecology and Obstetrics in Giessen, Germany. Ipsilateral trocar placement was used on the surgeon's side (Fig. 3).

The TLH followed a standardized procedure with following key steps:

1. Sealing and transecting the round ligament
2. Transecting the ovarian ligament and the uterine tube

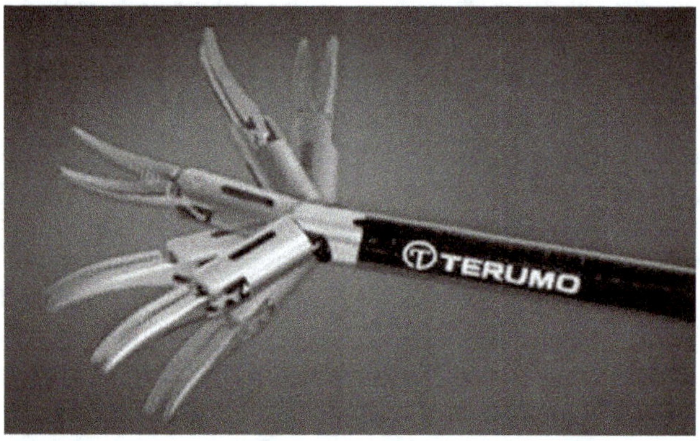

Fig. 2 The possible articulated and rotated instrument tip

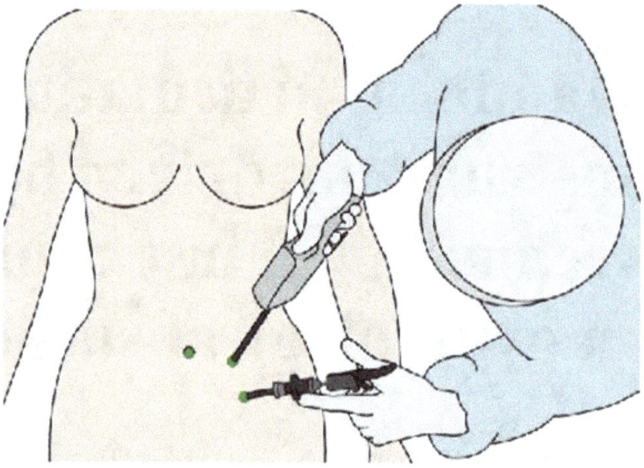

Fig. 3 The ipsilateral placement of working trocars for the surgeon

3. Dissecting the broad ligament
4. Identifying the ureter (Fig. 4)
5. Exposing and sealing the uterine vessels
6. Skeletonizing the cervix (Fig. 5)
7. Resecting the uterus (Fig. 6)
8. Closing the vaginal cuff (Fig. 7)

The surgical procedure was performed without any intraoperative complications. Blood loss was <5 ml, surgical time from insertion of the Veres needle to closure of the skin, 90 min. After an uneventful postoperative course, the patient was discharged on postoperative day 3.

Findings

The first clinical use in gynecological laparoscopy proved to be feasible with the new robotic-driven, articulating

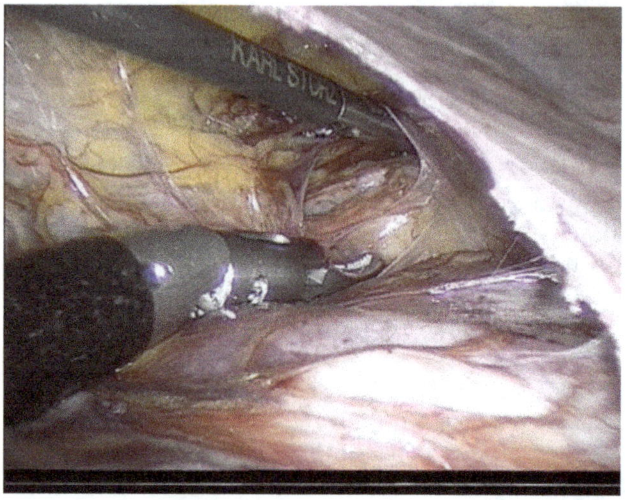

Fig. 4 The KYMERAX dissector is used to open the retroperitoneum and identify the ureter-uterine crossing

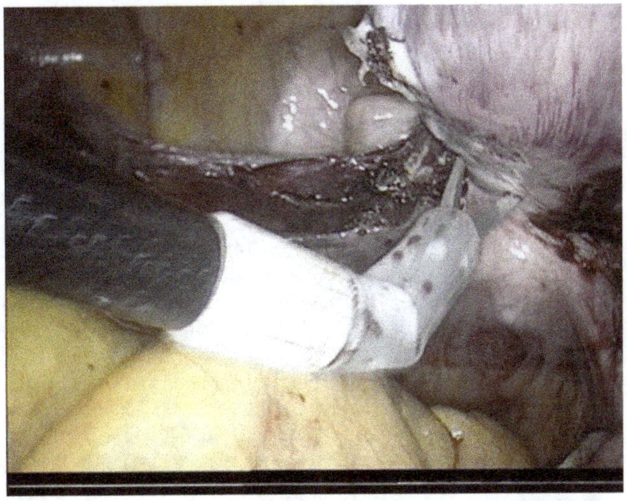

Fig. 5 The KYMERAX Monopolar Scissors are used for skeletonizing the uterine cervix

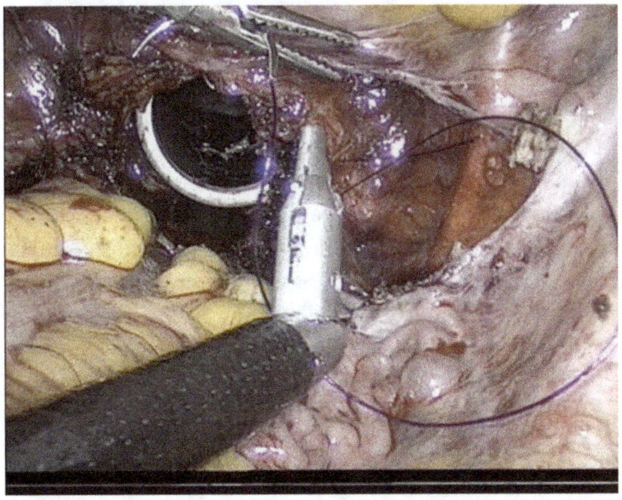

Fig. 7 The KYMERAX needle driver is used for suturing the vaginal cuff

instrument. Ipsilateral trocar placement was confirmed to be especially beneficial, as thee articulating tips of the KYMERAX instruments allowed for contralateral dissection of the broad ligament, the skeletonizing of the cervix, and transection and suturing of the vagina. There were no complications and the patient was discharged after an uneventful hospital stay of 3 days.

The idea of angled instruments for laparoscopy is not new [2]. Hand-manipulated angled instruments such as the Realhand or the Radius Surgical System have been proposed earlier, but never entered the market on a wide range [3, 4]. Advanced vision has also been introduced to the market and has shown a variety of possible benefits [5].

Though the KYMERAX System was previously used by the authors AH and MK extensively in bench studies, including animal and cadaver models, the first clinical use brightens the possible benefits. These may include more precise dissecting abilities while tissue can be manipulated three dimensionally, ease in identifying and dissecting hard to reach structures and compartiments with reduction of tissue trauma, advancing suture techniques within a limited space, possible reduction of shoulder strain experienced by the surgeon through ipsilateral trocar placement, and reduced number of abdominal incisions. Compared to other full robotic consoles, KYMERAX seems to be reasonably priced, therefore allowing for a wider spread distribution.

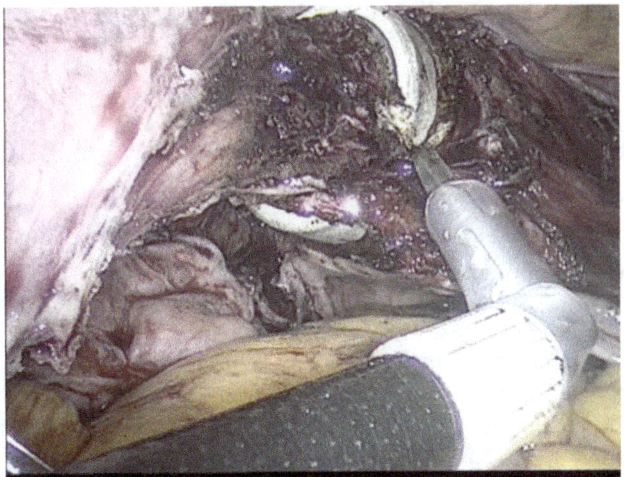

Fig. 6 The KYMERAX Monopolar Scissors are used for separating the vaginal cuff

However, as with all highly advanced new technical equipment, novices will experience a steeper learning curve when adapting to the articulation. The use of buttons placed on the instruments handle to drive the tip, requires familiarization. To increase patient safety and to reduce surgeon's efforts, a standardized curriculum for getting acquainted with the advances of triangulation should be mandatory for new users of the KYMERAX System. This may also reduce difficulties in directing the tip and support effectiveness of using the articulating branches.

Nowadays, surgeons have adapted to the drawbacks of conventional laparoscopy, such as limited maneuverability and two-dimensional vision, but are still able to perform highly advanced surgical procedures, such as pelvic and paraaortic lymphadenectomies. Patients requiring highly advanced surgical procedures, as well as those with procedures requiring extensive suturing (i.e., myomectomy, sacrocolpopexy), may benefit from a more precise and possibly faster surgery. Also, the surgeon may benefit, as shoulder and elbow strain may be reduced, when utilizing more comfortable and ergonomic trocar placement. This better trocar placement is the result of a shift of triangulation from the surgeon's upper extremities to the tip of the instrument.

Conclusion

KYMERAX, the new handheld robotic-driven technology with articulating instrument tips, is a long awaited development for minimally invasive surgery. This innovative device offers a path-breaking alternative between conventional laparoscopic surgery and the unrivaled Da Vinci Robotic system. Further clinical use and adequate clinical studies are necessary to highlight the instrument benefits. Independent from that, the uniqueness of allowing the surgeon to use his/her "wrist," offers a benefit that overcomes one of the major drawbacks of laparoscopic surgery.

Declaration of interest A. Hackethal and M. Koppan were actively involved in the development of KYMERAX as consultants for Terumo, Japan and received consulting fees or honoraria.

References

1. Wexner SD, Bergamaschi R, Lacy A, Udo J, Brolmann H, Kennedy RH, John H (2009) The current status of robotic pelvic surgery: results of a multinational interdisciplinary consensus conference. Surg Endosc 23:438–443
2. Usui S, Inoue H, Yoshida T, Kudo SE, Iwai T (2004) Preliminary report of multi degrees of freedom forceps for endoscopic surgery. Surg Laparosc Endosc Percutan Tech 14:66–72
3. Rettenmaier MA, Lopez K, Graham CL, Brown JV, John CR, Micha JP, Goldstein BH (2009) Realhand high dexterity instruments for the treatment of stage I uterine malignancy. JSLS 13:27–31
4. Waseda M, Inaki N, Torres Bermudez JR, Manukyan G, Gacek IA, Schurr MO, Braun M, Buess GF (2007) Precision in stitches: Radius Surgical System. Surg Endosc 21:2056–2062
5. Eskef K, Oehmke F, Tchartchian G, Muenstedt K, Tinneberg H-R, Hackethal A (2011) A new variable-view rigid endoscope evaluated in advanced gynecologic laparoscopy: a pilot study. Surg Endosc 25(10):3260–3265 [Record Supplied By Publisher]

Global–local anaesthesia: combining paracervical block with intramyometrial prilocaine in the fundus significantly reduces patients' perception of pain during radio-frequency endometrial ablation (Novasure®) in an office setting

Henrik Skensved

Abstract The aim of this study was to investigate the effectiveness of combining a paracervical block with an intramyometrial block of the uterine fundus on women's perception of pain during Novasure® radio-frequency impedance-controlled endometrial ablation. The study design was a case–control study. The study was conducted in private practice/office setting. The patients were 83 premenopausal women undergoing endometrial ablation due to heavy menstrual periods. The intervention used was hysteroscopic injection of local anaesthetic into the myometrium of the uterine fundus in addition to a paracervical block. There were no adverse events as a consequence of either the anaesthesia or the ablation procedure. All women were asked 60 s into the active ablation procedure to estimate their perception of pain on a scale from 0 to 10. Fifty-seven women (69%) scored a 0, and 77 (92%) scored 2 or less. None needed to use recovery room facilities after the procedure, and none made use of the access to performing surgeon the evening and night after the procedure. Combining a traditional paracervical block with a transhysteroscopic injection of local anaesthesia into the subendometrial myometrium of the fundus of the uterus significantly reduces women's perception of pain during radio-frequency impedance-controlled endometrial ablation.

Keywords Endometrial · Ablation · Local · Anaesthesia · Paracervical · Fundal · Pain · Ropivacaine

H. Skensved (✉)
Frederiksgade 2 A,
3400 Hillerod, Denmark
e-mail: henrik@gynaekologen.dk

Background

Second-generation endometrial ablation devices such as the Novasure® have been developed to enable clinicians to perform treatments under local anaesthesia in an office setting. However, a review of the literature on office-based Novasure® ablations reveals that an acceptable level of pain during active ablation has been difficult to achieve often necessitating simultaneous administration of general anaesthetics, sedatives or tranquillizers, which, in many hospitals and clinics, make the treatments unsuitable for the office setting for which they were originally intended.

Materials and methods

Between February 2002 and September 2011, premenopausal women referred from their general practitioner with heavy menstrual bleedings refractory to medical treatment or in whom such medical treatments were contraindicated were offered bipolar radio-frequency impedance-controlled endometrial ablation under local anaesthesia.

Women with large myomas, fibroids protruding into the cavity or a cavity depth exceeding 75 mm, were excluded from the study. Likewise, women with cavity depths of less than 35 mm and women in whom the distance from a caesarean scar to the fundus was less than 35 mm were not offered endometrial ablation. Furthermore, women with estimated cavity width of less than 30 mm were not offered endometrial ablation. Women with type 2 fibromas less than 40 mm in diameter with only marginal protrusion into the uterine cavity not disfiguring it were considered eligible for ablation. Women with known coagulation defects, inborn or iatrogenic, were not offered ablation under local anaesthesia.

Only women meeting the criteria of ASA group 1 and 2 were included in the study. To exclude intrauterine pathology and distorted cavities, a vaginoscopic microhysteroscopy was performed on all women at their first visit. A transvaginal ultrasound done immediately after the microhysteroscopy (with fluid still in the cavity) allowed measurement of length of the cervical canal, the cavity depth and an estimation of cavity width. The women were advised against fasting before surgery; on the contrary, they were recommended a light breakfast or lunch before treatment. Pre-emptive pain control consisted of 500 mg of naproxen 2 h before treatment; in women where NSAIDs were contraindicated, naproxen was replaced by 1 g of paracetamol.

In accordance with national Danish recommendations, all women received antibiotics as a prophylactic (cefalexin 500 mg twice daily for 5 days) commencing 12 h prior to surgery. After the woman had been placed in the dorsolithotomy position, a paracervical block (PCB) was established using a pudendal syringe with a 6-mm needle tip; repeated aspiration to avert intravascular injection was performed.

Until August 2008, women were treated under PCB only using alfentanil 0.2–0.4 mg intravenously on demand as rescue anaesthesia (Table 1). From September 2008 to March 2011, the PCB consisted of 10 ml of 0.25% of ropivacaine (Naropin®) at 3, 5, 7 and 9 o'clock, respectively (i.e., a total of 40 ml). Since March 2011, the concentration of ropivacaine has been reduced to 0.2% in a similar volume.

In addition, 0.5 ml of mepivacaine chloride was injected in the anterior lip to avoid pain from the later placement of a single-tooth Luer Vulsellum. To allow the paracervical block ample time to become fully effective, no uterine manipulation or instrumentation whatsoever was undertaken for 10 min after the injection of the last dose of ropivacaine. Subsequently, a hysteroscopy was performed using a 5.5-mm hysteroscope (Olympus Europa GmbH, Hamburg, Germany and Richard Wolf GmbH, Knittlingen, Germany) with a 5-F working channel.

Since September 2008, an additional 4 ml of Citanest® (30 mg prilocaine/0.54 μg felypressin per millilitre) was placed in the myometrium of the fundal wall through a 5-F Williams cystoscopic injection needle (Cook Medical Inc., Bloomington, IN, USA) (Fig. 1), under direct vision and after aspiration. One millilitre of local anaesthetic was placed medial to each of the tubal ostia; the remaining 2 ml was injected with 1 ml on either side of the midline of the fundus (Figs. 2, 3 and 4).

Table 1 Until August 2008, women were treated under PCB only using alfentanil 0.2–0.4 mg intravenously on demand as rescue anaesthesia

	Ropivacaine 0.5%	Ropivacaine 0.375%	Ropivacaine 0.25%
Number	25	25	27
VAS score (0–10)	4.1 (±1.7)	4.9 (±1.7)	4.0 (±1.6)
Rescue anaesthesia (*N*)	5	6	6

The 8-mm syringe at the end of the Williams needle was introduced at its full length into the myometrium at which stage aspiration was performed in order to confirm non-perforation. Applying pressure on the piston, the needle was subsequently retracted until there was a "loss of resistance", i.e. a decrease in resistance reflecting a position of the tip of the syringe at the superficial layer of the myometrium adjacent to the musculo-mucosal junction.

Link to video 1: http://www.youtube.com/watch?v=_I6gx4qAsWA

To avoid bleeding from obscuring the hysteroscopic view of the uterine cavity at the time of fundal injections, levonorgestrel-releasing intrauterine devices (LNG-IUDs) that where present were not removed until the fundal block had been established.

Link to video 1: http://www.youtube.com/watch?v=_I6gx4qAsWA

Hereafter, the cervical canal was dilated to Hegar number 8 and the Novasure® device placed according to the manufacturer's instructions. All the ablation procedures were performed by one surgeon (H.S.). The women's oxygen saturation, heart rate, and blood pressure were monitored during the whole procedure, beginning as the paracervical block was established.

Sixty seconds into the active ablation, all the women were asked the same standardized question with regard to pain. The question was posed by the nurse assisting the surgeon, and the women scored their perception of pain on a scale from 0 to 10 (visual analogue scale (VAS) score).

After the completion of the ablation procedure, a hysteroscopy was performed in order to determine whether the

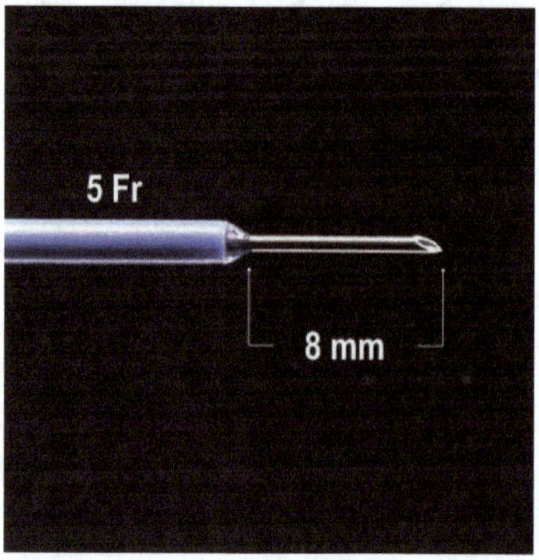

Fig. 1 William cystoscopic injection needle (Cook Medical Inc., Bloomington, IN, USA)

treatment could be categorized as complete and to exclude any trauma to the uterus. In all cases, the hysteroscopies before and after treatment were digitally recorded.

The women were asked to sit in the clinic's waiting room until they themselves felt fit to leave. The women had access to a stretcher in a separate room if necessary. At departure from the office, the women were encouraged to contact the surgeon on a mobile number on which they could reach him at any time during the first 24 h after surgery, if so needed. Postoperatively, the women were instructed to take naproxen 250 mg (or 1 g of paracetamol) 4 and 8 h after the procedure, respectively. All of the women were contacted by phone the following morning by the same nurse assistant who was present during the ablation procedure. The women included in the study were the first to whom the hysteroscopic fundal block was applied in this clinic.

Findings

In 99 women, the shape and size of the uterus fulfilled the inclusion criteria. Five women had medical illnesses preventing treatment in an office setting. Two women insisted on a hysterectomy, and nine women did not want treatment under local anaesthesia and thus were referred to a tertiary unit for a transcervical resection of the endometrium under general anaesthesia. Hence, 83 women were included in the study. Twenty-three women (27.7%) had a retroverted uterus, and 24 women (28.9%) had an LNG-IUD (Mirena®) correctly placed in the uterine cavity at their first visit. All of the ablation procedures were completed with no intra- or postoperative complications. None of the women had any adverse reaction to the paracervical block; ten (12.0%) described a slight dizziness or light-headedness after the injection of prilocaine into the fundal myometrium, five of them experienced an additional tingling of the tongue, but in all ten cases, blood pressure, pulse rate and oxygen saturation remained stable and within normal limits. In none of the 83 cases did aspiration after placing the tip of the William needle in the fundal myometrium give suspicion of perforation.

The VAS scores 60 s into the ablation procedure are presented in Table 2. The average VAS score of 0.6 is significantly lower than the score of 4.0 using a 0.25% ropivacaine PCB only ($p<0.0001$). None of the 83 women in the present study asked for alfentanil during the active ablation or immediately after.

None of the 83 women needed to use the surgery's recovery room, and none of the women spent more than 20 min sitting in the waiting room having tea or coffee after the termination of the Novasure® procedure. During the first evening and night after the procedure, 3 women did not use any pain relief at all, 9 women used paracetamol only, 50 used the 250 mg of naproxen that was prescribed to them prior to surgery, and 21 women used paracetamol and naproxen in combination. None of the women made use of the access to the performing surgeon that was made available to them by mobile phone during the first 24 h after surgery.

Twenty women returned to work the day after the ablation procedure; the remaining 63 women returned to work 1–3 days after treatment. At 1-month follow-up, none had experienced genital infection. Three of the women (3.6%) developed haematometra which was easily resolved by dilatation under an intracervical block in the office. All of the 83 women (100%) stated that they would recommend the Novasure® procedure as performed above to a friend.

One of the women scoring a 7 had a distorted uterine cavity following resection of the left cornua due to a tubal pregnancy, a (failed) laparoscopic sterilization and a caesarean section including a resection of the remaining right tube. As a consequence, it was very difficult to reach the left corner of the cavity during preablative hysteroscopy, and hence, the block of the left cornua was insufficient.

The other woman with a score of 7 and the woman scoring 5 had completely normal, anteverted uteruses, and there were no problems in placing the intramyometrial injections. They both completed the ablation procedure without needing rescue anaesthesia, and their vital functions did not change during the active ablation.

The additional expense using the cystoscopic needle and 4 ml of Citanest for the fundal block amounted to €33 for each patient as compared to the cost of the Novasure device of €840 (Gothia Medical, Bildal, Sweden).

Discussion

Scientific data on bipolar radio-frequency ablations under local anaesthesia are equivocal. Several trials describing the use of local anaesthesia for Novasure® ablation include use of conscious sedation in addition to the intra- or paracervical block [2–4], making an evaluation of the specific contribution of the local anaesthesia in a single accumulated pain score impossible.

Most studies did not report specific pain scores [2–6], and therefore, the conclusions that Novasure® under local anaesthesia was *feasible* could not be supported by specific and comparable data. This again makes it difficult to establish whether the protocol reported is broadly and not only locally acceptable to the women and hence the results generalizable to and reproducible in other settings than the one tested.

One study [7] reported an average VAS score of 5.1 (out of 10) which, however, was obtained 4 h after the ablation procedure was terminated, making an evaluation of the women's perception of pain during the active endometrial destruction process arbitrary. This is also the case with the latest published study, in which the participating women were not asked until 30 min after the end of the procedure when the average VAS score was 4.18 (out of 10) [8]. The latter result is in line with the VAS scores we obtained using a PCB as the sole anaesthetic (Table 1).

Only one study reported VAS scores obtained during the actual ablation procedure [9], and the average VAS score here was 7.7 (±2.0) (out of 10). This result was achieved despite the use of a deep intracervical block in which the local anaesthetic was placed at the level of the internal os.

The cervix and the lower two thirds of the corpus are innervated from the sacral S1–3 nerves, whereas the upper part of the uterus including the fundus receives its innervation from the thoracic nerves T8–10 [1].

All studies included here [2–4, 6–9] used local anaesthesia injected by the intra- or paracervical route only, thus leaving the nerves from T8–10 in the upper part of the uterus unanaesthetized and hence susceptible to noxious stimuli during the ablation which can explain the high VAS scores in women treated under para- or intracervical block only.

The significance of the separate innervation of the fundus as a key to understanding the insufficient pain relief during intracavitary surgery under PCB is underpinned by results obtained during hysteroscopic sterilization under a paracervical block (which provided effective pain relief for cervical manipulations but did not reduce the pain associated with upper uterine/tubal manipulation when placing the devices) [10] as well as during vacuum aspiration under PCB after incomplete miscarriage [11]. These results are in line with conclusions in the latest Cochrane review on PCB for uterine interventions [12].

Investigators have sought to solve the above dilemma by intrauterine installation of local anaesthetics in the form of liquid, aerosol, or gel, but positive effects of such procedures have not been demonstrated in practice [13]. Thurkow (2005, personal communication) speculated that one way of addressing the above problem could be transhysteroscopically injected local anaesthesia in the fundus as a means of blocking the nerves to the upper part of the uterus.

This is the first published study where the paracervical block is combined with a hysteroscopically guided, submucosal, intramyometrially injected local anaesthetic into the upper part of the body of the uterus as the sole anaesthesia for endometrial ablation.

Ropivacaine was selected for the PCB because it is low toxic and long acting covering the first 3–4 h of the postoperative period when risk of painful uterine cramping

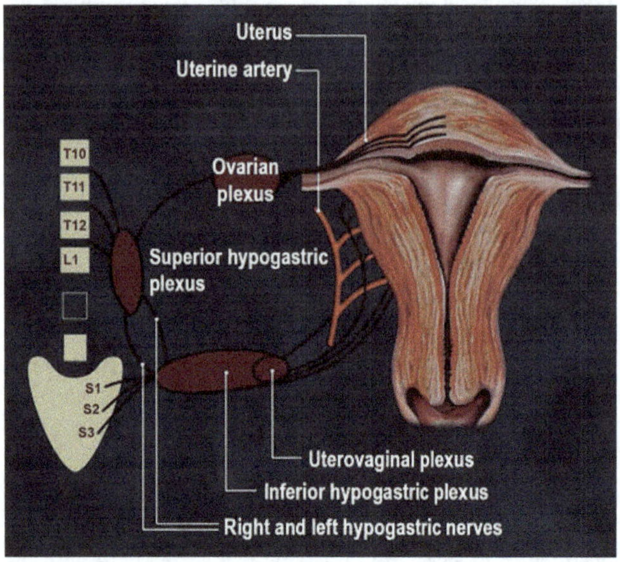

Fig. 2 The innervation of the uterus

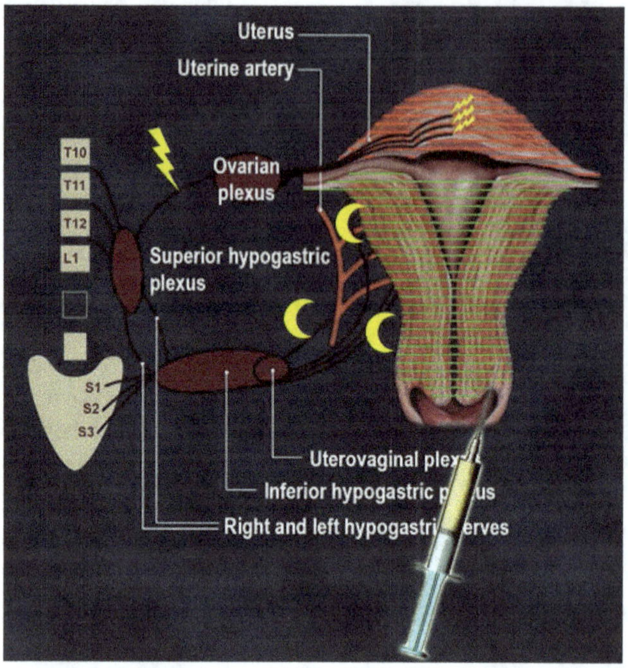

Fig. 3 Anaesthetic coverage of an intra- or paracervical block only

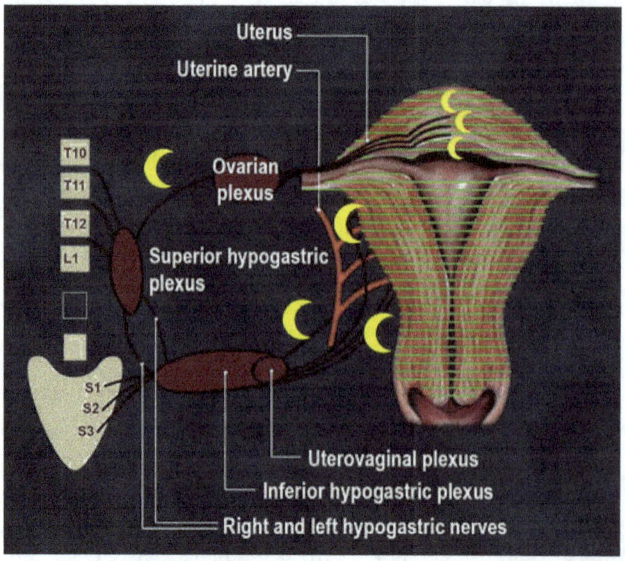

Fig. 4 Anaesthetic coverage of the global–local anaesthesia

Table 2 VAS score (0–10) 60 s into active Novasure endometrial ablation

Results from 83 consecutive ablations September 2008 to September 2011
Pain score 0 (zero) 57 (69%)
Pain score 1 (one) 14 (17%)
Pain score 2 (two) 5 (6%)
Pain score 3 (three) 5 (6%)
Pain score 7 (seven) 2 (2%)

is at its highest. Ropivacaine at high concentrations produces vasodilation, but a study of infiltration anaesthesia demonstrated that 0.25% ropivacaine decreases skin blood flow in man [14]. Hence, it is possible that ropivacaine has a similar vasoconstrictive effect on the uterine vessels, but no studies exist to support (or contradict) this. In order to avoid systemic side effects in case of accidental intravasal injection, no epinephrine or any other vasoconstrictor was added to the ropivacaine.

Whereas a high-volume/low-concentration ropivacaine solution was chosen for the PCB, the high-concentration/low-volume prilocaine solution was chosen for the fundal block in order to minimize the risk of larger subendometrial depots of liquid interfering with the registration of tissue impedance on which the control of the radio-frequency ablation is based.

Maximum dose recommendations concerning local anaesthetics should ideally, as stressed by Scott [15], take into consideration factors such as varying absorption at different injection sites (such as the parametrium) as well as patient characteristics (e.g. age). However, no such ideal recommendations exist.

Compared to the maximum dose of ropivacaine of 300 mg officially recommended in Finland, Japan and the USA and the maximum dose of prilocaine of 400 mg officially recommended in Finland and Sweden [16], the doses of 100 mg of ropivacaine (subsequently 80 mg) and 135 mg of prilocaine used in the present study are well within the limits of these guidelines.

Breuninger et al. [17] used up to 150 ml of a mixture of 50 ml 1% ropivacaine, 50 ml of 2% prilocaine and 400 ml of Ringer's solution as local anaesthesia in 2,257 patients undergoing minor surgical procedures (excision of dermal tumours and scars as well as transplantations in the head and neck region) without a single major or minor incident involving the local anaesthesia. This result further indicates that the combination of ropivacaine and prilocaine used here is safe.

The results of the present study deviate significantly from the studies on pain during and after bipolar radio-frequency endometrial ablation hitherto published [7–9]. It should be emphasised that this conclusion is based on findings of a non-randomised controlled study and therefore may not reliably support the effectiveness and use of intramyometrial anaesthesia in the fundus during endometrial ablation.

Aside from the block of the nerves supplying the fundal region of the uterine cavity used only in this study, part of this difference might also be ascribable to the difference in anaesthetic compound used for paracervical and intracervical block in the studies. The popular use of prilocaine might be attributable to its faster onset of action compared to ropivacaine. However, the study by Breuninger et al. [17] demonstrated that a mixture of prilocaine and ropivacaine, albeit decreasing the median duration of action, at the same time increased the speed of onset.

Consequently, future trials should test various mixtures of prilocaine and ropivacaine for the PCB in order to determine the most optimal combination with regard to onset as well as duration of action. Furthermore, tests of different concentrations of prilocaine for the fundal block can establish the most effective volume and concentration of local anaesthetic.

Conclusion

The results of this study indicate that through a combination of a high-volume/low-concentration paracervical block and a fundal block, the latter placed in the submucosal myometrium during the preoperative hysteroscopy, it is possible to establish a globally active local anaesthesia—*the global–local*—which makes procedures such as the Novasure® endometrial ablation safely performable in a low-tech out-of-hospital office setting with very little discomfort to the patient and without need of additional anaesthetics, sedatives and tranquillizing agents, anaesthesiological support or recovery facilities. Obviously, further studies particularly in the form of randomised controlled trials on a larger scale are necessary.

References

1. Campbell I (2005) Uterine physiology. Anaesth intensive care med 6:76
2. Cooper J, Gimpelson R, Laberge P, Galen D, Garza-Leal JG, Scott J, Leyland N, Martyn P, Liu J (2002) J Am Assoc Gynecol Laparosc 9:418–428
3. Laberge P, Sabbah R, Fortin C, Gallinat A (2003) J Am Assoc Gynecol Laparosc 10:223–232
4. Baskett TF, Clough H, Scott TA (2005) NovaSure bipolar radiofrequency endometrial ablation: report of 200 cases. J Obstet Gynecol Can 27:473–476
5. Bongers MY, Bourdrez P, Mol BWJ, Heintz APM, Brölmann HAM (2004) Randomised controlled trial of bipolar radio-frequency endometrial ablation and baloon endometrial ablation. BJOG 111:1095–1102

6. Samuel NC, Karragianniadou E, Clark TJ (2009) Outpatient versus day-case endometrial ablation using the Novasure impedance-controlled ablative system. Gynecol Surg 6:3–9
7. Penninx JPM, Mol BW, Bongers MY (2009) Endometrial ablation with paracervical block. J Reprod Med 54:617–620
8. Kalkat RK, Cartmill SV (2011) Novasure endometrial ablation under local anaesthesia in an outpatient setting: an observational study. J Obstet Gynaecol 31:152–155
9. Clark TJ, Samuel N, Malick S, Middleton LJ, Daniels J, Gupta JK (2011) Bipolar radiofrequency compared with thermal baloon endometrial ablation in the office. Obstet Gynecol 1:109–118
10. Chudnoff S, Einstein M, Levie M (2010) Paracervical block efficacy in office hysteroscopic sterilization: a randomized controlled trial. Obstet Gynecol 115:26–34
11. Gomez PI, Gaitán H, Nova C, Paradas A (2004) Paracervical block in incomplete abortion using manual vacuum aspiration: randomized clinical trial. Obstet Gynecol 103:943–951
12. Tangsiriwatthana T, Sangkomkamhang US, Lumbiganon P, Laopaiboon M. (2009) Paracervical local anaesthesia for cervical dilatation and uterine intervention. Cochrane Database of Systematic Reviews 2009, Issue 1. Art. No.: CD005056. doi:10.1002/14651858.CD005056.pub2
13. Hassan L, Gannon MJ (2005) Anaesthesia and analgesia for ambulatory hysteroscopic surgery. Best Pract Clin Obstet Gynaecol 19:681–691
14. Cederholm I, Evers H, Löfström JB (1991) Effect of intradermal injection of saline or a local anaesthetic agent on skin blood flow—a methodological study in man. Acta Anaesthesiol Scand 35:208–215
15. Scott DB (1989) Maximum recommended doses of local anaesthetic drugs. Br J Anaesth 63:373–374
16. Rosenberg PH, Veering BT, Urmey WF (2004) Maximum recommended doses of local anesthetics: a multifactorial concept. Reg Anesth Pain Med 29:564–575
17. Breuninger H, Schimek F, Heeg P (2000) Subcutaneous infusion anaesthesia with diluted mixtures of prilocain and ropivacain. Langenbeck's Arch Surg 385:284–289
18. Kalkat RK, Cartmill SV (2011) Novasure endometrial ablation under local anaesthesia in an outpatient setting: an observational study. J Obstet Gynaecol 31:152–155

8

Clinical indices and histological changes over time in ovarian torsion related to ovarian tumors

Mitsuru Shiota • Yasushi Kotani • Masahiko Umemoto • Takako Tobiume • Hiroshi Hoshiai

Abstract In some emergency surgeries for ovarian torsion, the ovary cannot be conserved because of necrosis. Ovarian necrosis and the time from the onset of symptoms to surgery are likely to be directly correlated. In this study, we retrospectively evaluated the clinical indices from the time of onset of acute abdomen to surgery at our hospital, in patients with tumor-related ovarian torsion. Among cases diagnosed preoperatively with benign ovarian tumors between 1995 and 2010, there were 54 patients who developed acute abdomen that was surgically diagnosed as ovarian torsion. For evaluation, these patients were divided into two groups according to the time from the onset of acute abdomen to surgical intervention as follows: <10 and ≥10 h. C-reactive protein (CRP) levels, leukocyte counts, body temperature, tumor size, and degree of torsion were compared between the two patient groups. Ovarian status based on postoperative histopathology was classified as necrotic, congestive, or normal, and was also evaluated. The mean CRP level was significantly higher in the ≥10-h patient group than in the patients undergoing surgery in <10 h. No differences were observed between the two groups for leukocyte counts, body temperature, tumor size, and mean degree of torsion. Ovarian necrosis was only observed only in patients undergoing surgery at ≥10 h. When tumor-related ovarian torsion is suspected, surgery should be performed within 10 h after the onset of acute abdomen to conserve ovarian function.

Keywords Ovarian tumor · Acute abdomen · Torsion · Emergency surgery · Necrosis

M. Shiota (✉) · Y. Kotani · M. Umemoto · T. Tobiume · H. Hoshiai
Department of Obstetrics and Gynecology,
Kinki University Faculty of Medicine,
377-2 Ohno-higashi, Osaka-sayama Osaka 589-8511, Japan
e-mail: shiota@med.kindai.ac.jp

Background

Ovarian tumor is one of the most common gynecological diseases. Among complications of ovarian tumors, ovarian torsion causes acute abdomen and is an indication for emergency surgery. Torsion has been reported to occur in 6.9–11% of ovarian tumor patients [1, 2]. In general, when ovarian torsion develops, venous blood flow to the ovary is first blocked, followed by abrupt onset of abdominal pain, and then, the arterial blood flow is blocked, then in some cases the ovary becomes necrotic [3] over time. In addition, ovarian tumors can rupture in some patients, resulting in peritonitis and even disseminated intravascular coagulation (DIC) [4]. In the event of necrosis, sometimes the ovary cannot be conserved and oophorectomy is required, and in other cases, even if the ovary can be conserved, ovarian function is lost. However, Mashiach et al. [5] have shown that black-blue ovaries can be preserved with no damage, maintaining future ovarian function. From the aspect of fertility, it is especially important to preserve ovarian function in pubescent and sexually mature patients with torsion.

Mazouni et al. reported that necrosis was significantly more frequently observed in patients undergoing surgery more than 10 h from the onset of abdominal pain [6]. However, there has been no definitive report on the relationship between the time to surgery and ovarian function in tumor-related ovarian torsion. In this study, we retrospectively examined patients with tumor related ovarian torsion who had undergone surgery at our hospital, and evaluated their clinical indices from the time of onset of acute abdomen until surgery.

Methods

There were 1,723 patients (1,224 laparoscopies and 499 laparotomies) who were preoperatively diagnosed with benign ovarian tumor and underwent surgery at our hospital from January 1995 to December 2010. Among these, there were 54 patients (25 laparoscopies and 29 laparotomies, 29 adnexectomies and 25 ovarian tumorectomies) who underwent surgery because of acute abdomen and who were diagnosed with tumor-related ovarian torsion based on the intraoperative findings.

These patients were divided into the following two groups according to the time from the onset of acute abdomen to surgery: <10 and ≥ 10 h until surgery. C-reactive protein (CRP) levels (upper limit of normal, ≤ 0.3 mg/dl), leukocyte counts (reference range, $3.5–8.5 \times 10^3/\mu l$), body temperature, tumor size, and degree of torsion were compared between the two groups. The degree of torsion was estimated at 90° intervals intraoperatively. Blood samples and body temperatures were obtained approximately 1 h before surgery.

Based on postoperative histopathological examinations of excised ovaries, the subjects were also classified into the following three groups for evaluation: a group in which necrosis was observed in at least some of the ovarian tumor tissues (Fig. 1), a group in which necrosis was not found but congestion was observed, and a normal group in which neither necrosis nor congestion was observed. The two patient groups characterized by time to surgery were compared in relation to the distribution of histopathological classifications.

For statistical analysis, the Student *t*-test was used to evaluate comparisons between the two groups. P values <0.05 were considered statistically significant.

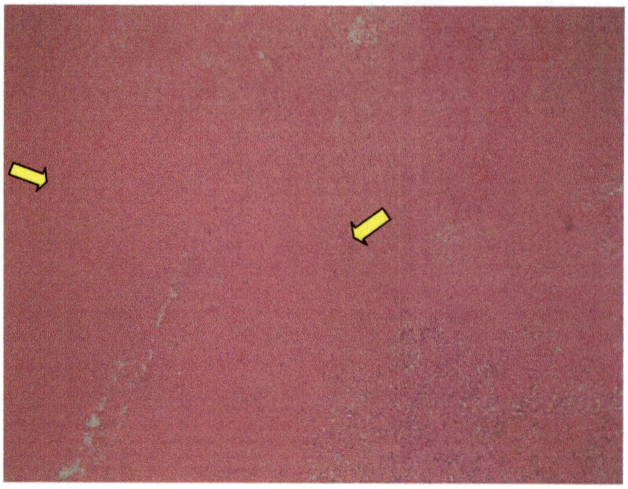

Fig. 1 Pathologic necrosis (H&E, ×40)

Findings

The values of the assessed parameters are shown in Table 1. The mean CRP levels in the patients who underwent surgery 10 h or more after symptom onset were 1.7 mg/dl, and 0.1 mg/dl in patients who underwent surgery in less than 10 h, which was significant. No differences were observed in mean leukocyte counts at $10.1 \times 10^3/\mu l$ and $10.0 \times 10^3/\mu l$; in mean body temperatures, at 36.7°C and 37.1°C; in mean tumor sizes, at 8.3 and 9.5 cm; and mean degrees of ovarian torsion, at 506° and 667°, respectively, for the group of less than 10 h and the group of 10 h or more. Regarding histopathlogical findings, there were ten normal and ten congestive histological tissue specimens in the group of patients undergoing surgery less than 10 h after symptoms, whereas there were nine normal, 12 congestive, and 13 necrotic specimens in the patients undergoing surgery at 10 h or more. Necrotic ovaries were only seen in the $\geq$10-h group. Among the 13 necrotic specimens, there were 11 with partial necrosis and two with complete necrosis, in which the entire tissue was necrotic. The delay was due to transportation from the referring clinic to our hospital (Table 2).

Discussion

Preoperative diagnosis of ovarian torsion caused by ovarian tumor is difficult, and the condition must be differentiated from other emergent gynecological diseases that present with abdominal pain, such as rupture of ovarian tumor, ovarian hemorrhage, uterine adnexitis and ectopic pregnancy. Ovarian torsion has been found

Table 1 Comparisons of data on the two groups of patients classified by time to surgery

	Overall (n=54)	Time <10 h (n=20)	Time ≥10 h (n=34)	P value
CRP[a] (mg/dl)	1.1±2.9 (0–2.9)	0.1±0.3 (0–1.4)	1.7±3.6 (0–12.9)	<0.01
WBC[b] (10^3/μl)	10.1±3.1 (3.2–17.3)	10.1±2.8 (4.7–13.4)	10.0±3.2 (4.2–17.3)	n.s.
Temperature (°C)	36.9±0.7 (35.9–38.7)	36.7±0.5 35.9–37.7)	37.1±0.7 (35.6–38.7)	n.s.
Tumor diameter (cm)	9.1±3.3 (3.6–20.0)	8.3±2.8 (4.5–15.0)	9.5±3.6 (3.6–20.0)	n.s.
Degree of torsion (°)	607±309 (120–1260)	506±258 (120–900)	667±325 (180–1,260)	n.s.

n.s. no significant difference

[a] CRP upper limit of normal: ≤ 0.3 mg/dl

[b] White blood cell count reference range: 3.5–8.5×10^3/μl

to represent between 2.5% and 7.4% of surgical cases of acute abdomen [7, 8]. Thus, it is not uncommon for the diagnosis to be made only after emergency diagnostic laparoscopy [9, 10]. Currently, there is no specific blood biomarker for tumor-related ovarian torsion [11, 12]. In suspected torsion, it is of primary importance to diagnose the torsion as soon as possible for emergent surgery, but it is also important to determine whether the affected ovary can be conserved by assessing for necrosis. However, determining the necrotic status of an ovary preoperatively is difficult. Mazouni et al. reported that necrosis was more frequently observed in cases in which more than 10 h had passed since the onset of abdominal pain [6]. On the other hand, Bar-On et al. reported that patients undergoing operations less than 10 h after admission were statistically more likely to have ovarian torsion [13]. In this study, the mean CRP level was significantly higher in the group undergoing surgery at 10 h or more than in the group undergoing surgery at less than 10 h. Histologically confirmed necrosis was only observed in the group undergoing surgery at 10 h or more. Some studies have reported that ovarian torsion could occur following ovarian stimulation [14–16]. In this study, however, all ovarian torsion cases were associated with ovarian tumor.

Therefore, ovarian necrosis caused by ovarian torsion associated with an ovarian tumor tends to develop when more than 10 h have elapsed since the onset of acute abdomen, and development of necrosis leads to an elevated CRP level. The results of this study also indicate that if ovarian torsion is suspected, surgery should be performed as soon as possible at least within 10 h after the onset of acute abdomen to conserve ovarian function. In our hospital, surgery is performed promptly for an inpatient when ovarian torsion is suspected. The cases that were delayed were primarily those cases transported from other hospitals. Therefore, if the hospital does not have the appropriate operating facilities, prompt arrangement of transportation is necessary for a patient with suspected ovarian torsion.

Table 2 Number of cases according to histopathological status in the two groups of patients classified by time to surgery

	<10 h (range)	≥10 h (range)	Total
Normal	10 (3–9 h)	9 (10–31 h)	19
Congestive	10 (4–6 h)	12 (10–27 h)	22
Necrotic	0	13 (10–264 h)	13
Total	20	34	54

Conclusion

In all the cases in this study that were classified in the necrotic group for evaluation, necrosis was seen in least a part of the tissue specimen. Although we cannot conclude from our findings that ovarian function would be lost in every patient in the necrotic group, if torsion is suspected, we believe that immediate action is necessary to preserve ovarian function. Also, in any cases where the torsion is suspected, surgery should be performed as soon as possible.

The limit of this present study is that 10 h was taken as cut-off reference time on the basis of the result indicated in the study by Mazouni et al. However, time to surgery is a continuous variable, and the cases should have been investigated at different time points especially regarding the torsion of ovary. We will address this issue more precisely in the future study, taking the time parameter as a continuous variable.

Conflicts of interest The authors report no conflicts of interest. The authors alone are responsible for the content and writing of the paper.

References

1. Lee CH, Raman S, Sivanesaratnam V (1989) Torsion of ovarian tumors: a clinicopathological study. Int J Gynaecol Obstet 28:21–25
2. Sommerville M, Grimes DA, Koonings PP, Campbell K (1991) Ovarian neoplasms and the risk of adnexal torsion. Am J Obstet Gynecol 164:577–578
3. Nichols DH, Julian PJ (1985) Torsion of the adnexa. Clin Obstet Gynecol 28:375–380
4. Ishikawa M, Tamate K (1999) Comprehensive handbook of women's medicine 8. In: Taketani Y (ed) Emergency gynecologic and obstetric cases. Nakayama Shoten, Tokyo, p 40
5. Mashiach S, Bider D, Moran O, Goldenberg M, Ben-Rafael Z (1990) Adnexal torsion of hyperstimulated ovaries in pregnancies after gonadotropin therapy. Fertil Steril 53:76–80
6. Mazouni C, Bretelle F, Ménard JP, Blanc B, Gamerre M (2005) Diagnosis of adnexal torsion and predictive factors of adnexal necrosis. Gynecol Obstet Fertil 33:102–106 (in French)
7. Hibbard LT (1985) Adnexal torsion. Am J Obstet Gynecol 152:456–461
8. Anteby SO, Schenker JG, Polishuk WZ (1975) The value of laparoscopy in acute pelvic pain. Ann Surg 181:484–486
9. Mage G, Canis M, Manhes H, Pouly JL, Bruhat MA (1989) Laparoscopic management of adnexal torsion. A review of 35 cases. J Reprod Med 34:520–524
10. Porpora MG, Gomel V (1997) The role of laparoscopy in the management of pelvic pain in women of reproductive age. Fertil Steril 68:765–779
11. Chiou SY, Lev-Toaff AS, Masuda E, Feld RI, Bergin D (2007) Adnexal torsion: new clinical and imaging observations by sonography, computed tomography, and magnetic resonance imaging. J Ultrasound Med 26:1289–1301
12. Descargues G, Tinlot-Mauger F, Gravier A, Lemoine JP, Marpeau L (2001) Adnexal torsion: a report on forty-five cases. Eur J Obstet Gynecol Reprod Biol 98:91–96
13. Bar-On S, Mashiach R, Stockheim D et al (2010) Emergency laparoscopy for suspected ovarian torsion: are we too hasty to operate? Fertil Steril 93:2012–2015
14. Bider D, Mashiach S, Dulitzky M, Kokia E, Lipitz S, Ben-Rafael Z (1991) Clinical, surgical and pathologic findings of adnexal torsion in pregnant and nonpregnant women. Surg Gynecol Obstet 173:363–366
15. Oelsner G, Bider D, Goldenberg M, Admon D, Mashiach S (1993) Long-term follow-up of the twisted ischemic adnexa managed by detorsion. Fertil Steril 60:976–979
16. Shalev E, Peleg D (1993) Laparoscopic treatment of adnexal torsion. Surg Gynecol Obstet 176:448–450

9

Laparoscopic sacrocolpopexy: impact of the learning curve

Céline Castellier · Lucie Bresson · Michel Cosson · Jean-Philippe Lucot

Abstract Genital prolapse is one of the most frequent reasons for gynaecologic consultations. Laparoscopic sacrocolpopexy (LSC) became the gold standard since laparoscopy was developed. We retrospectively compared two groups of patients: 82 who undergone LSC from January 1996 to December 2002 (group A) and 169 from January 2002 to December 2009 (group B), always by the same team. Suspension was reinforced with two strips of synthetic mesh. Laparoscopy was performed in 93 women of group A and 169 of group B. They all had symptomatic uterine prolapse. Conversion to laparotomy because of technical difficulties was significantly lower in the second than the first period (1 vs. 11, $p<0.001$). We performed less culdoplasty, levator myorrhaphy and Burch colposuspension ($p<0.001$) but more associated cure of urinary stress incontinence in the second period. Peri-operative complications (7.3% vs. 1.8%, $p=0.006$), post-operative complications (21% vs. 5%), and surgical length decreased (231 to 191 min, $p<0.001$). Six patients (7%) in group A had re-intervention, 15 (9%) in group B. LSC is a reproducible technique. A learning curve shortens the length of intervention and operative and post-operative complications and rate of conversion to laparotomy.

Keywords Laparoscopy · Sacrocolpopexy · Complications · Learning curve

C. Castellier (✉) · L. Bresson · M. Cosson · J.-P. Lucot
Pôle de chirurgie gynécologique, Hôpital Jeanne de Flandre,
Avenue Eugène Avinée,
59 037 Lille Cedex, France
e-mail: celine.castellier@yahoo.fr

Background

Genital prolapse is one of the most frequent reasons for gynaecological consultation. In their lifetime, women have an 11% risk to be surgically treated for altered pelvic statics. Prolapse is linked to urinary incontinence in 38% of cases and one third of patients will have further intervention [1], the risk growing with age. Life is longer, quality of life is better, and women's demands for surgery increase. Prolapse surgery is an anatomical reconstruction but, above all, a functional surgery.

Nowadays, several techniques using several surgical routes are possible to treat prolapse (vaginal, laparotomy and laparoscopy). The operator may freely choose which are according to his experience and his skills, the type of the prolapse, the age of the patient, her characteristics and her wishes. However, the use of one technique over another is still subject to discussion.

Sacrocolpopexy remains the reference in this prolapse surgery. Described by laparotomy by the Huguier and Scali team in 1957 [2, 3], the technique has evolved. It has since been adapted to laparoscopy [4] with gestures now standardised [5, 6]. Laparoscopic surgery of prolapse with mesh began more than 10 years ago [7, 8]. Laparoscopy, which is less invasive, allows more precise and complete dissection of the different spaces with more precise view of anatomical landmarks.

In the same way, procedures associated with sacrocolpopexy have changed; Burch has been replaced by suburethral transobturator strips (TVT®) and culdoplasty has disappeared.

We wanted to compare two groups of patients treated for prolapse by the same laparoscopic sacrocolpopexy (LSC) technique, the same team, at two different periods. We could thus assess the evolution of associated procedures, peri- and post-surgical complications, and rate of re-interventions.

Methods

Patients

We realised a retrospective study of patients who had a laparoscopic sacrocolpopexy for genital prolapse, by the same team, from January 1996 to December 2009. There were divided in two groups: group A, 1996–2002 at Paul Gellé maternity ward of Roubaix Hospital and group B: 2002–2009 in medico-surgical gynaecologic service of Hospital Jeanne de Flandre (CHRU, LILLE).

Surgical indication for symptomatic prolapse largely depended on the patient's demand and wishes which were discussed with her. When clinical examination also found urinary incontinence, it was treated in the same surgical time.

Surgical technique

Keyhole interventions were done under general anaesthesia, in dorsal decubitus, an in Trendelenburg position. Surgical technique used was described by Cosson [9]. Four trocars were used: a 10-mm transumbilical trocar for the laparoscope, two reusable 5-mm trocars inserted lateral to the umbilicus and epigastric vessels on either side, and finally a 10-mm trocar placed in the suprapubic position. Associated procedures, such as supracervical hysterectomy with or without adnexectomy, were performed first, using bipolar coagulation and scissors. The cervix was sectioned with monopolar scissors. After supracervical hysterectomy, the uterus was morcellated using a morcellator (STORZ®). We dissected the vaginal fornices by mobilising the bladder anteriorly and the rectum and sigmoid posteriorly. Anterior and posterior lengths of non-resorbable synthetic mesh were sutured to the vaginal wall. When conservation of the uterus was required, the anterior strip was Y-shaped, its two arms going through the broad ligament before reaching the sacral promontory. The peritoneum overlying the sacrum was opened, and the areolar tissue was carefully dissected to expose the anterior longitudinal sacral ligament. Two permanent O sutures were placed in the anterior longitudinal sacral ligament to suspend the mesh. Tension was applied via extra-abdominal knots and checked by the surgeon. The mesh was then trimmed and implanted by closing the peritoneum with a resorbable continuous non-locking running suture. Meshes used were made of polyester (PARIETEX®) or of knitted polypropylene monofilament (SURGIPRO®, GYNEMESH®).

When necessary, a BURCH colposuspension was performed. The retropubic space was dissected transperitoneally after opening the peritoneum. The ureterovaginal junction and Cooper's ligament were exposed. One non-resorbable suture was placed on either side of the urethra in the vaginal wall, taking care not to transfix the vagina, and suspended on Cooper's ligament. The peritoneum was then closed with resorbable 2/0 using a running suture. Burch colposuspension was performed except in cases of previous surgery for incontinence without recurrence.

Vaginal myorrhaphy of the levator muscles was carried out as in Huguier's description [10]. A 4-cm longitudinal incision of the vaginal mucosa was made over the posterior fourchette. The edges of the incision were held with Allis clamps and the peri-rectal fascia was dissected, revealing the margins of the levator ani. A heavy number 1 absorbable synthetic suture was passed through the levator ani near the posterior fourchette. The posterior vaginal wall was closed with a resorbable running suture. Myorrhaphy of the levator muscles was performed when clinically indicated.

Urinary incontinence was cured with suburethral strips (TVT®, TVT-O®)[11, 12]. With the patient in lithotomy position, suburethral vaginal wall was infiltrated with xylocain. After a medial incision, we dissected laterally to ischiopubic ramus. The obturator membrane was perforated with scissors. The mesh was then placed and tension was regulated. Vaginal closure was effected with a running suture of resorbable thread 3/0.

Data were stored retrospectively in patient's files. Operation length was estimated on laparoscopic time only. Patients with concomitant laparoscopic rectopexy were excluded from the study.

Statistical analysis was realised with Excel Microsoft and Epi-Info (6.4 version). Student's t test was used to analyse quantitative variables. Qualitative variables were analysed with χ^2 test, odds ratio or bilateral Fischer's test for values inferior to 5. Results are considered significant when $p<0.005$.

Findings

During the period of the study, 93 patients underwent surgery in group A (1996–2002) and 169 in group B (2002–2009). The characteristics of patients and their antecedents are summed up in Table 1. The only significant difference is the women's age which is higher in group B. History of hysterectomy and cure of prolapse are not significantly different between the two groups.

Associated procedures with laparoscopic sacrocolpopexy are detailed in Table 2. There is a significant decrease of culdoplasties and transvaginal myorrhaphy of elevators. Burch's colposuspension was replaced by synthetic sub-urethral strips. Indications of curing urinary incontinence

Table 1 Characteristics of patients with their main gynaecologic surgical antecedents

	Group A N=82	Group B N=168	p value	Odds ratio (IC at 95%)
Age	47±8.6	51±8.6	<0.001	NA
BMI	25±5.0	24±3.9	0.25	NA
Parity	3.2±1.9	2.8±1.4	0.05	NA
Menopausal	20 (24%)	60 (36%)	0.07	0.58 (0.31–1.09)
Substitutive hormonal treatment	9 (11%)	11 (7%)	0.23	1.76 (0.64–4.82)
Surgical gynaecologic history	29 (35%)	41 (24%)	0.07	1.69 (0.92–3.13)
Cure of prolapse	7 (9%)	21 (13%)	0.35	0.65 (0.24–1.72)
Cure of urinary incontinence	7 (9%)	15 (9%)	0.92	0.95 (0.34–2.62)
Hysterectomy	9 (11%)	13 (8%)	0.40	1.47 (0.55–3.88)

NB. Some patients had several interventions for prolapse and/or urinary incontinence and several procedures were sometimes concomitant

NA not applicable, *BMI* body mass index

remain stable at 9% in both study periods. Mean surgical length is significantly shorter, 231 to 191 min (p<0.001). Hospitalisation length remains identical in the two groups: 3.2±1.5 days in group A vs. 3.0±1.1 days in group B (p=0.21).

Post-surgical complications are shown in Table 3. There was no mortality or major peri-operative complication. Post-surgical complications did not decrease enough to be significant (7.3% in group A and 1.8% in group B, p= 0.06). Most frequent complication was bladder injury. Diagnosis was always made during intervention, with immediate laparoscopic suture and permanent urinary catheterization for 7 days. After-effects were straightforward. In group A, bladder was wounded when threading the needle of retropubic TVT®. Diagnosis was achieved by cystoscopy, the needle removed then replaced without further complication. A vaginal lesion happened at time of dissection in group B. Laparoscopic suture, then fixing of a polypropylene mesh, was straightforward without infection or prosthetic exposure. Omental haematoma was noted when sigmoid was suspended to abdominal wall. The after-effects were straightforward. Subcutaneous emphysema did not prevent laparoscopy.

Laparotomy conversion rates were significantly different between the two groups, from 12% to 0.6%. In group A, indications of 11 laparoconversions were adhesions (four cases), hypercapnia (three cases), difficult access to promontory (two cases), or bleeding (two cases). In group B, the only conversion was due to adhesions.

Early post-surgical complications were four times less frequent in group B (5%) than in group A, p<0001 (Table 4.). These complications were mainly lower urinary tract infections. Their frequency in the two periods changed from 15% to 4%. In group A, we had two haematomas, one in Retzius space was surgically drained and another was medically treated. Two women had a urinary retention, while re-intervention and section of TVT strip was necessary in one case. In group B, three haematomas were seen at trocar port, one needed a re-intervention for drainage. All in all, two patients in group A and one in group B had a re-intervention for early post-surgical complications.

Table 2 Procedures associated with laparoscopic sacrocolpopexy

	Group A N=82	Group B N=168	p value	Odds ratio (IC at 95%)
Supracervical hysterectomy	57 (70%)	100 (60%)	0.13	1.55 (0.85–2.83)
Adnexectomy	26 (32%)	72 (43%)	0.09	0.62 (0.34–1.12)
Culdoplasty	67 (82%)	42 (25%)	<0.001	13 (6.62–27.47)
Posterior perineorraphy	36 (44%)	0	<0.001	NA
Burch	45 (55%)	0	<0.001	NA
TVT-O®	0	57 (34%)	<0.001	NA
TVT®	4 (5%)	1 (0, 6%)	0.002	8.56 (0.88–205)
Mini-Arc®	0	1 (0, 6%)		
Tubal ligation	2 (2%)	8 (5%)	0.38	0.50 (0.07–2.62)
Perineoplasty	0	2 (1.2%)		
Anal sphincteroplasty (Musset)	2 (2%)	0		
Richter	1 (1%)	0		

Table 3 Peri-surgical complications

	Group A N=82	Group B N=168	p value	Odds ratio (IC at 95%)
Total (except laparoconversion)	6 (7.3%)	4 (1.8%)	0.06	3.24 (0.78–14)
Bladder injury	3	1		
Subcutaneous emphysema	3	1		
Vaginal breach	0	1		
Omental haematoma	0	1		
Laparoconversion	11 (12%) on 93 patients	1 (0, 6%) on 169 patients	<0.001	22 (3.15–971)

Table 5 gives the detail of long-term re-intervention (secondary complications, relapse). The global rate of long-term re-interventions is similar in both groups, around 8%.

The rate of prosthetic exposure was identical in both groups, around 3%. They were only polyester meshes. In group A, three cases of vaginal exposure of sacrocolpopexy mesh were systematically medically treated before re-intervention. In one case, mesh had been fixed by clips, which were taken away as well as exposed mesh. In group B, two posterior prosthetic exposures were mentioned. In the first case, diagnosis was made at post-surgical consultation and resection realised at 2 months. In the other case, the diagnosis of exposure was achieved very early, and conservative treatment was tried first, but infection at 4 months imposed prosthetic resection.

Otherwise, there were three cases of vaginal exposure of TVT-O® mesh in 41 patients of group B. Two patients (6%) had re-intervention at 2 months and resection of exposed strip.

There were, only in group B, three re-interventions for prolapse: two sacrocolpopexies by laparotomy, one sub-vesical mesh by vaginal route according to PROLIFT® technique and one antefixation of the uterus with partial cervical resection. One patient had two re-interventions (sacrocolpopexy by laparotomy then uterine antefixation).

Re-intervention for urinary incontinence remained around 4% in the two groups. These re-interventions were carried out after de novo urinary incontinence, significant pre-existing urinary incontinence more important after laparoscopic sacrocolpopexy, or relapse in patients who already had a cure of urinary incontinence.

Only one patient from group B had a hysterectomy for menorrhagia at 34 months of LSC.

Discussion

Many authors have published papers on keyhole surgery and laparoscopic sacrocolpopexy; very few have followed up chronologic analysis of results in the same team. To our knowledge, only Claerhout fixed at 60, the number of LSC necessary to improve the learning curve, guided by the rate of laparotomy conversion and the number of peri-surgical complications [13]. Akladios saw a significant reduction of intervention length after around 20 procedures [14]. These data are important as certain publications include initial phase of this learning curve and so overestimate complications and may limit indications of a technique. Our aim was to compare two consecutive periods in the same team. The limit between the two periods is the time when the surgical team moved from one hospital to another. The judgement criteria to evaluate the control of this technique were the rate of conversion to laparotomy and the peri- and early post-surgical complications. Long-term anatomic and functional results are also probably highly relevant in this analysis, this surgery being functional. One of our limitations

Table 4 Early post-surgical complications

	Group A N=82	Group B N=168	p value	Odds ratio (IC at 95%)
Early post-surgical complications	17 (21%)	9 (5%)	<0.001	4.62 (1.83–12)
Lower urinary tract infection	12 (15%)	6 (4%)		
Haematoma	2	0		
Urinary retention	2	0		
Thromboembolic complication	1	0		
Haematoma at trocar port	0	3		
Re-intervention for early complication	2 (2.4%)	1 (0.6%)	0.25	4.14 (0.21–247)

Table 5 Late re-interventions

	Group A N=82	Group B N=168	p value	Odds ratio (IC at 95%)
Vaginal exposure of sacrocolpopexy mesh	3 (3.7%)	2 (1.2%)	0.33	3.13 (0.35–38)
Vaginal exposure of TVT-O® mesh	–	2 on 41 patients		
Prolapse (relapse or de novo)	0	3 (1.7%)	0.55	NA
Stress urinary incontinence	3 (3.7%)	7 (4.2%)	1	0.87 (0.14–3.96)
among which a patient with TVT-O®	–	1		
Menorrhagias of remaining uterus	0	1		
Total of re-interventions	6 (7%)	15 (9%)	0.67	0.81 (0.27–2.33)

is probably the consecutive evaluation with different stand-back in both groups. We could not use retrospectively international classification POP-Q, which was proposed in 1996 by Bump [15].

The rate of laparotomy conversion decreased greatly from 12% to 0.6%. These rates are similar in literature (0–11%) as well as reasons for conversion (adhesions, difficult access to promontory and hypercapnia) [7, 8, 16–18]. This may be due to better mastery and standardisation of techniques for surgeons but also anaesthetists and all the operating staff [5, 6]. Hypercapnia and difficult access to the promontory are no more an indication for conversion in group B. This may also be due to better selection of patients: vaginal route immediately chosen in case of surgical antecedent or foreseeable surgical difficulties. In case of difficult access to promontory, alternative techniques, such as Dubuisson's, with lateral suspension, will be used which avoids laparotomy conversion and gives good anatomic results [19].

Peri-surgical complications are significantly less frequent in the more recent group, 1.8% vs. 7.3% in group A. This may be compared to the rates reported in the literature between 2.2% and 17.4% [18, 20–25]. Bladder wounding is the most frequent complication: 0.8–3% in our study vs. 1–7% in literature [8, 9, 18–21, 26–31]. Diagnosis was always made during intervention with immediate suture and simple after-effects. Certain authors report rectal or vaginal wounding [8, 9, 18, 32]. Certain technical devices such as a vaginal valve may allow easier vaginal dissection and reduce surgical risk. After vaginal injury, a polypropylene mesh seems imperative to limit ulterior risk of infection. We have had no major complications in both study periods. Since 2009, we had noted only once a wound of left common iliac vein when dissecting promontory. An emergency laparotomy and a suture by a vascular surgeon allowed to control bleeding (haemorrhage of nearly 3.5 L). Follow-up was straightforward. Sacrocolpopexy was not realised and the cure of prolapse by vaginal route was done later.

Post-surgical complications were significantly divided into four. They were essentially lower urinary tract infections with probably multifactorial genesis. One limitation of our study is its retrospective character. Certain complications may not have been written up in files or only when the team began this study. In group A, one haematoma of Retzius space was probably linked to Burch's intervention associated. Evolution to suburethral strips limits this risk, which is still non-existent with retropubic route [33]. Other complications are reported in literature such as small intestine occlusion sometimes imposing digestive resection [8, 21, 28]. For us, it seems of utmost importance to peritonize the mesh and suture aponeurosis for trocars superior to 10 mm to limit this risk.

Our rate of early post-surgical complications decreased from 2.4% to 0.6%, but not in a significant way (p=0.25), similar to Ganatra's review who demonstrated an average rate of 1.6% [17]. There was a slight increase in re-interventions for prolapse relapse, without statistical significance (0–1.7%, NS). Patients were treated by an experienced senior in 90% in group A vs. 75% in group B. This slight difference of relapse might be explained by the learning curve of operators. Our results are similar to those found in literature: 4% in our team in 2002 and 6.2% for Ganatra [9, 17].

Average surgery length was reduced from 213 to 191 min, slightly superior to literature data (average, 158 min; extremes, 96–286 min) [17]. However, it is difficult to determine precisely the surgical duration, as there are associated procedures. For example, subtotal hysterectomy, very often performed by our team, lasts 30 to 60 min (hysterectomy and dissection). If our interventions become shorter, that may be due to better surgical technique but also to technical devices and more efficient material (electrocoagulation techniques, needle holder, knot pushers, etc.). Akladios showed a significant reduction of surgery length for each surgeon after around 20 procedures [14]. Our results seem to show that time saving seemed to last longer with more significant techniques even if indications were extended and certain surgeons of the second group were beginning their training experience. These conclusions may come from a fellowship teaching and new devices that make learning shorter.

These conclusions, learning from colleagues and quitting certain procedures (such as culdoplasty or Burch), may also explain why surgical times were reduced between the two groups.

Conclusion

Our study shows that LSC technique can be reproduced with a low rate of complications. There is, though, a learning curve with significant impact on length of interventions, rate of conversion to laparotomy, and peri- and post-surgical complications. The threshold seems quite high since we saw a real difference after the 93 first cases. This parameter must be considered when analysing the results of publications not to overestimate complications. We might also think on the ways to teach these surgical techniques to young doctors, who need to master these techniques

Conflicts of interest The authors report no conflicts of interest. The authors alone are responsible for the content and writing of the paper.

References

1. Olsen AL, Smith VJ, Bergstrom JO, Colling JC, Clark AL (1997) Epidemiology of surgically managed pelvic organ prolapse and urinary incontinence. Obstet Gynecol 89(4):501–506. doi:10.1016/S0029-7844(97)00058-6
2. Ameline A, Huguier J (1957) Posterior suspension to the lumbosacral disk; abdominal method of replacement of the utero-sacral ligaments. Gynecol Obstet (Paris) 56(1):94–98
3. Huguier J, Scali P (1958) Posterior suspension of the genital axis on the lumbosacral disk in the treatment of uterine prolapse. Presse Med 66(35):781–784
4. Nezhat C, Nezhat F (1992) Operative laparoscopy (minimally invasive surgery): state of the art. J Gynecol Surg 8(3):111–141
5. Wattiez A, Boughizane S, Alexandre F, Canis M, Mage G, Pouly JL, Bruhat MA (1995) Laparoscopic procedures for stress incontinence and prolapse. Curr Opin Obstet Gynecol 7(4):317–321
6. Wattiez A, Canis M, Mage G, Pouly JL, Bruhat MA (2001) Promontofixation for the treatment of prolapse. Urol Clin North Am 28(1):151–157
7. Cosson M, Bogaert E, Narducci F, Querleu D, Crepin G (2000) Laparoscopic sacral colpopexy: short-term results and complications in 83 patients. J Gynecol Obstet Biol Reprod (Paris) 29(8):746–750
8. Cheret A, Von Theobald P, Lucas J, Dreyfus M, Herlicoviez M (2001) Laparoscopic promontofixation feasibility study in 44 patients. J Gynecol Obstet Biol Reprod (Paris) 30(2):139–143
9. Cosson M, Rajabally R, Bogaert E, Querleu D, Crepin G (2002) Laparoscopic sacrocolpopexy, hysterectomy, and burch colposuspension: feasibility and short-term complications of 77 procedures. JSLS 6(2):115–119
10. Huguier J (1957) [Posterior colpo-perineo-myorraphy]. Bull Fed Soc Gynecol Obstet Lang Fr 9(1):28–31, discussion 31–24
11. de Leval J (2003) Novel surgical technique for the treatment of female stress urinary incontinence: transobturator vaginal tape inside-out. Eur Urol 44(6):724–730
12. Ulmsten U, Petros P (1995) Intravaginal slingplasty (IVS): an ambulatory surgical procedure for treatment of female urinary incontinence. Scand J Urol Nephrol 29(1):75–82
13. Claerhout F, De Ridder D, Roovers JP, Rommens H, Spelzini F, Vandenbroucke V, Coremans G, Deprest J (2009) Medium-term anatomic and functional results of laparoscopic sacrocolpopexy beyond the learning curve. Eur Urol 55(6):1459–1467. doi:10.1016/j.eururo.2008.12.008
14. Akladios CY, Dautun D, Saussine C, Baldauf JJ, Mathelin C, Wattiez A (2010) Laparoscopic sacrocolpopexy for female genital organ prolapse: establishment of a learning curve. Eur J Obstet Gynecol Reprod Biol 149(2):218–221. doi:10.1016/j.ejogrb.2009.12.012
15. Bump RC, Mattiasson A, Bo K, Brubaker LP, DeLancey JO, Klarskov P, Shull BL, Smith AR (1996) The standardization of terminology of female pelvic organ prolapse and pelvic floor dysfunction. Am J Obstet Gynecol 175(1):10–17
16. Nezhat CH, Nezhat F, Nezhat C (1994) Laparoscopic sacral colpopexy for vaginal vault prolapse. Obstet Gynecol 84(5):885–888
17. Ganatra AM, Rozet F, Sanchez-Salas R, Barret E, Galiano M, Cathelineau X, Vallancien G (2009) The current status of laparoscopic sacrocolpopexy: a review. Eur Urol 55(5):1089–1103. doi:10.1016/j.eururo.2009.01.048
18. Bui C, Ballester M, Chereau E, Guillo E, Darai E (2010) Functional results and quality of life of laparoscopic promontofixation in the cure of genital prolapse. Gynecol Obstet Fertil 38(10):563–568. doi:10.1016/j.gyobfe.2010.06.001
19. Dubuisson JB, Jacob S, Chapron C, Fauconnier A, Decuypere F, Dubernard G (2002) Laparoscopic treatment of genital prolapse: lateral utero-vaginal suspension with 2 meshes. Results of a series of 47 patients. Gynecol Obstet Fertil 30(2):114–120
20. Antiphon P, Elard S, Benyoussef A, Fofana M, Yiou R, Gettman M, Hoznek A, Vordos D, Chopin DK, Abbou CC (2004) Laparoscopic promontory sacral colpopexy: is the posterior, recto-vaginal, mesh mandatory? Eur Urol 45(5):655–661. doi:10.1016/j.eururo.2004.01.004
21. Rozet F, Mandron E, Arroyo C, Andrews H, Cathelineau X, Mombet A, Cathala N, Vallancien G (2005) Laparoscopic sacral colpopexy approach for genito-urinary prolapse: experience with 363 cases. Eur Urol 47(2):230–236. doi:10.1016/j.eururo.2004.08.014
22. Rivoire C, Botchorishvili R, Canis M, Jardon K, Rabischong B, Wattiez A, Mage G (2007) Complete laparoscopic treatment of genital prolapse with meshes including vaginal promontofixation and anterior repair: a series of 138 patients. J Minim Invasive Gynecol 14(6):712–718. doi:10.1016/j.jmig.2007.06.017
23. Agarwala N, Hasiak N, Shade M (2007) Laparoscopic sacral colpopexy with Gynemesh as graft material–experience and results. J Minim Invasive Gynecol 14(5):577–583. doi:10.1016/j.jmig.2007.03.005
24. Misrai V, Chartier-Kastler E, Cour F, Mozer P, Almeras C, Richard F (2006) Surgical management of chronic refractory pain after TVT treatment for stress urinary incontinence. Prog Urol 16(3):368–371
25. North CE, Ali-Ross NS, Smith AR, Reid FM (2009) A prospective study of laparoscopic sacrocolpopexy for the management of pelvic organ prolapse. BJOG 116(9):1251–1257. doi:10.1111/j.1471-0528.2009.02116.x
26. Weng SS, Liu CY (2008) Laparoscopic pelvic floor repair using polypropylene mesh. Taiwan J Obstet Gynecol 47(3):312–317. doi:10.1016/S1028-4559(08)60130-8
27. Descargues G, Collard P, Grise P (2008) Surgical management of pelvic organ prolapse in women: laparoscopic or vaginal sacrocolpopexy? Gynecol Obstet Fertil 36(10):978–983. doi:10.1016/j.gyobfe.2008.05.007
28. Ross JW, Preston M (2005) Laparoscopic sacrocolpopexy for severe vaginal vault prolapse: five-year outcome. J Minim Invasive Gynecol 12(3):221–226. doi:10.1016/j.jmig.2005.03.017
29. Gadonneix P, Ercoli A, Salet-Lizee D, Cotelle O, Bolner B, Van Den Akker M, Villet R (2004) Laparoscopic sacrocolpopexy with two separate meshes along the anterior and posterior vaginal walls

for multicompartment pelvic organ prolapse. J Am Assoc Gynecol Laparosc 11(1):29–35
30. Sarlos D, Brandner S, Kots L, Gygax N, Schaer G (2008) Laparoscopic sacrocolpopexy for uterine and post-hysterectomy prolapse: anatomical results, quality of life and perioperative outcome—a prospective study with 101 cases. Int Urogynecol J Pelvic Floor Dysfunct 19 (10):1415–1422. doi:10.1007/s00192-008-0657-0
31. Higgs PJ, Chua HL, Smith AR (2005) Long term review of laparoscopic sacrocolpopexy. BJOG 112(8):1134–1138. doi:10.1111/j.1471-0528.2005.00646.x
32. Bruyere F, Rozenberg H, Abdelkader T (2001) Laparoscopic sacral colpopexy: an attractive approach for prolapse repair. Prog Urol 11(6):1320–1326
33. Novara G, Artibani W, Barber MD, Chapple CR, Costantini E, Ficarra V, Hilton P, Nilsson CG, Waltregny D (2010) Updated systematic review and meta-analysis of the comparative data on colposuspensions, pubovaginal slings, and midurethral tapes in the surgical treatment of female stress urinary incontinence. Eur Urol 58(2):218–238. doi:10.1016/j.eururo.2010.04.022

10

Patient safety risk factors in minimally invasive surgery

Sharon P. Rodrigues · Moniek ter Kuile ·
Jenny Dankelman · Frank W. Jansen

Abstract This study was conducted to adapt and validate a patient safety (PS) framework for minimally invasive surgery (MIS) as a first step in understanding the clinical relevance of various PS risk factors in MIS. Eight patient safety risk factor domains were identified using frameworks from a systems approach to patient safety. A questionnaire was drafted containing 34 questions. Three experts in the field of patient safety critically reviewed the questionnaire on clinical relevance and completeness. The questionnaire was distributed among known patient safety experts in person and also sent electronically. A total of 41 questionnaires were distributed and the response rate was 71%. The intraclass correlation coefficient was 0.42 representing moderate agreement. For seven of nine risk domains, Cronbach's alpha was sufficient (α>0.7). Mean scores of the risk domains showed the following order of influence on patient safety from high to low: surgeon's experience [6.6, standard deviation (SD) 0.5], technical skills surgeon (6.6, SD 0.7), technology (5.9, SD 1.1), complications (5.9, SD 1.2), social interaction (5.0, SD 1.0), leadership surgeon (5.4, SD 1.2), blood loss (5.0, SD 1.2), length of surgery (5.0, SD 1.3), surgical team (4.9, SD 1.3), fallibility (4.9, SD 1.3), patient (4.5, SD 1.5), safety measures (4.4, SD 1.5), and finally environment(3.9, SD 1.5). This study is an initiative to give insight into clinical relevance of the maze of PS risk factors in MIS. All investigated risk domains were considered to be of noticeable influence on PS. Nevertheless, it is possible to prioritize various risk domains. In fact, experience and technical skills of the surgeon, technology, and complications are rated as the most important risk factors, closely followed by social interaction and leadership of the surgeon. Patient, safety measures, and environment are rated as the least important risk factors.

Keywords Patient safety · Risk factors · Risk domains · MIS · Laparoscopy · Systems approach

Background

Over the past years, society has become more quality driven. Also, in health care, the demand for the highest quality possible has become an important center of attention, especially in the operating room. This urgent request for high quality has made patient safety (PS), as a quality parameter, a very important research topic. Research concerning "patient safety" has expended explosively since 1999 and "patient safety" in the "operating room" has been increasing since 2004. Research concerning "patient safety" combined with "laparoscopy" only recently started to increase, whereas research on "laparoscopy" alone has been increasing fairly stable. All the while, research with the keyword "operating room" as well as the total number of yearly publications has been stable for years.

Recently, many PS issues considering minimally invasive surgery (MIS), especially laparoscopy, have been brought to our attention. In The Netherlands, PS issues

S. P. Rodrigues · M. ter Kuile · F. W. Jansen (✉)
Department of Gynecology, K6-76,
Leiden University Medical Center,
PO Box 9600, 2300 RC Leiden, The Netherlands
e-mail: F.W.Jansen@lumc.nl

S. P. Rodrigues
e-mail: s.p.rodrigues@lumc.nl

J. Dankelman · F. W. Jansen
Department of BioMechanical Engineering,
Delft University of Technology,
Delft, The Netherlands

about MIS (especially laparoscopy) brought to the attention by the Dutch Inspectorate of Healthcare even led to a discussion in the Dutch parliament about the desirability of MIS [1]. Despite the great amount of research about PS and laparoscopy in general, only a few publications concern both items.

In general, patient safety is a complex multidimensional concept and the clinical relevance of its various dimensions is not clearly understood. To comprehend the clinical relevance of various PS risk factors in surgery, the degree to which a patient is exposed to all of these risk factors during surgery should be studied. Yet, studies that try to measure risk factors during surgery usually focus on specific parts of the multidimensional concept. Nonetheless, it has been widely accepted that a wide range of factors influence PS in surgery and a number of important studies [2–5] have addressed this by developing frameworks according to the systems approach to quality and safety in surgery. The aim of this study is to adapt and validate these frameworks for MIS as a first step in understanding the clinical relevance of various PS risk factors in MIS.

Methods

Existing frameworks that were developed according to a systems approach to quality and safety in surgery [2–5] were adapted for MIS. The adapted framework consisted of the following risk domains:

1. Surgeon: risk factors regarding functioning of the surgeon,
2. Surgical team: risk factors regarding functioning of the scrub or circulating nurse,
3. Technology: risk factors regarding the availability and functioning of technology,
4. Social interaction: risk factors regarding teamwork and communication,
5. Environment: risk factors that potentially cause distraction or disruptions of the surgical process,
6. Patient: patient-related risk factors,
7. Fallibility: risk factors regarding factors that influence the fallibility of the surgeon,
8. Safety measures: items regarding (compliance of) safety protocols, and
9. Result: items regarding the result of the procedure.

For each risk domain, risk factors were defined and incorporated in a questionnaire (Table 1). At the end of the questionnaire, there was free space for comments on missing risk factors or other issues. The questionnaire was critically reviewed on clinical relevance and completeness by three independent experts, who did not participate in the development of the questionnaire, i.e., the president of the commission on patient safety of the Dutch society of obstetrics and gynecology, the president of the commission on patient safety of the association of surgeons of the Netherlands who is also a pioneer in MIS, and the president of the Dutch society of endoscopic surgery who is also a gynecologist with a research line in patient safety in MIS. This led to a minor addition to the questionnaire.

Next, a sample of international gynecological PS experts was asked to rate all PS risk factors. A PS expert was defined as a gynecologist specialized in laparoscopic surgery, who is well recognized by their peers and that had either published a minimum of two articles on PS-related topics and/or is actively involved in a commission on PS. All experts were members of the European Society for Gynaecological Endoscopy and/or the American Association of Gynecologic Laparoscopists. The questionnaire was distributed internationally both directly among PS experts during a gynecological MIS conference ($N=12$) and electronically by email ($N=29$). The risk factors were rated according to their potential impact on PS in MIS on a 6-cm Visual Analogue Scale (VAS) with at the endpoints "no impact" and "huge impact". Because of technological restrictions, the electronic version of the VAS was converted to a 13-point scale with, similar to the VAS, at the endpoint 0 "no impact" and at the endpoint 12 "huge impact" and every intermediate point corresponded with half a centimeter on the VAS. For conventional reasons and ease of interpretation, both scales were converted to a seven-point scale after all data were collected. The mean scores of the VAS and 13-point scale were first analyzed separately showing similar results for both rating scales. As such, it was decided to combine the two rating scales to report the results of this study.

Data analysis

All data were analyzed with SPSS 16.0 software package (SPSS, Chicago, IL, USA). An overall inter-rater agreement was determined for the complete questionnaire with the intraclass correlation coefficient (ICC). The ICC is exactly identical to the weighted kappa with quadratic weights [6] and is an appropriate method to determine an inter-rater agreement between multiple raters of multiple questions with a large rating scale as is the case in the current study. The ICC values were interpreted according to Landis and Koch's [7] guidelines for the interpretation of kappa (kappa values <0 poor; 0 to 0.2 slight; 0.2 to 0.4 fair; 0.4 to 0.6 moderate; 0.6 to 0.8 substantial; and >0.8 almost perfect agreement).

Table 1 Categorization of risk factors

Risk domains	Risk factors
Surgeon	Experience of the surgeon
	Technical skills of the surgeon
	Leadership of the surgeon
Surgical team	Qualified staffing
	Experience of the scrub nurse
	Scrub nurse's knowledge of the procedure
	Experience of the circulating nurse
Technology	All instruments are present
	All instruments work properly
	It is known how to handle all instruments
	All equipment is present
	All equipment works properly
	The OR team knows how to handle all equipment
	The surgeons knows how to handle all equipment
Social interaction	Communication between OR team members
	Failure of professional communication
	Communication of important issues at shift changes
	Collaboration between OR team members
Environment	Disruptions of the surgical process
	Distractions (e.g., questions not relating to the patient)
	Number of people in the OR
Patient	Patient's BMI
	Patient's ASA score
	Previous surgeries
Fallibility	Time of day surgery takes place (e.g., daytime, nighttime)
	Workload
	Number of procedure (e.g., first or last of that day)
	Fatigue
Safety measures	Universal safety protocols
	Briefing according to WHO checklist
	Compliance of safety measures (protocol)
Result	Intraoperative complications
	Amount of blood loss
	Length of surgery

BMI body mass index, *OR* operating room, *ASA score* American Society of Anesthesiologists Physical Status Scores

For each PS risk factor domain (containing a number of separate risk factors), internal consistency was determined using Cronbach's alpha. If internal consistency of a PS risk factor domain was accepted (Cronbach's alpha >0.7) [8], further analysis was performed for that domain as a whole. If internal consistency was insufficient (Cronbach's alpha <0.7), further analysis was performed for every risk factor separately. Mean scores and 95% confidence intervals (95% CI) were calculated per PS risk domain (or single risk factors if internal consistency was insufficient) and plotted. Statistical significant difference between PS risk domains was determined with one-way analysis of variance (ANOVA) and Bonferroni post hoc analysis (p value<0.05).

Findings

A total of 41 questionnaires were distributed of which 29 were completed and returned, resulting in a response rate of 71%. Out of the 29 questionnaires, 28 were filled out completely and one incomplete (five items at the last page were not completed). An agreement over the complete questionnaire was moderate (ICC=0.42). The internal consistency of PS risk domains surgical team, technology, social interaction, environment, patient, fallibility, and safety measures were all acceptable (Cronbach's alpha >0.7) (Table 2). The PS risk domains surgeon and result did not reach sufficient internal consistency (Cronbach's alpha 0.54 and 0.14, respectively) and therefore further analysis

Table 2 Cronbach's alpha per risk domain

Patient safety risk domain	Cronbach's alpha	
1	Surgeon	0.54
2	Surgical team	0.74
3	Technology	0.90
4	Social interaction	0.81
5	Environment	0.78
6	Patient	0.70
7	Fallibility	0.72
8	Safety measures	0.93
9	Result	0.14

was done for every risk factor separately. ANOVA analysis showed significant differences between groups ($p<0.001$). Further analysis with Bonferroni post hoc test will be described in more detail below.

Mean ratings and 95% CIs are plotted in Fig. 1. This figure illustrates the relative importance of the PS risk factor domains towards each other and shows that on average the experience and technical skills of the surgeon are rated highest [6.6, standard deviation (SD) 0.5 and 6.6, SD 0.7, respectively], whereas leadership of the surgeon was rated significantly less important (mean 5.4, SD 1.2). Although all risk factors are rated relatively high (right side of the seven-point scale), the mean rating of the PS risk domain environment (3.9, SD 1.5) is significantly lower than all other risk domains except for the mean rating of patient and safety measures (4.5, SD 1.5 and 4.4, SD 1.5, respectively). Both technology and social interaction are rated among the most important risk domains (mean 5.9, SD 1.1 and mean 5.5, SD 1.0, respectively). Within the risk domain result, both length of surgery and blood loss were rated relatively lower [mean 5.0, SD 1.3 and 5.0, SD 1.2, respectively] than complications (mean 5.9, SD 1.2), although not significant. On average, the risk domains surgical team (4.9, SD 1.3), fallibility (4.9, SD 1.3), patient, and safety measures did not differ significantly.

There were no missing risk factors reported in the free space section. There were a few comments, which will be further discussed in the next section.

Discussion

In this study, an adapted framework of PS risk factors in MIS was validated as a first step in understanding the clinical relevance of various PS risk factors in MIS. All investigated risk domains were rated of noticeable influence on PS, confirming the multidimensionality of the concept PS. This also implies that in order to completely assess PS in MIS, all of the proposed risk factors should be considered.

The results of this study should be interpreted carefully. The selection of PS experts comprises only gynecologists who specialize in MIS; therefore, the results can only be interpreted as valid for gynecological MIS. Further research is needed to examine whether these results can be extrapolated to other specialisms and whether other professionals that participate in MIS (i.e., anesthesiologists and OR nurses) share this opinion. Furthermore, it should be taken into account that there are differences in agreement on the importance of various risk factors. This is illustrated

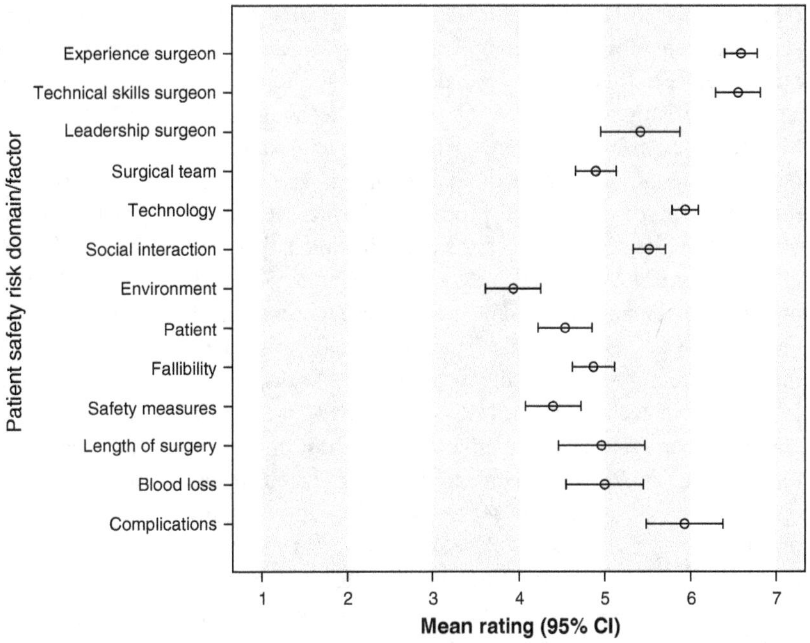

Fig. 1 Mean scores and 95% confidence interval (95% CI) per risk domain

by the differences in width of the 95% CI of mean (Fig. 1). A small 95% CI should be interpreted as strong agreement and a wide 95% CI should be interpreted as weak agreement. As such, agreement on the importance of technology, experience of the surgeon, and social interaction is strongest and therefore the average rating can be interpreted as more reliable than the average rating of length of surgery, leadership of the surgeon, complications, and blood loss, of which the 95% CIs are wider (e.g., agreement is less strong). Yet, overall agreement of the complete questionnaire was moderate (ICC=0.42) and the widest 95% CI is 1.0 point wide. Together with the response rate of 71%, this is considered satisfactory.

The free space section in the questionnaire gave experts the possibility to comment on the questionnaire. There were no missing risk factors reported; however, there were few relevant comments made. There was one comment on the importance of the first assistant's experience by directly affecting safety and by adding experience to a difficult procedure. We agree, however, we considered this as part of the qualified staff. Another expert commented that the 13-point scale in the electronic version of the questionnaire gives too much choice and could lead to clustering of the answers in the middle of the scale. Because of software restrictions, converting the VAS to a Likert-type scale for the electronic questionnaire was imperative. We chose to let every half a centimeter on the VAS correspond to a point on the Likert-type scale, hence the origin of the 13-point scale. Furthermore, the results show an arrangement of the risk domains in given rating; therefore, it can be stated that clustering of the answers due to the large scale is no issue in the current questionnaire.

It is possible to prioritize certain risk domains over others. As such, experience and technical skills of the surgeon, technology, and complications have the highest ratings, closely followed by social interaction and leadership of the surgeon. The use of advanced technology in MIS easily explains the experts' view on the importance of good functioning instruments and equipment. The magnitude of technology-related problems during MIS has previously been illustrated in several studies [9, 10]. Also, in gynecological MIS procedures, many technology-related problems, with potentially dangerous consequences, have been observed [11]. In these studies, technology-related incidents mainly led to delay and extra work. The importance of technology in MIS is supported by the fact that the experts rate this domain among the most important risk domains in MIS. Surgeons could be facilitated in the optimal use of advanced technology in laparoscopic operating units by checklists. Checklists have already been shown to improve the use of the available technology and reduce technology-related incidents [9, 12]. Problems in social interaction (such as communication and teamwork) have also been shown to occur frequently during surgery [13, 14]. For example, communicational difficulties have been reported to occur in approximately 30% of team exchanges [13]. About a third of these communicational failures resulted in visible effects that can influence PS [14]. The importance of social interaction for PS in MIS is supported by the fact that the experts also rate this domain among the most important risk domains in MIS.

Many studies concerning PS in the operating room have been focusing on disruptions and distractions from the surgical process (environment) because they are believed to influence the surgeon's concentration or are perceived as stressful events [15–20]. Remarkably, the experts rated this risk domain (environment) as the least influential of all risk domains. The results of an observational study are in line with the experts' opinion as they found frequent disruptions, however, the stressfulness of disruptions were least severe compared to other (e.g., technical) incidents [16].

Conclusion

This study is an initiative to give insight into clinical relevance of the maze of PS risk factors in MIS. All investigated risk domains were considered to be of noticeable influence on PS. Nevertheless, it is possible to prioritize various risk domains. In fact, experience and technical skills of the surgeon, technology, and complications are rated as the most important risk factors, closely followed by social interaction and leadership of the surgeon. Although in general, patient safety measures and environment are among the most widely studied risk factors, experts in the field rate them as the least important risk factors. Although the effect of environmental factors should not be underestimated, experts in the field indicate that it should not be overestimated as well.

More research is needed to give us better insight in the pitfalls of patient safety as perceived in clinical practice to guide us in future research. As the results of this study can only be interpreted as valid for gynecological MIS, it would be interesting to examine whether experts of other specialisms (i.e., surgeons, anesthesiologists, and OR nurses) share the same view on patient safety. A focal group session including experts from different specialisms could give us more insight in the real need and concerns of experts on patient safety in minimally invasive surgery.

Acknowledgments The authors are grateful to all experts that participated in this study.

Conflicts of interest The authors report no conflicts of interest. The authors alone are responsible for the content and writing of the paper.

References

1. Inspectie voor de gezondheidszorg (2007) Risico's minimaal invasieve chirurgie onderschat, kwaliteitssysteem voor laparoscopische operaties ontbreekt. IGZ, Den Haag
2. Calland JF, Guerlain S, Adams RB, Tribble CG, Foley E, Chekan EG (2002) A systems approach to surgical safety. Surg Endosc 6:1005–1014
3. Vincent C, Moorthy K, Sarker SK, Chang A, Darzi AW (2004) Systems approaches to surgical quality and safety: from concept to measurement. Ann Surg 4:475–482
4. Leake PA, Urbach DR (2010) Measuring processes of care in general surgery: assessment of technical and nontechnical skills. Surg Innov 17(4):332–339
5. Dankelman J, Grimbergen CA (2005) Systems approach to reduce errors in surgery. Surg Endosc 8:1017–1021
6. Steiner DL, Norman GR (2008) Health measurement scales: a practical guide to their development and use. Oxford University Press, New York
7. Landis JR, Koch GG (1977) The measurement of observer agreement for categorical data. Biometrics 1:159–174
8. Nunnaly JC (1967) Psychometric theory. McGraw Hill, New York
9. Verdaasdonk EG, Stassen LP, Hoffmann WF, van der Elst M, Dankelman J (2008) Can a structured checklist prevent problems with laparoscopic equipment? Surg Endosc 10:2238–2243
10. Wubben I, van Manen JG, van den Akker BJ, Vaartjes SR, van Harten WH (2010) Equipment-related incidents in the operating room: an analysis of occurrence, underlying causes and consequences for the clinical process. Qual Saf Health Care 19:1–7
11. Courdier S, Garbin O, Hummel M, Thoma V, Ball E, Favre R, Wattiez A (2009) Equipment failure: causes and consequences in endoscopic gynecologic surgery. J Minim Invasive Gynecol 1:28–33
12. Buzink SN, van Lier L, de Hingh I, Jakimowicz JJ (2010) Risk-sensitive events during laparoscopic cholecystectomy: the influence of the integrated operating room and a preoperative checklist tool. Surg Endosc 8:1990–1995
13. Lingard L, Regehr G, Espin S, Whyte S (2006) A theory-based instrument to evaluate team communication in the operating room: balancing measurement authenticity and reliability. Qual Saf Health Care 6:422–426
14. Lingard L, Espin S, Whyte S, Regehr G, Baker GR, Reznick R, Bohnen J, Orser B, Doran D, Grober E (2004) Communication failures in the operating room: an observational classification of recurrent types and effects. Qual Saf Health Care 5:330–334
15. Wiegmann DA, ElBardissi AW, Dearani JA, Daly RC, Sundt TM III (2007) Disruptions in surgical flow and their relationship to surgical errors: an exploratory investigation. Surgery 5:658–665
16. Arora S, Hull L, Sevdalis N, Tierney T, Nestel D, Woloshynowych M, Darzi A, Kneebone R (2010) Factors compromising safety in surgery: stressful events in the operating room. Am J Surg 1:60–65
17. Healey AN, Primus CP, Koutantji M (2007) Quantifying distraction and interruption in urological surgery. Qual Saf Health Care 2:135–139
18. Sevdalis N, Forrest D, Undre S, Darzi A, Vincent C (2008) Annoyances, disruptions, and interruptions in surgery: the Disruptions in Surgery Index (DiSI). World J Surg 8:1643–1650
19. Sevdalis N, Healey AN, Vincent CA (2007) Distracting communications in the operating theatre. J Eval Clin Pract 3:390–394
20. Zheng B, Martinec DV, Cassera MA, Swanstrom LL (2008) A quantitative study of disruption in the operating room during laparoscopic antireflux surgery. Surg Endosc 10:2171–2177

11

Is adenomyosis the neglected phenotype of an endomyometrial dysfunction syndrome?

Ivo Brosens · Georg Kunz · Giuseppe Benagiano

Abstract Since the dissociation between adenomyoma and endometriosis in the 1920s and the laparoscopic progress in the diagnosis and surgery of endometriosis, the literature has been greatly focused on the disease endometriosis. The study of adenomyosis, on the other hand, has been neglected as the diagnosis remained based on hysterectomy specimens. However, since the introduction of magnetic resonance and sonographic imaging techniques in the 1980s, the myometrial junctional zone has been identified as a third uterine zone and interest in adenomyosis was renewed. This has also been the start for the interest in the role of the myometrial junctional zone dysfunction and adenomyosis in reproductive and obstetrical disorders.

Keywords Adenomyosis · Endometriosis

Introduction

Endometriosis and adenomyosis are both defined by the presence of ectopic endometrial-like tissue, respectively outside the uterus and in the myometrium. Although both disorders were described under the common name of "adenomyoma" by early authors [1] and extensively studied by Cullen [2] as one condition, today they are considered two different diseases. The dissociation practiced in the 1920s by Frankl [3] and Sampson [4] is largely a consequence of the limitations in diagnostic tools that have existed up to the mid-1980s. Today, new insights in the structural and functional characteristics of the endometrium and myometrial junctional zone (the "endomyometrium"), in women with adenomyosis and endometriosis, provide increasing evidence that they are frequently associated and both are characterized by an aberrant function of the endomyometrium. Data indicating that they could well represent two phenotypes of a similar endomyometrial dysfunction syndrome rather than two different diseases have been accumulated—thanks to current imaging techniques, functional, and molecular investigations. In addition, evidence has also been gathered that the endomyometrial dysfunction has major repercussion on reproductive functions. The present review first describes the history and clinical background of the two anomalies; subsequently, it outlines reproductive dysfunctions existing in both disorders and, finally, tries to define clinical features of the syndrome.

Historical diagnostic bias

Glandular inclusions in a number of pelvic sites were identified during the second part of the nineteenth century; their presence created a controversy that continued for decades. It was Cullen [5] that, in 1896, unequivocally stated that these pelvic inclusions were derived from the "mucous membrane of the uterus". Then, in 1920, he provided a detailed description of a number of ectopic sites where the inclusions could be present, including the outer myometrium, the rectovaginal septum, uterine ligaments, the muscular wall of bladder and bowel, and other abdominal structures and coined the lesions

I. Brosens (✉)
Leuven Institute for Fertility and Embryology,
Leuven, Belgium
e-mail: ivo.brosens@med.kuleuven.be

G. Kunz
Department of Obstetrics and Gynaecology, St-Johannes-Hospital,
Dortmund, Germany

G. Benagiano
Department of Gynaecology, Obstetrics and Urology,
University of Rome,
Sapienza, Italy

adenomyomas [2, 6] (Fig. 1). In 1927, Sampson [4] formulated the hypothesis that "peritoneal endometriosis" was "due to the menstrual dissemination of endometrial tissue into the peritoneal cavity". From there on, uterine adenomyosis, which could not be explained by regurgitation of menstrual elements, was coined in 1925 by Frankl [3] adenomyosis; and endometriosis, with its separate pathogenesis, became widely regarded as a disease entity distinct from adenomyosis.

Although already in the 40s, Novak and de Lima [7] linked again adenomyosis and endometriosis, stating "one cannot resist the feeling that there is some common denominator between endometrial hyperplasia and adenomyosis, and possibly also pelvic endometriosis", it was only over the last two decades that the search for the underlying link between endometriosis and adenomyosis received a major booster. The development that provided the first important lead was the introduction of magnetic resonance (MR) imaging; using this technique, the "myometrial junctional zone" (JZ) was identified as a functional uterine zone to form with the endometrium

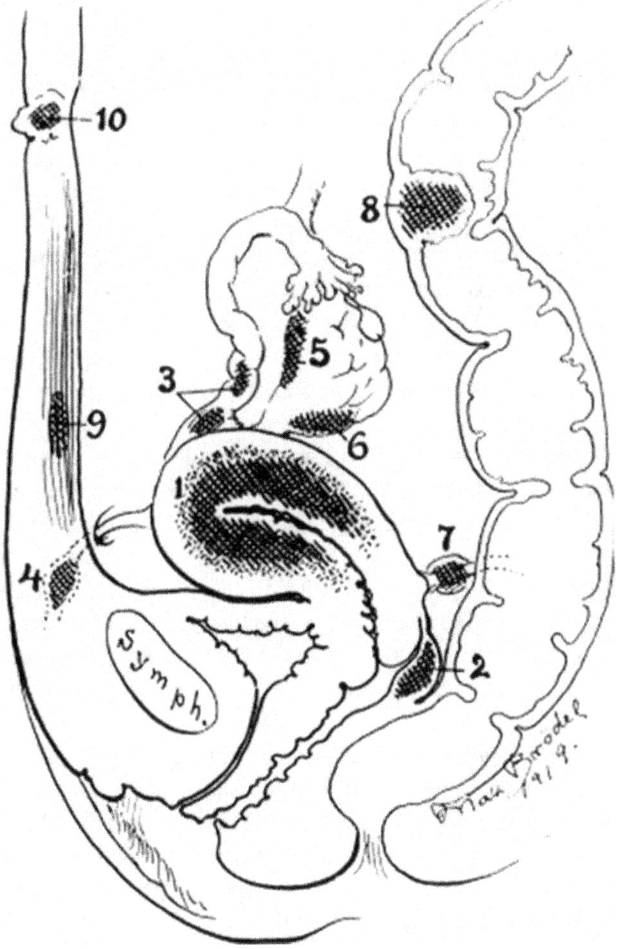

Fig. 1 Diagram showing localizations of ectopic endometrial tissue (indicated as adenomyomas): *1*, uterine wall; *2*, rectovaginal septum; *3*, fallopian tubes; *4*, round ligament; *5*, hilum of ovary; *6*, utero-ovarian ligament; *8*, colon; *9*, musculus rectus; *10*, umbilicus. From Cullen [2] with permission

the endomyometrium unit [8]. Shortly after, numerous molecular studies showed that the endometrium in endometriosis and adenomyosis is characterized by impaired cellular responses to ovarian sex steroids [9], as well as by a number of other metabolic aberrations.

Notwithstanding, these important developments, a major stumbling block remained since the histological diagnosis of endometriosis is based on a simple biopsy obtained at the time of laparoscopy or laparotomy, while the diagnosis of adenomyosis traditionally required a hysterectomy specimen. Indeed, to this day, almost all studies involving adenomyosis have been carried out on uteri removed at surgery. This has major scientific consequences. First, according to Scopus, the number of publications in 2011 on endometriosis is 22,730 and on adenomyosis 2,368, a tenfold difference. Secondly, endometriosis is frequently diagnosed in its early stage by the presence of variable or scarred peritoneal endometriosis, while adenomyosis is rarely diagnosed during the early reproductive life, its identification being made only after the appearance, in older women, of symptoms of abnormal menstrual bleeding and/or dysmenorrhea, severe enough to necessitate hysterectomy. Consequently, endometriosis risks to be overdiagnosed, while adenomyosis is neglected or overlooked.

The endomyometrium link

Aberrant eutopic endometrium

Although histologically normal, a series of biochemical evaluations of the endometrium in women with endometriosis and adenomyosis has, already in the late 1990s, revealed profound disturbances. The eutopic endometrium in women with these conditions is characterized by a large range of abnormalities including alterations in immune cell population [10], aberrant expression of aromatase [11], dysregulation of IL-6 production [12], impaired temporal expression of beta3-integrin [13], and HOX genes [14] and reduced spontaneous apoptosis [15]. During the last decade, many more molecules and functions have been found to be altered in endometriosis [16] and adenomyosis [17].

An additional problem in any attempt at comparatively analyzing endometrial abnormalities is given by the diagnostic modality utilized for endometriosis. On one hand, endometrial biopsies are easily obtained at the time of laparoscopy for the diagnosis of endometriosis; on the other, the contemporary presence of adenomyosis cannot be excluded in the vast majority of these studies due to the absence of a hysterectomy specimen or imaging scan. As a consequence, most studies on the endometrium in endometriosis have failed to exclude the presence of adenomyosis, whereas, as it will be detailed below, several studies—although disagreeing on the percentage—have shown that the two conditions coexist in a significant proportion of cases; therefore, a major bias persists in the biochemical evaluation of the eutopic endometrium in women with endometriosis when adenomyosis is not excluded.

Aberrant myometrial junctional zone

Since the junctional zone myometrium started to be investigated by MR imaging, every abnormality observed has been described as indicative of the presence of endometrium in the outer myometrium or adenomyosis sensu stricto. In fact, however, distinction should be made between junction zone abnormalities and adenomyosis. Tocci et al. [18] have now proposed that the "endometrial–subendometrial myometrium unit (or junctional zone myometrium) disruption disease" be considered as a new entity distinguished from adenomyosis. The diagnosis of which is feasible and straightforward on imaging. This condition is expressed mainly by a pathological thickening or abnormality of the subendometrial myometrium (myometrial halo or junctional zone). Clearly, there is a need for uniform terminology and classification [19] and until this is agreed upon, confusion will persist.

Although it is generally accepted that adenomyosis develops as a result of downward growth of the endometrium into the myometrium, MR imaging studies suggest that smooth muscle proliferation and hyperplasia in the junctional zone may precede the outgrowth of endometrial cells [20]. Leyendecker et al. [21] speculated that disruption of the specific uterine microenvironment in the basal endometrium may explain the structural and functional abnormalities of the junctional zone, such as hyperperistalsis, dysperistalsis, and inordinate smooth muscle proliferation associated with endometriosis and adenomyosis.

In a case–control-blinded comparison, Mehasseb et al. [22] studied the morphometric features of the myometrium in uteri from pre- and postmenopausal women with and without uterine adenomyosis as the sole pathology. Uteri were also divided according to the phase of the cycle and examined using immunohistochemistry and image analysis. The authors found clear differences between the inner myometrium and the outer myometrium, but the transition is gradual, with no distinct "zonation". Adenomyosis is characterized by reduced cell density and increased nuclear size and features of hyperplasia and hypertrophy that are not confined to the inner myometrium.

In a previous study, the same authors [23] found that smooth muscle cells from uteri with adenomyosis are ultrastructurally different from smooth muscle cells of normal uteri. They suggested a possible effect of these distinct features on myometrial contractility, together with hypertrophy.

Asssociation between endometriosis and adenomyosis

Using MR imaging, Kennedy et al. [24] found a high correlation between the presence of endometriosis and of adenomyosis in first degree relatives, suggesting that both are phenotypes of a single disorder rather that two distinct disease entities. Pelvic endometriosis, especially in severe stages, is strongly associated with JZ thickening [25–27]. In 2005, Kunz et al. [26] tested the hypothesis of a strong association between endometriosis and adenomyosis with adenomyosis playing a role in causing infertility in women with endometriosis. Using magnetic resonance imaging, they found that the posterior junctional zone (PJZ) was significantly thicker in women with endometriosis than in those without the disease. The MR imaging method as described in their previous publication [28] allowed them to identify alterations of the junctional zone that were interpreted as signs of focal and diffuse adenomyosis, respectively, according to the guidelines provided by Reinhold et al. [29]. A threshold value of more than 10 mm was chosen, above which with additional signs up to 12 mm, diffuse adenomyosis was assumed. There was a positive correlation of the diameter of the PJZ with the stage of the disease and the age of the patients. The prevalence of adenomyotic lesions in all 160 women with endometriosis was 79%. In women with endometriosis below an age of 36 years and fertile partners, the prevalence of adenomyosis was 90% ($p<0.01$). Kunz et al. [26] concluded that with a prevalence of up to 90%, uterine adenomyosis is significantly associated with pelvic endometriosis and constitutes an important factor of sterility in endometriosis presumably by impairing uterine sperm transport.

With respect to the effect of uterine contractions as creating thickening of the JZ, Kunz et al. [26] clarified that these contractions only exceeded those of healthy women during the late menstrual and early follicular phase, whereas the study was not restricted to these phases of the menstrual cycle. Moreover, these contractions were never confined to the posterior wall myometrium or prevailed as compared to the anterior wall contractions, hence always comprising the anterior as well as the posterior uterine myometrium within one contraction wave. But only the PJZ showed this highly significant difference in relation to the incidence of adenomyosis. They concluded that a possible bias with uterine wall contractions influencing the findings obtained from the 227 patients cannot be absolutely excluded, but appears to be negligible.

Traditionally, the diagnosis of adenomyosis is obtained from women in their fourth to fifth decade of life. However, recent MR imaging data suggest that adenomyosis may develop much sooner in life, particularly in women with endometriosis. In order to test this hypothesis, Kunz et al. [30] performed MR imaging of the uterus in 227 women with and without endometriosis and related the results to the age of the subjects (age groups, 17–24, 25–29, 30–34, and >34 years). The study revealed that the process of development of adenomyosis, represented by an increased diameter of the dorsal junctional zone of the uterus (the imaging feature indicative of the invasion of basal endometrium into the junctional zone), had already commenced early in the third decade of life and progressed steadily during the fourth decade in women with endometriosis. Women without endometriosis showed almost no signs of adenomyosis up to the age of 34 years. Surprisingly, in both groups of women, a parallel marked increase in the incidence of adenomyosis could be observed beyond the age of 34 years, thus representing a common phenomenon in the age-related pathophysiological continuum of adenomyosis.

Furthermore, in a prospective study of 70 patients presenting with severe dysmenorrhea, Kissler et al. [31] found that dysmenorrhea of long duration in patients who have had endometriosis for over a threshold value of 11 years is significantly related to adenomyosis. Hence, evaluation of adenomyosis using MRI should become a standard procedure in cases of severe dysmenorrhea associated with endometriosis and, if of long duration, this symptom should always pose a suspicion of adenomyosis. Finally, in 2010, Mijatovic et al. [32], in a retrospective study of 74 infertile patients with surgically proven endometriosis (90.4% of them with endometriosis rASRM stages III–IV), found also the presence of adenomyosis in 27% of them, predominantly located in the posterior wall of the uterus.

Recently Larsen et al. [33] correlated the degree of adenomyotic infiltration with the degree of infiltration and stage of endometriosis. MR imaging of the uterus was performed in 153 women with suspected deeply infiltrating endometriosis and planned surgery, and in a reference group of 129 women without endometriosis, verified during hysterectomy. Diagnosis of adenomyosis at MR imaging was based on optimal criteria derived from the hysterectomy control group, while the stage of endometriosis (rAFS stage) was determined during surgery. The authors found that in the group of women with endometriosis, 34.6% had adenomyosis compared with 19.4% in the reference group ($p<0.05$). More women with endometriosis (39.9%) had an irregular JZ compared to 22.5% in the reference group ($p<0.01$). Among women with severe endometriosis (AFS stage IV), 42.8% had adenomyosis compared to 29.4% in the women with other stages of endometriosis (AFS stages I + II + III) ($p=0.10$). More women with severe endometriosis (AFS stage IV) had deeper wall invasion of adenomyosis ($p>0.05$), but the presence of deep infiltrative rectovaginal endometriosis and the size of infiltration were not correlated to adenomyosis or to the depth of infiltration of adenomyosis. The authors concluded that, based on a systematic evaluation of the junctional zone by MR imaging, severe symptomatic endometriosis is in one third of the cases associated with uterine adenomyosis. For some reason, however, "deep endometriosis" and "deep adenomyosis" correspond only to a limited degree.

The potential role of endomyometrial dysfunction in reproductive and obstetrical disorders

In the normal human pregnancy, the remodeling of the spiral arteries involves both their myometrial and decidual segments. There is growing evidence that a pre-pregnancy disorder of the myometrial junctional zone is at the basis of defective deep placentation which, in turn, is associated with major reproductive and obstetrical complications [34]. Comparative studies on placentation show that the human is not unique among primates in showing deep trophoblast invasion [35], although recent investigations indicate that the baboon, with no appreciable trophoblast invasion of the myometrium is not an appropriate model for the study of either endometriosis [36] or preeclampsia [35]. On the other hand, there are case reports showing that preeclampsia may occur in chimpanzees and gorillas where trophoblast invasion and spiral artery remodeling are basically similar to the human [37, 38].

Today, the investigation of reproductive outcomes in young women with junctional zone abnormalities and/or adenomyosis has become possible—thanks to MR imaging and ultrasonography; using these techniques, an improved and clinically useful correlation with histology-based diagnosis for adenomyosis has been accomplished [39, 40]—thanks also to the analysis of the myometrial junctional zone. The importance of myometrial junctional zone research in reproductive medicine is frequently underestimated: indeed, the inner myometrium is the critical zone for the adequate transformation of spiral arteries supplying maternal blood to intervillous spaces of the placenta and a defective transformation of myometrial spiral arteries in the placental bed has been associated with major obstetrical syndromes [41].

The disappearance of the distinct myometrial zonal anatomy very early during pregnancy on MR imaging has also been observed in a unique case report by Turnbull et al. [42]. This may correspond to the early decidualization process of the myometrial spiral arteries in the placental bed well before the zone is colonized by intravascular and interstitial trophoblast [43, 44].

Impaired follicular function

A recent MR imaging study by Kunz and Beil [45] suggests that the uterine junctional zone may be of significance with respect to the early process of human reproduction. In 113 infertile women, the diameter of the anterior and posterior JZ myometrium was documented by MR imaging prior to the use of in vitro fertilization (IVF)/intracytoplasmic sperm injection (ICSI). Each group of women was also subdivided according to the presence [metaphase I (MI)/germinal vesicle (GV) >0%] or absence (MI/GV=0%) of MI and GV oocytes. The MRI measurements were related to these and further parameters like expansion of the cumulus oophorus, pronuclei stages, embryo morphology, and pregnancy rates. The authors found that in all women with MI/GV=0%, the JZ myometrium was significantly enlarged ($p<0.004$) and the clinical pregnancy rate was significantly lower ($p<0.025$) compared to that of women with MI/GV >0%. The authors suggested that the JZ, as documented by MR imaging, might interfere with follicular function.

Implantation failure and miscarriage

In a prospective clinical-imaging study including 152 patients, Maubon et al. [46] have explored the influence of the uterine junctional zone thickness (as measured on pelvic MR imaging), on implantation rates during IVF. They measured average and maximal junctional zone thickness values and implantation outcomes were correlated with these values and with infertility subtypes (endometriosis, tubal, dysovulation, male, and unexplained). A junctional zone thickness increase was significantly correlated with implantation failure at IVF: implantation failure rate was 95.8% for patients with an average junctional zone greater than 7 mm and a maximal junctional zone greater than 10 mm, versus 37.5% in other patient groups ($p<0.0001$), independently from cause of infertility or patients' age. The authors concluded that a pelvic MR scan showing a thickened uterine junctional zone has a negative predictive factor for embryo implantation after IVF.

Tremellen and Russell [47] reported that in four women who had previously undergone multiple unsuccessful in vitro fertilization attempts, inactivation of adenomyosis by an ultra-long pituitary downregulation regime, promptly resulted in successful pregnancy for all four women. In women with endometriosis, Mijatovic et al. [32] found no significant differences for any of the IVF/ICSI outcomes between women with and without concomitant adenomyosis after pretreatment with GnRH agonist for 3 to 26 months. Clearly, further prospective controlled studies are required to clarify the impact of adenomyosis on implantation following IVF.

Martinez-Conejero et al. [48] evaluated the effect of adenomyosis on endometrial gene expression and reproductive outcome in an oocyte donation program. The clinical and molecular data indicate that implantation is not affected by adenomyosis, but higher rates of miscarriage were associated with this condition leading to lower term pregnancies.

Major obstetrical syndromes

On the basis of pre-pregnancy imaging, Juang et al. [49] reported that adenomyosis is an important risk factor for spontaneous preterm delivery. Other recent studies have shown that endometriosis is associated with preterm delivery and other major obstetrical syndromes, such as small for gestation age in the absence of hypertension, preterm delivery, and obstetrical abnormal bleeding [50–52]. In evaluating the significance of these investigations, once again the question arises whether adenomyosis may not be a critical confounding factor in the endometriosis studies as long as adenomyosis or junctional zone hyperplasia is not systematically excluded by imaging scan. In addition, advanced maternal age is not only an important confounding factor for the likelihood of pregnancy complications, but is also associated with structural changes in JZ anatomy as demonstrated by Kunz et al. [30]. Indeed, observational studies suggest that perturbations in JZ structure or functions prior to conception predispose towards impaired deep trophoblast invasion that underpins a spectrum of obstetrical complications, including preterm birth [53–55]

Conclusions

While the link between endometriosis and endometriosis has been puzzling, the role of the myometrial junctional zone appears in both conditions to be associated with several pathologically and clinically recognizable features. Therefore, the presence of either endometriosis or adenomyosis should alert the physician to the possible presence of the other. Both tend to have a range of possible etiologies that could create a set of reproductive and obstetrical disorders. Although the reason that they occur together has not yet been discovered, they have several molecular aberrations of the endometrium and myometrial junction zone in common. As a consequence, these features can justify the introduction of the endomyometrium dysfunctional syndrome.

Finally, there are several practical implications for research and clinical management. It is clear that, from now on, biochemical and clinical studies of the eutopic endometrium in women with endometriosis need to document the presence or absence of myometrial junctional zone abnormalities and uterine adenomyosis.

Conflicts of interest The authors report no conflicts of interest. The authors alone are responsible for the content and writing of the paper.

References

1. Benagiano G, Brosens I (2011) Who identified endometriosis? Fertil Steril 95(1):13–16

2. Cullen TS (1920) The distribution of adenomyomata containing uterine mucosa. Arch Surg 1:215–283
3. Frankl O (1925) Adenomyosis uteri. Am J Obstet Gynecol 10:680–684
4. Sampson JA (1927) Peritoneal endometriosis due to the menstrual dissemination of endometrial tissue into the peritoneal cavity. Am J Obstet Gynecol 14:422–469
5. Cullen TS (1896) Adeno-myoma Uteri diffusum benignum. Johns Hopkins Hosp Rep 6:133
6. Kuligowska E, Deeds L 3rd, Lu K 3rd (2005) Pelvic pain: overlooked and underdiagnosed gynecologic conditions. Radiographics 25(1):3–20
7. Novak E, de Lima OA (1948) A correlative study of adenomyosis and pelvic endometriosis, with special reference to the hormonal reaction of ectopic endometrium. Am J Obstet Gynecol 56:634–644
8. Hricak H, Alpers C, Crooks LE, Sheldon PE (1983) Magnetic resonance imaging of the female pelvis: initial experience. Am J Roentgen 141(6):1119–1128
9. Brosens IA, Brosens JJ (2000) Endometriosis. Eur J Obstet Gynecol Reprod Biol 90(2):159–164
10. Bulmer JN, Jones RK, Searle RF (1998) Intraepithelial leukocytes in endometriosis and adenomyosis: comparison of eutopic and ectopic endometrium with normal endometrium. Hum Reprod 13 (10):2910–2915
11. Noble LS, Takayama K, Zeitoun KM, Putman JM, Johns DA, Hinshelwood MM, Agarwal VR, Zhao Y, Carr BR, Bulun SE (1997) Prostaglandin E2 stimulates aromatase expression in endometriosis-derived stromal cells. J Clin Endocrinol Metab 82 (2):600–606
12. Tseng JF, Ryan IP, Milam TD, Murai JT, Schriock ED, Landers DV, Taylor RN (1996) Interleukin-6 secretion in vitro is upregulated in ectopic and eutopic endometrial stromal cells from women with endometriosis. J Clin Endocrinol Metab 81(3):1118–1122
13. Ota H, Tanaka T (1997) Integrin adhesion molecules in the endometrial glandular epithelium in patients with endometriosis or adenomyosis. J Obstet Gynaecol Res 23(5):485–491
14. Taylor HS, Bagot C, Kardana A, Olive D, Arici A (1999) HOX gene expression is altered in the endometrium of women with endometriosis. Hum Reprod 14(5):1328–1331
15. Dmowski WP, Steele RW, Baker GF (1981) Deficient cellular immunity in endometriosis. Am J Obstet Gynecol 141(4):377–383
16. Carvalho L, Podgaec S, Bellodi-Privato M, Falcone T, Abrão MS (2011) Role of eutopic endometrium in pelvic endometriosis. J Minim Invasive Gynecol 18(4):419–427
17. Benagiano G, Brosens I (2011) Adenomyosis and endometriosis have a common origin. J Obstet Gynecol India 61:27–31
18. Tocci A, Greco E, Ubaldi FM (2008) Adenomyosis and 'endometrial-subendometrial myometrium unit disruption disease' are two different entities. Reprod BioMed Online 17(2):285–291
19. Gordts S, Brosens JJ, Fusi L, Benagiano G, Brosens I (2008) Uterine adenomyosis: a need for uniform terminology and consensus classification. Reprod Biomed Online 17(2):244–248
20. Brosens JJ, de Souza NM, Barker FG (1995) Uterine junctional zone: function and disease. Lancet 346(8974):558–560
21. Leyendecker G, Kunz G, Noe M, Herbertz M, Mall G (1998) Endometriosis: a dysfunction and disease of the archimetra. Hum Reprod Update 4(5):752–762
22. Mehasseb MK, Bell SC, Brown L, Pringle JH, Habiba M (2011) Phenotypic characterisation of the inner and outer myometrium in normal and adenomyotic uteri. Gynecol Obstet Invest 71 (4):217–224
23. Mehasseb MK, Bell SC, Pringle JH, Habiba MA (2010) Uterine adenomyosis is associated with ultrastructural features of altered contractility in the inner myometrium. Fertil Steril 93(7):2130–2136
24. Kennedy S, Hadfield R, Westbrook C, Weeks DE, Barlow D, Golding S (1998) Magnetic resonance imaging to assess familial risk in relatives of women with endometriosis. Lancet 352(9138): 1440–1441
25. Devlieger R, D'Hooghe T, Timmerman D (2003) Uterine adenomyosis in the infertility clinic. Hum Reprod Update 9(2):139–147
26. Kunz G, Beil D, Huppert P, Noe M, Kissler S, Leyendecker G (2005) Adenomyosis in endometriosis - Prevalence and impact on fertility. Evidence from magnetic resonance imaging. Hum Reprod 20(8):2309–2316
27. Landi S, Mereu L, Pontrelli G, Stepniewska A, Romano L, Tateo S, Dorizzi C, Minelli L (2008) The influence of adenomyosis in patients laparoscopically treated for deep endometriosis. J Minim Invasive Gynecol 15(5):566–570
28. Kunz B, Beil D, Huppert P, Leyendecker G (2000) Structural abnormalities of the uterine wall in women with endometriosis and infertility visualized by vaginal sonography and magnetic resonance imaging. Hum Reprod 15(1):76–82
29. Reinhold C, Tafazoli F, Mehio A, Wang L, Atri M, Siegelman ES, Rohoman L (1999) Uterine adenomyosis: endovaginal US and MR imaging features with histopathologic correlation. Radiographics 19:S147–S160
30. Kunz G, Herbertz M, Beil D, Huppert G, Leyendecker G (2007) Adenomyosis as a disorder of the early and late human reproductive period. Reprod Biomed Online 15(6):681–685
31. Kissler S, Zangos S, Kohl J, Wiegratz I, Rody A, Gätje R, Vogl TJ, Kunz G, Leyendecker G, Kaufmann M (2008) Duration of dysmenorrhoea and extent of adenomyosis visualised by magnetic resonance imaging. Eur J Obstet Gynecol Reprod Biol 137(2):204–209
32. Mijatovic V, Florijn E, Halim N, Schats R, Hompes P (2010) Adenomyosis has no adverse effects on IVF/ICSI outcomes in women with endometriosis treated with long-term pituitary down-regulation before IVF/ICSI2010. Eur J Obstet Gynecol Reprod Biol 151(1):62–65
33. Larsen SB, Lundorf E, Forman A, Dueholm M (2011) Adenomyosis and junctional zone changes in patients with endometriosis. Eur J Obstet Gynecol Reprod Biol 157(2):206–211
34. Brosens I, Derwig I, Brosens J, Fusi L, Benagiano G, Pijnenborg R (2010) The enigmatic uterine junctional zone: the missing link between reproductive disorders and major obstetrical disorders? Hum Reprod 25(3):569–574
35. Carter AM, Pijnenborg R (2011) Evolution of invasive placentation with special reference to non-human primates. Best Pract Res Clin Obstet Gynaecol 25(3):249–257
36. Dehoux J-P, Defere S, Squifflet J, Donnez O, Polet R, Mestdagt M, Foidart J-M, Van Langendonckt A, Donnez J (2011) Is the baboon model appropriate for endometriosis studies? Fertil Steril 96 (3):728–733.e3
37. Pijnenborg R, Vercruysse L, Carter AM (2011) Deep trophoblast invasion and spiral artery remodelling in the placental bed of the lowland gorilla. Placenta 32(8):586–591
38. Pijnenborg R, Vercruysse L, Carter AM (2011) Deep trophoblast invasion and spiral artery remodelling in the placental bed of the chimpanzee. Placenta 32(4):400–408
39. Bazot M, Darai E, Clement de Givry S, Boudghene F, Uzan S, Le Blanche AF (2003) Fast breath-hold T2-weighted MR imaging reduces interobserver variability in the diagnosis of adenomyosis. Am J Roentgenol 180(5):1291–1296
40. Lone FW, Balogun M, Khan KS (2006) Adenomyosis: not such an elusive diagnosis any longer. J Obstet Gynaecol 26(3):225–228
41. Brosens I, Pijnenborg R, Vercruysse L, Romero R (2011) The "Great Obstetrical Syndromes" are associated with disorders of deep placentation. Am J Obstet Gynecol 204:193–201
42. Turnbull LW, Manton DJ, Horsman A, Killick SR (1995) Magnetic resonance imaging changes in uterine zonal anatomy during a conception cycle. Brit J Obstet Gynaecol 102(4):330–331

43. Brosens IA (1977) Morphological changes in the utero-placental bed in pregnancy hypertension. Clin Obstet Gynaecol 4(3): 573–593
44. Pijnenborg R, Bland JM, Robertson WB, Brosens I (1983) Uteroplacental arterial changes related to interstitial trophoblast migration in early human pregnancy. Placenta 4(4):397–414
45. Kunz G, Kunz G, Beil D (2010) Characterization of the uterine junctional zone prior to IVF/ICSI: an observational study (2010). Archiv Gynecol Obstet 281(5):945–953
46. Maubon A, Faury A, Kapella M, Pouquet M, Piver P (2010) Uterine junctional zone at magnetic resonance imaging: a predictor of in vitro fertilization implantation failure. J Obstet Gynaecol Res 36(3):611–618
47. Tremellen K, Russell P (2011) Adenomyosis is a potential cause of recurrent implantation failure during IVF treatment. Aust NZ J Obstet Gynaecol 51(3):280–283
48. Martínez-Conejero JA, Morgan M, Montesinos M, Fortuño S, Meseguer M, Simón C, Horcajadas JA, Pellicer A (2011) Adenomyosis does not affect implantation, but is associated with miscarriage in patients undergoing oocyte donation. Fertil Steril 96(4):943–950.e1
49. Juang C-M, Chou P, Yen M-S, Twu N-F, Horng H-C, Hsu W-L (2007) Adenomyosis and risk of preterm delivery. Brit J Obstet Gynaecol 114(2):165–169
50. Fernando S, Breheny S, Jaques AM, Halliday JL, Baker G, Healy D (2009) Preterm birth, ovarian endometriomata, and assisted reproduction technologies. Fertil Steril 91(2):325–330
51. Stephansson O, Kieler H, Granath F, Falconer H (2009) Endometriosis, assisted reproduction technology, and risk of adverse pregnancy outcome. Hum Reprod 24(9):2341–2347
52. Healy DL, Breheny S, Halliday J, Jaques A, Rushford D, Garrett C, Talbot JM, Baker HWG (2010) Prevalence and risk factors for obstetric haemorrhage in 6730 singleton births after assisted reproductive technology in Victoria Australia. Hum Reprod 25(1):265–274
53. Arias F, Victoria A, Cho K, Kraus F (1997) Placental histology and clinical characteristics of patients with preterm premature rupture of membranes. Obstet Gynecol 89(2):265–271
54. Kim YM, Chaiworapongsa T, Gomez R, Bujold E, Yoon BH, Rotmensch S, Thaler HT, Romero R (2002) Failure of physiologic transformation of the spiral arteries in the placental bed in preterm premature rupture of membranes. Am J Obstet Gynecol 187 (5):1137–1142
55. Kim YM, Bujold E, Chaiworapongsa T, Gomez R, Yoon BH, Thaler HT, Rotmensch S, Romero R (2003) Failure of physiologic transformation of the spiral arteries in patients with preterm labor and intact membranes. Am J Obstet Gynecol 189(4):1063–1069

12

A multidisciplinary evidence-based guideline for minimally invasive surgery: Part 1 - entry techniques and the pneumoperitoneum

Claire F. la Chapelle · Willem A. Bemelman · Bart M. P. Rademaker · Teus A. van Barneveld · Frank Willem Jansen · on behalf of the Dutch Multidisciplinary Guideline Development Group Minimally Invasive Surgery

Abstract The Dutch Society for Endoscopic Surgery together with the Dutch Society of Obstetrics and Gynecology initiated a multidisciplinary working group to develop a guideline on minimally invasive surgery to formulate multidisciplinary agreements for minimally invasive surgery aiming towards better patient care and safety. The guideline development group consisted of general surgeons, gynecologists, an anesthesiologist, and urologist authorized by their scientific professional association. Two advisors in evidence-based guideline development supported the group. The guideline was developed using the "Appraisal of Guidelines for Research and Evaluation" instrument. Clinically important aspects were identified and discussed. The best available evidence on these aspects was gathered by systematic review. Recommendations for clinical practice were formulated based on the evidence and a consensus of expert opinion. The guideline was externally reviewed by members of the participating scientific associations and their feedback was integrated. Identified important topics were: laparoscopic entry techniques, intra-abdominal pressure, trocar use, electrosurgical techniques, prevention of trocar site herniation, patient positioning, anesthesiology, perioperative care, patient information, multidisciplinary user consultation, and complication registration. The text of each topic contains an introduction with an explanation of the problem and a summary of the current literature. Each topic was discussed, considerations were evaluated and recommendations were formulated. The development of a guideline on a multidisciplinary level facilitated a broad and rich discussion, which resulted in a very complete and implementable guideline.

Keywords Guideline · Minimally invasive surgery · Multidisciplinary · Laparoscopy · Access · Entry · Pneumoperitoneum

C. F. la Chapelle (✉) · F. W. Jansen
Department of Gynecology, Leiden University Medical Center, K6 room 76, P.O. Box 9600, 2300 RC Leiden, the Netherlands
e-mail: c.f.la_chapelle@lumc.nl

W. A. Bemelman
Department of Surgery, Academic Medical Center, Amsterdam, the Netherlands

B. M. P. Rademaker
Department of Anesthesiology, Onze Lieve Vrouwe Gasthuis, Amsterdam, the Netherlands

T. A. van Barneveld
Department of Quality in Healthcare, Dutch Association of Medical Specialists, Utrecht, the Netherlands

Introduction

Since the early 1990s, "minimally invasive surgery" (MIS) or laparoscopic surgery has been rapidly implemented into a variety of surgical disciplines. Accordingly, new risks have emerged and complications of laparoscopic surgery are constantly being evaluated. The Dutch Healthcare Inspectorate conducted a study of the risks presented by MIS procedures and observed many unsubstantiated differences between general surgery, gynecology, and urology. Although the basic knowledge and skills are identical regardless of specialism, multidisciplinary agreements were lacking. The Dutch Healthcare Inspectorate encouraged different specialties performing laparoscopy to work together and develop a multidisciplinary guideline for MIS.

This guideline represents a review of the evidence and consensus clinical opinion. The objective of this guideline is to provide guidance for MIS in daily practice. By formulating multidisciplinary agreements, the aim is to increase patient safety in MIS. It is intended primarily for all specialists performing laparoscopic surgery or those directly involved. This guideline can also be used as a standard by patients, patients' organizations, hospital organizations, health insurances, and government agencies. The scope of this guideline is laparoscopy in general, specific laparoscopic procedures are not addressed. Different aspects in MIS are described, including laparoscopic entry techniques, pneumoperitoneum, trocar use, electrosurgical techniques, prevention of trocar site herniation, patient positioning, anesthesiology, perioperative care, patient information, multidisciplinary user consultation, and the registration of complications.

In this first of three series papers on the multidisciplinary guideline, we present our literature reviews, conclusions, and practical recommendations for entry techniques and the pneumoperitoneum.

Methods

The Dutch Society for Endoscopic Surgery together with the Dutch Society for Obstetrics and Gynecology initiated a multidisciplinary working group to develop a guideline on MIS. Two general surgeons, two gynecologists, an urologist, and an anesthesiologist participated in the guideline working group. All were authorized by their scientific professional association (the Dutch Society of Surgery, the Dutch Urological Association, and the Dutch Association of Anesthesiologists, respectively). Because of the surgical technical contents, patients were not involved in the guideline development.

The guideline was developed consistent with the "Appraisal of Guidelines for Research and Evaluation" instrument [1]. Initially, the working group performed a problem analysis to define the scope and topics of the guideline. These problem topics were translated into clinical key questions and the scientific literature was searched for answering the key questions. Separate search strategies were developed for each problem topic. Searches were conducted in collaboration with information specialists. Studies were limited to English and Dutch language in view of the limitations on time and resources. The search strategies are appended (see Appendix). The developers selected relevant literature. The bibliographies of relevant articles were hand searched for other valuable references. The characteristics and methodological quality of the studies were assessed using the checklists from the Dutch Cochrane Center [2]. The evidence was summarized in evidence tables and in the guideline text. The grading system of the Dutch Institute for Healthcare improvement CBO was used to level the evidence (Table 1). The guideline text is structured according to a prescribed Evidence-Based Guideline Development (EBGD) format. Each defined key question has its own text-section that comprises the clinical key question followed by a summary of the literature and a conclusion including the level of evidence. Then, considerations (including: patient preferences, availability of services, organization of care, impact on costs, legal consequences) are discussed and each section ends with recommendations. The recommendations are the practical answer to the key question. They are based on 'evidence' (the summary of literature) and balanced with 'experience' (the paragraph considerations). An illustrative overview of the EBGD process is shown in Fig. 1.

Background

The incidence of laparoscopic complications described in the literature varies considerably. Reported complication rates vary from 1.0 to 12.5 per 1,000, depending on the retrospective or prospective nature of the study, the definition of "complication", the experience of the surgeons, the characteristics of the study participants, and the complexity of the procedure. The largest reported studies on complication rates in laparoscopy are based on gynecologic procedures. The Finish National Insurance Association registered a total of 256 complications in 70,607 gynecologic laparoscopic procedures (3.6/1,000). The incidence of gastrointestinal injuries was 0.6/1,000, of urological injuries 0.3/1,000 and of vascular injury 0.1/1,000 [3]. A Dutch prospective multicenter study reported 145 complications in a total of 25,764 gynecologic laparoscopies (5.7/1,000). Two fatal cases were described and in 84 procedures a complication resulted in conversion to laparotomy. The incidence of gastrointestinal injuries was 1.13/1,000, and of intra-abdominal vessels 1.05/1,000. Fifty-seven percent of the complications were entry related (closed- and open-entry techniques were included). Women who had undergone a prior history of laparotomy had an increased risk for complications [4].

Other complications in laparoscopy are a pneumothorax or subcutaneous emphysema, with reported incidences of 1.9% and 2.3%, respectively [5]. Pneumothorax is frequently seen together with subcutaneous emphysema and associated with inadequate insufflation of CO_2 through an improperly placed trocar or Veress needle [6, 7]. Subcutaneous emphysema may also occur when pressurized CO_2 moves into pre-existing or iatrogenic defects in the diaphragm or retroperitoneum. Due to its good solubility, CO_2 is rapidly absorbed in the blood circulation and may lead to an increase in hypercapnia and acidosis. Subcutaneous emphysema located in the head and neck area can lead to airway obstruction. The airways should therefore be secured until all emphysema has been dissolved [8].

Table 1 Grading system for level of evidence

Level	Studies on therapy/prevention	Studies on diagnostic accuracy	Studies on harm, etiology or prognosis
A1	Systematic review/meta-analysis of at least two independent studies of A2 level with consistent results		
A2	Double-blind randomized controlled trial of good quality and sufficient power	Study with respect to a reference test (gold standard) with pre-defined cut-off values, among large series consecutive persons that received both the index and the reference test and adequate blinding of interpretation of test results	Prospective cohort study of sufficient power and follow-up, adequate control for confounding and selective follow up
B	Randomized controlled trial of modest quality or insufficient power, or other analytic study (e.g., case–control study, cohort study)	A comparison with a reference standard that does not meet the criteria required for level A2 evidence	Prospective cohort study that does not meet the criteria required for level A2 evidence. Or retrospective cohort study or case–control study
C	Non-analytic study		
D	Expert opinion		
Level	Conclusion based on		
1	One systematic review (A1) or at least two independent randomized controlled trials of level A2		
2	One study of level A2 or at least 2 independent studies of level B		
3	One study of level B or C		
4	Expert opinion		

Grading system used at the Dutch Institute for Healthcare Improvement CBO

The incidence of complications related to laparoscopy is low; however, they can be very severe. More than 50% of laparoscopic complications are entry related and these occasionally require emergency surgery. Basically, two different

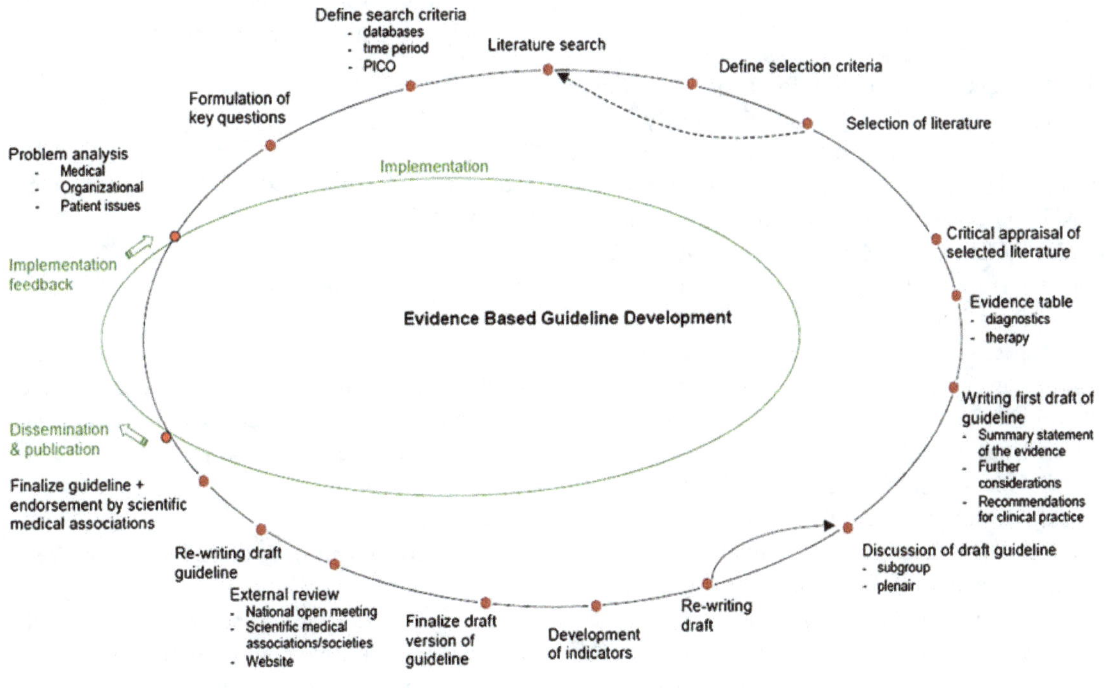

Source: Dutch Institute for Healthcare Improvement CBO

Fig. 1 Overview of the developmental process in EBGD

entry techniques can be distinguished the open- and closed-entry technique. Surgeons and urologists often use the open technique with Hasson trocar (also called the Hasson technique) [9] while gynecologists often use the closed technique with blind introduction of the Veress needle and primary trocar. The risks associated with the two different techniques are investigated and can be variously interpreted. The text below describes the strategies for a safe application of entry techniques in laparoscopy.

Key question

Which entry technique, open or closed, is associated with the lowest risks for complications?

Summary of the literature

Injuries of the intra-abdominal vessels and bowel are known entry-related complications. Since the incidences of these complications are low, a randomized controlled trial (RCT) would not be the appropriate design to detect risk differences. To detect a risk difference for bowel injury from 0.3% to 0.2%, over 800,000 patients would be needed for inclusion in an RCT [10].

In a Cochrane review, different entry techniques were compared in terms or their influence on intraoperative and postoperative complications [11]. The outcomes were divided into major complications (mortality, vascular injury, bladder injury, bowel injury, gas embolism, and solid organ injury) and minor complications (e.g., extraperitoneal insufflation, trocar site bleeding). Two RCTs were included (a total of 210 patients enrolled) wherein open- and closed-entry techniques were compared. No significant risk differences were found for major and minor complications, neither in more specified analyses. In 2001, the Australian College of Surgeons systematically reviewed the effectiveness and safety of entry techniques for establishing a pneumoperitoneum in laparoscopic surgery. Besides RCTs, other relevant studies with different study designs were included. The outcome data for bowel injury and vascular injury in five nonrandomized prospective and retrospective comparative studies were pooled. A higher risk of bowel injury showed for the open-compared to the closed-entry technique (RR 2.17, 95% CI: 1.14–4.10). No statistical significant risk difference was found comparing the open-versus closed-entry technique for vascular injury (RR 0.68, 95% CI: 0.16–2.84) [12].

Interpreting these results, the potential for selection bias should be taken into account. For example, the open-entry technique would often be the preferred technique in patients with previous abdominal surgery. This selection bias may result in an increased relative risk of bowel injury for the open-entry technique compared to the closed-entry technique.

Conclusion

Level 1	No significant risk differences have been found for bowel and vascular injuries, when comparing the open-entry to the closed-entry technique. *Evidence level A1* [11]

Considerations

Theoretically, it could be claimed that retroperitoneal vascular injury can be prevented by using the open-entry technique and thereby eliminating the potential for abrupt and uncontrolled introduction of the primary trocar that may result in a deeper penetration than needed. This risk is inherent in the closed-entry technique and thus vigilance is needed. In practice, it shows that the risk for uncontrolled introduction reduces by gaining experience. No robust conclusions can be drawn from the results of nonrandomized studies because of insufficient power and a high risk of bias.

Recommendations

- In general, no completely safe entry technique can be recommended. Specialists should preferably practice the technique they have learned and with which they are familiar. According to expert opinion, experience with a particular entry technique will reduce the risks of complications. Exceptions to this rule are: patients with prior abdominal surgery, obese patients, very thin patients and pregnant patients (see key question 1.7).

Key question

How should the closed- and open-entry techniques be performed?

Summary of the literature

There are no comparative studies of good methodological quality about differing aspects in specifically closed- and open-entry techniques. The majority of the studies are descriptive and based on expert opinions.

Closed-entry technique: placement of the Veress needle

The Veress needle will be checked for its potency and spring action before inserting it into the abdomen. This is to ensure a free flow of CO_2 and the protective function of the blunt tip. The blunt tip emerges out of the sharp end to protect the bowel and other intra-abdominal organs from inadvertent puncture.

The abdominal wall is lifted until a 45° angle to the horizontal. This can be done by lifting the skin at the umbilicus by hand or with a towel clip. In the Cochrane review on laparoscopic entry techniques, one RCT was included comparing abdominal wall lifting versus not lifting for placement of the Veress needle. Not lifting the abdominal wall showed less failed entries, with no difference in complication rate. According to the experts however, abdominal wall lifting is aimed to prevent compression and thereby reduction of distance between instruments and retroperitoneal structures. The Veress needle is inserted perpendicular to the fascia and then directed towards the surgical field, avoiding the major vessels.

There are several tests to verify the correct position of the Veress needle tip. Different tests were evaluated in an observational study and it was concluded that a low initial gas pressure (<10 mmHg) followed by a free influx of CO_2 is the only valuable measure to reflect correct intraperitoneal Veress needle placement [13].

Conclusions

Level 3	A low initial gas pressure (<10 mmHg), followed by a free influx of CO_2, is a reliable indicator of correct intraperitoneal Veress needle placement
	Evidence level B [13]
Level 4	There are insufficient high-quality comparative studies on safety and effectiveness of the different aspects in the specific open- and closed-entry techniques
	Evidence level D (*opinion of the guideline development group*)

Considerations

In practice, for selected patients, only specific entry techniques are applied. An adequate selection is required, which is discussed among key question 1.7.

During every laparoscopic procedure, instruments to perform a laparotomy should be available. These could be necessary in the event that an injury occurs for which a conversion is required. Prior to the closed-entry technique, the patient is catheterized or an indwelling catheter is inserted. A nasogastric tube can be used. A filled stomach or bladder may hinder the placement of laparoscopic instruments or these structures can be damaged. Positioning the patient in Trendelenburg prior to the insertion of laparoscopic instruments could theoretically increase the risk for inadvertent aortic puncture. In most cases, the primary incision is preferred in the umbilicus because it overlies the location where the skin, fascia, and parietal peritoneum converge and fuse. Consequently, the distance between skin and abdominal cavity is short and an umbilical incision generally has a good cosmetic result. The skin incision should be large enough to prevent overshoot injury. In lean patients, initial skin incision should not involve the fascia. One should avoid stab incision. These precautions are not sufficiently investigated, but are considered common sense.

Closed-entry technique: insertion of the primary trocar

After the pneumoperitoneum is achieved and the Veress needle is removed, the primary trocar is inserted through the umbilical incision in the same directions as the Veress needle. When using a normal intra-abdominal pressure (IAP; 12–16 mmHg), the umbilicus should be lifted and fixated as with the insertion of the Veress needle. Every move associated with introduction of the instrument should be well controlled. It is recommended to open the valve of the trocar to hear if the tip is located in the abdominal cavity. After inserting the laparoscope, visual inspection is intended to check for iatrogenic injuries and intraperitoneal aberrations.

Open-entry technique: insertion of the primary trocar

In the open-entry technique, the introduction of sharp instruments is avoided. A small incision is created and the layers of the abdominal wall are incised. The peritoneum is opened bluntly or sharply. When reaching the peritoneal cavity this is often visible and can be verified by palpation with a finger. The primary trocar is then inserted and CO_2 is inflated to create the pneumoperitoneum. Today, balloon blunt-tip trocars are commonly used. The distal end of the sleeve has an inflatable balloon to create an air-tight fixation of the trocar.

Trocar removal

At the end of each laparoscopic procedure, the removal of all trocars should be under direct vision. As yet, unnoticed injuries, e.g., tamponaded hemorrhage or bowel perforation, can be detected. Thereby, trocar site herniation can possibly be prevented by avoiding bowel or omental tissue is pulled into the trocar site.

Recommendations for the closed-entry technique

- Prior to continuing the insufflation, the initial IAP should be <10 mmHg (measured via Veress needle).
- Prior to the closed-entry technique, it is preferable to insert a nasogastric tube and to empty the urinary bladder.

General recommendations for primary entry

- Instruments to perform an emergency laparotomy should be available at close hand. These could be necessary in the event that a complication occurs for which conversion is required.
- During primary entry, the patient must be positioned horizontally until the primary trocar is safely inserted. The umbilicus can be stabilized by lifting it this can prevent compression and consequent reduction of the distance between the instruments and retroperitoneal structures.
- After opening the peritoneum and prior to the introduction of the (blunt) primary trocar, it is important to ensure that the peritoneal cavity has been reached.
- The primary trocar must be introduced in a controlled manner, at an angle of 90° to the fascia. Once the peritoneal cavity has been reached, the insertion must be stopped immediately.
- After introduction of the laparoscope, the abdomen must be inspected for adjacent bowel by rotating the laparoscope 360°. If adjacent bowel is observed, it must be inspected for (signs of) hemorrhage, lesion, or retroperitoneal hematoma.
- The removal of all trocars should under direct vision, to recognize a tamponaded hemorrhage or a bowel perforation that has not been noticed, and to prevent bowel or omental tissue being pulled into the trocar site.

Key questions

Closed-entry technique and IAP:

1 What IAP should be achieved prior to insertion of the primary trocar?
2. What IAP should be applied once the insertion of trocars is complete?

Summary of the literature

When applying "peritoneal hyperdistention", the abdomen is insufflated to 25–30 mmHg before inserting the primary trocar. After introduction of the trocars, the IAP is reduced to a normal pressure (12–16 mmHg).

Prospective observational studies have shown that the increased size of the "gas bubble" has a splinting effect and allows the trocar to be more easily inserted through the layers of the abdominal wall. Furthermore, when force is applied to a hyperdistended abdomen (25 mmHg), the depth under the umbilicus is larger, compared to a normally distended abdomen (10 mmHg) [14]. An increased IAP induces a hemodynamic stress response. The venous return from the lower extremities alters, cardiac output decreases and there is an increase in mean arterial pressure (MAP) systemic, pulmonary and vascular resistances [15–17]. In a prospective observational study, significant hemodynamic changes were observed when the IAP was elevated above 12 mmHg. There was a decrease in stroke volume and cardiac output and an increase in MAP and systemic vascular resistance [18].

No studies were found that analyzed for the upper limit of IAP. Neither systematic reviews nor RCTs evaluating the clinically relevant consequences of "peritoneal hyperdistention" were found. In a prospective cohort study including 100 women undergoing gynecological laparoscopy, hemodynamic changes were analyzed. High pressures (25–30 mmHg) resulted in minimal changes in heart rate and blood pressure and a statistical significant decrease of pulmonary compliance, all without clinically relevant consequences [19]. This study was conducted in healthy women with classified American Society of Anesthesiologists scores (ASA) I and II. The hemodynamic and pulmonary consequences of "peritoneal hyperdistention" has not been studied in men and patients with higher ASA scores. A larger prospective cohort study (1,150 consecutive ASA I patients undergoing gynecological laparoscopy) investigated the safety of the pressure technique for insertion of the primary trocar. No insertion complications or adverse clinical effects were noted during hospital stay [20].

In a Cochrane review, the harms and benefits of the low pressure pneumoperitoneum (<12 mmHg) compared with standard pressure pneumoperitoneum (12–16 mmHg) were assessed in patients undergoing laparoscopic cholecystectomy [21]. A total of 15 RCTs were included (690 patients), all with high risk of bias. There was no difference in mortality, postoperative complications, or conversion to open cholecystectomy between the groups. None of the trials reported any cardiopulmonary complications. Only patients with ASA I scores were included in the trials, together with a low overall incidence of cardiopulmonary complications (0.5% in a case series of 400 patients, 70% of the patients were scored ASA I) [22] the meta-analysis was under powered. In seven trials, the outcome data were incomplete: reasons for conversion were not reported. This caused a high risk of bias and thus the safety of the low-pressure pneumoperitoneum could not be ascertained [21].

Conclusions

Level 1	The safety of low pressure pneumoperitoneum (<12 mmHg) has only been studied in patients undergoing cholecystectomy. It is uncertain whether low pressures in comparison with conventional pressures, result in equal risks of morbidity and conversion to open surgery. *Evidence level A1* [21]
Level 2	Elevated IAP above 12 mmHg is associated with significant hemodynamic effects. These effects did not demonstrate any clinically relevant consequences *Evidence level A2* [18]

Level 3	"Peritoneal hyperdistention" has only been studied and found to be safe in healthy female patients with ASA scores I or II *Evidence level C* [19, 20]
Level 3	"Peritoneal hyperdistention" (insufflation to IAP 25–30 mmHg), results in an increased size or "gas bubble" and a splinting effect of the abdominal wall, compared to the traditional, limited-volume pneumoperitoneum *Evidence level C* [14]

Considerations

The abdominal wall cannot be lifted when the abdomen is hyperdistended. Thus when using the "peritoneal hyperdistention" technique, the primary trocar is inserted perpendicular to the abdominal wall.

"Peritoneal hyperdistention" can result in hemodynamic changes and compromise the respiratory ventilation of the patient. The anesthesiologist should therefore be informed when changing the IAP. "Peritoneal hyperdistention" should last no longer than necessary: after introduction of the trocars, the IAP should be reduced to a normal pressure (12–16 mmHg). High pressures did not result in any clinical relevant compromises in healthy patients but could possibly have more clinically significant effects in patients with ASA III and IV scores.

RCTs have shown that the use of a low pressure pneumoperitoneum results in less hemodynamic changes [22], less shoulder pain [23, 24], less postoperative pain [25], and less use of analgesics [24, 25]. However, main criticism of low pressure pneumoperitoneum is its ability to provide adequate surgical exposure and its safety.

Recommendations for IAP

- Before blind introduction of the primary trocar, the IAP must be at least 12–16 mmHg. The "pressure technique" to 25–30 mmHg may be applied briefly in selected patients.
- After introduction of the trocars, the IAP must be reduced to a normal pressure (12–16 mmHg, depending on patient characteristics) creating sufficient distension to perform laparoscopy and where the anesthesiologist can provide safe and effective pulmonary ventilation.

Key question

What alternative entry techniques are available?

Summary of the literature

Direct trocar entry

The direct trocar entry has been described as an alternative to the Veress needle technique. The primary entry is initiated with one blind step instead of two (Veress needle and trocar). The direct trocar entry is faster than any other method of entry [26]. In the Cochrane review on laparoscopic entry techniques, a meta-analysis was performed comparing direct trocar entry to Veress needle entry. A total of 1,909 participants in six RCTs were included and no major complications occurred with both techniques [27–32]. There were however, statistically significant reductions in the risk of extraperitoneal insufflation and failed entry in the direct-entry group (OR 0.06; 95% CI: 0.02–0.023 and 0.22; 95% CI: 0.08–0.56, respectively) [11].

Other entry systems

Different entry-systems have been developed to reduce the risk for entry-related complications: direct-vision entry systems [33, 34], radially expanding trocars [35], tapered blunt tipped trocars (TrocDoc, second generation Endotip®) [36]. For the Cochrane review, no RCTs comparing direct-vision versus Veress needle entry were identified. There were no other observational studies with sufficient power to demonstrate a risk reduction for major complications when direct-vision entry was used. The Cochrane review on laparoscopic entry techniques concludes that radially expanding access trocars offer advantages in terms of reduced trocar site bleedings, less extraperitoneal insufflations, and failed entries [11, 34, 37, 38]. RCTs and other observational studies comparing tapered blunt tip systems with the conventional Veress needle or open-entry technique did have insufficient power to demonstrate risk reductions for any complication.

Needlescopes are optical Veress needles with 1–2 mm diameter [39]. There is as yet no evidence for their superiority compared to the conventional Veress needle entry.

Conclusions

Level 1	Direct trocar entry leads to fewer extraperitoneal insufflations and failed entries when compared with Veress needle entry *Evidence level A1* [11, 27–32]
Level 1	For primary entry, radially expanding access trocars reduce the risks for trocar site bleedings, extraperitoneal insufflations and failed entries compared to conventional trocars *Evidence level A2* [11, 34, 37, 38]
Level 3	There is no evidence that use of direct vision systems, a tapered blunt tipped trocar or a needlescope for primary entry is safer than the conventional open- or closed-entry techniques *Evidence level C* [26, 40]

Considerations

Some RCTs excluded specific patient groups, e.g., patients with previous abdominal surgery, obese patients, or patients at risk for sub-umbilical adhesions. Therefore, the results of these RCTs do not apply for the complete laparoscopic patient population. For a select patient group, the direct trocar entry seems a safe and fast method with a lower risk for extraperitoneal insufflation and failed entry compared to Veress needle entry. This technique is not widely used in laparoscopic practice, probably because extensive experience is required for its use.

Moreover, high costs of newly developed systems could be a limiting factor for their use. Studies on cost effectiveness should be conducted to make informed choices for the use of specific instruments in laparoscopic practice.

Recommendations for alternative entry techniques

- The guideline development group does not recommend the use of direct trocar entry, since a high level of experience is needed for the safe application of this technique.
- The use of visual entry systems is only recommended when an adequate pneumoperitoneum (with the Veress needle) has been created.
- Radially expanding trocars are an expensive alternative to standard trocars. The use of these trocars may reduce trocar site bleedings and extraperitoneal insufflations.

Key question

What alternative sites can be safely used for insertion of the Veress needle and primary trocar?

Summary of the literature

The rate of adhesion formation at the umbilicus may occur up to 50% in patients following midline laparotomy and 23% following low transverse incision [41]. A Veress needle or trocar should never be blindly inserted at a site where adhesions may be expected. In those cases, the umbilicus is not the appropriate site for closed-entry. The most usual alternative site following laparotomy is in the left upper quadrant via Palmer's point. Palmer's point is located 3 cm below the costal margin in the midclavicular line. Adhesions are rarely formed in this area, though, in cases of previous surgery in this area or splenomegaly, Palmer's point may as well be inappropriate.

It remains unclear what rates of adhesion formation are found in patients following laparoscopy and thus which entry location is most suitable following a prior laparoscopy.

Conclusion

Level 3	When periumbilical adhesions may be expected, Palmer's point is the appropriate site for insertion of the Veress needle and primary trocar *Evidence level C* [41]

Considerations

When periumbilical adhesions are suspected, either an open entry technique or a closed entry at a different location (preferably Palmers' point) must be performed. It could be an option to insert the primary trocar sub-umbilical, after first having excluded periumbilical adhesions with a needlescoop [42].

Other sites for insertion of the Veress needle and trocar have been described (suprapubic, through the uterine fundus or posterior fornix) but, given the greater risks of complications, are to be avoided.

Recommendation for alternative entry site

- In the event of doubt or suspected periumbilical adhesions, the Veress needle and primary trocar should not be introduced at the umbilicus. An alternative technique (e.g., the open entry technique or insufflation at the point of Palmer) should be chosen.

Key question

How should secondary ports be created?

Summary of the literature

The safety of different methods to create secondary ports has not systematically been studied. A prospective observational study showed that 64% of the superficial epigastric vessels could be identified with transillumination. Laparoscopic visualization successfully identified 82% of the inferior epigastric vessels. Both methods were less effective as patient's weight increased [43].

The insertion of secondary ports should be visualized laparoscopically, taking care to avoid injury to the vessels and viscera. Suprapubic insertion of a trocar puts the bladder at risk of damage; therefore, the bladder should be visualized. If the margins of the bladder are unclear, the bladder can be filled retrograde.

Conclusion

Level 3	Superficial epicastric vessels can be visualized with transillumination. Deeper epigastric vessels can be visualized laparoscopically *Evidence level B* [43]

Considerations

Secondary ports are inserted perpendicular to the skin to minimize the iatrogenic defect in the fascia. Once the tip has passed the peritoneum, it is directed towards the surgical field. The inferior epigastric vessels should be visualized laparoscopically to ensure that the entry site is away from the vessels. The deep epigastric arteries and venae comitantes are located lateral to the lateral umbilical ligaments. The visualization can be difficult in obese patients. Then, the incision should be placed lateral to the rectus sheath, taking care to avoid injury of the pelvic side wall.

Recommendations for secondary ports

- The superficial epigastric vessels should be visualized by translumination prior to the insertion of secondary trocars. Deeper epigastric vessels should be visualized laparoscopically.
- When inserting the secondary trocars, this must be under direct vision and with the presence of an adequate pneumoperitoneum. The trocars should be inserted perpendicular to the fascia and then directed towards the surgical site.
- When a suprapubic port is inserted, attention must be paid to the localization of the bladder. Retrograde filling of the bladder is possible.

Key question

What entry techniques should be applied for laparoscopy in a pregnant patient, a patient who is very thin or a patient with morbid obesity?

Summary of the literature

No trials that compare different entry techniques in pregnant patients or very thin patients or patients with morbid obesity have been described. There is some descriptive literature for these specific patient groups.

The pregnant patient

Concerning pregnant patients, there are specific concerns for a higher likelihood of injury to the uterus or other intra-abdominal organs. From 12 weeks of gestation, the fundal height of the uterus increases rapidly. The Society of American Gastrointestinal and Endoscopic Surgeons (SAGES) published a guideline on laparoscopy in pregnancy [44, 45]. In this guideline, the authors recommend that in the second and third trimesters of pregnancy, the site of entry should be adapted to the fundal height: from the umbilicus towards subcostal regions [46]. In their opinion, through this adjustment together with elevation of the abdominal wall during insertion, both the Hasson technique and Veress needle entry could be safely and effectively utilized.

The very thin patient

In children and extremely thin patients (BMI <18 kg/m^2), the aorta may lie less than 2.5 cm under the skin [47]. These patients are at particular risk for retroperitoneal vascular injury during primary entry and for this reason, the open entry technique or closed entry at Palmer's point are preferable

The obese patient

The site for primary entry, umbilicus or Palmer's point, in obese patients should depend on the body habitus and distribution of fat. The location where the thinnest subcutis is expected is best used for inserting the Veress needle or trocar. The open as well as the closed-entry technique can be applied. If the Veress needle is inserted vertically downward at the umbilicus, the mean distance from the lower margin of the umbilicus to the peritoneum is 6 cm (with a standard deviation of 3 cm). In this way, it is possible to use a Veress needle with standard length, even in extremely obese patients.

Conclusion

Level 4	There is insufficient qualitative data comparing the safety of different entry techniques in pregnant patients, very thin patients and patients with morbid obesity *Evidence level D (opinion of the MIS guideline development group)*

Considerations

In a pregnant patient, blind insertion of a Veress needle or trocar gives an additional risk for injury of the uterus. The SAGES describes a closed entry can be considered, however, in our opinion, an open-entry technique is preferable. Since the fundal height can be increased in the first trimester due to a twin pregnancy or myomas, the open techniques is recommended in all trimesters. Attention should be paid to other aspects of laparoscopy in pregnancy as well: positioning, IAP, fetal monitoring, and possibly medicinal tocolysis.

Recommendations for specific patient groups

- In pregnant patients, the open-entry technique or closed-entry technique via Palmers' point is preferred.
- In underweight patients (BMI <18 kg/m^2 and children), the open-entry or closed-entry technique via Palmers' point is preferred.
- In patients with morbid obesity (BMI >40 kg/m^2), the closed-entry technique via the umbilicus or Palmers' point is preferred.

Acknowledgments The authors thank all members of the guideline development group Minimally Invasive Surgery for their critical contributions in the discussions on the aspects described in this article. The Dutch Ministry of Health together with the Dutch Association of Medical Specialists supported the development of this guideline.

Declaration of interest The authors report no conflicts of interest.

Appendix

Table 2 Literature search for entry techniques

Subject	Database	Search terms
Entry	Medline (OVID) 1950-Aug.2010	1. Laparoscopy/
		2. exp *Laparoscopy/
		3. Surgical Procedures, Minimally Invasive/
		4. "lapar*scop*".m_titl.
		5. "minimal invasive*".m_titl.
		6. or/1–5
		7. ("laparoscopic injur*" or "laparoscopic entr*" or "laparoscopic adj2 complication*" or "closed laparoscop*" or "open laparoscop*" or "direct-entry adj2 laparoscop*").ti,ab.
		8. 6 and 7
		9. limit 8 to yr="2006 -Current"
		10. RCT (filter)
		11. SR (filter)
		12. exp epidemiological studies/
	Embase	laparoscop*:ti OR 'laparoscopy'/exp/mj OR 'minimal invasive':ti OR 'laparoscopic surgery'/exp AND ((laparoscopic NEAR/1 injur*):ab,ti OR (laparoscopic NEAR/1 entr*):ab,ti OR (laparoscopic NEAR/1 complication*):ab,ti OR (closed NEAR/1 laparoscop*):ab,ti OR (open NEAR/1 laparoscop*):ab,ti OR 'direct entry':ab,ti) AND [embase]/lim AND [2006–2011]/py
Pneumo-peritoneum	Medline (OVID) 1950-March 2010	1. exp *Laparoscopy/
		2. Surgical Procedures, Minimally Invasive/
		3. "lapar*scop*".m_titl.
		4. "minimal invasive*".m_titl.
		5. or/1–5
		6. Pneumoperitoneum, Artificial/ae [Adverse Effects]
		7. 6 and 7
	Embase	laparoscop*:ti OR 'laparoscopy'/exp/mj OR 'minimal invasive':ti OR 'laparoscopic surgery'/exp AND (intraperitoneal NEAR/5 pressure OR intraperitoneal NEAR/5 insufflation) NOT [animals]/lim)
		Searchfilter RCTs

The literature search for entry techniques was based on the search strategy of the Green-top Guideline "Preventing entry-related gynecological laparoscopic injuries" from the Royal College of Obstetricians and Gynaecologists. Medline and Embase were searched for relevant randomized controlled trials, systematic reviews and meta-analyses. The search was restricted to articles published in Dutch and English from 1966 to Augustus 2010

References

1. AGREE Collaboration (2003) Development and validation of an international appraisal instrument for assessing the quality of clinical practice guidelines: The AGREE project. Qual Saf Health Care 12:18–23
2. http://dcc.cochrane.org/beoordelingsformulieren-en-andere-downloads
3. Harkki-Siren P, Kurki T (1997) A nationwide analysis of laparoscopic complications. Obstet Gynecol 89(1):108–112
4. Jansen FW, Kapiteyn K, Trimbos-Kemper T, Hermans J, Trimbos JB (1997) Complications of laparoscopy: a prospective multicentre observational study. Br J Obstet Gynaecol 104(5):595–600
5. Murdock CM, Wolff AJ, Van GT (2000) Risk factors for hypercarbia, subcutaneous emphysema, pneumothorax, and pneumomediastinum during laparoscopy. Obstet Gynecol 95 (5):704–709
6. Ko ML (2010) Pneumopericardium and severe subcutaneous emphysema after laparoscopic surgery. J Minim Invasive Gynecol 17 (4):531–533
7. Perko G, Fernandes A (1997) Subcutaneous emphysema and pneumothorax during laparoscopy for ectopic pregnancy removal. Acta Anaesthesiol Scand 41(6):792–794
8. Badawy SZ, Dalpe C, Romano DJ (2002) Pneumomediastinum and subcutaneous emphysema during carbon dioxide laser laparoscopy for tuboplasty. J Gynecol Surg 18:159–163
9. Hasson HM (1984) Open laparoscopy. Biomed Bull 5(1):1–6
10. Garry R (1999) Towards evidence-based laparoscopic entry techniques: clinical problems and dilemmas. Gynaecol Endosc 8:315–326
11. Ahmad G, Duffy JM, Phillips K, Watson A (2008) Laparoscopic entry techniques. Cochrane Database Syst Rev (2): CD006583
12. Merlin T, Jamieson G, Brown A, Maddern G, Hiller J, Kolbe A (2001) A systematic review of the methods used to establish laparoscopic pneumoperitoneum. ASERNIP-S report
13. Teoh B, Sen R, Abbott J (2005) An evaluation of four tests used to ascertain Veres needle placement at closed laparoscopy. J Minim Invasive Gynecol 12(2):153–158
14. Phillips G, Garry R, Kumar C, Reich H (1999) How much gas is required for initial insufflation at laparoscopy? Gynaecol Endosc 8:369–374
15. Galizia G, Prizio G, Lieto E, Castellano P, Pelosio L, Imperatore V et al (2001) Hemodynamic and pulmonary changes during open, carbon dioxide pneumoperitoneum and abdominal wall-lifting cholecystectomy. A prospective, randomized study. Surg Endosc 15(5):477–483
16. Henny CP, Hofland J (2005) Laparoscopic surgery: pitfalls due to anesthesia, positioning, and pneumoperitoneum. Surg Endosc 19 (9):1163–1171
17. Joris JL, Chiche JD, Canivet JL, Jacquet NJ, Legros JJ, Lamy ML (1998) Hemodynamic changes induced by laparoscopy and their endocrine correlates: effects of clonidine. J Am Coll Cardiol 32 (5):1389–1396
18. Borg IR Mertens zur, Lim A, Verbrugge SJ, IJzermans JN, Klein J (2004) Effect of intraabdominal pressure elevation and positioning on hemodynamic responses during carbon dioxide pneumoperitoneum for laparoscopic donor nephrectomy: a prospective controlled clinical study. Surg Endosc 18(6):919–923
19. Abu-Rafea B, Vilos GA, Vilos AG, Ahmad R, Hollett-Caines J, Al-Omran M (2005) High-pressure laparoscopic entry does not adversely affect cardiopulmonary function in healthy women. J Minim Invasive Gynecol 12(6):475–479
20. Tsaltas J, Pearce S, Lawrence A, Meads A, Mezzatesta J, Nicolson S (2004) Safer laparoscopic trocar entry: it's all about pressure. Aust N Z J Obstet Gynaecol 44(4):349–350
21. Gurusamy KS, Samraj K, Davidson BR (2009) Low pressure versus standard pressure pneumoperitoneum in laparoscopic cholecystectomy. Cochrane Database Syst Rev (2):CD006930
22. Dexter SP, Vucevic M, Gibson J, McMahon MJ (1999) Hemodynamic consequences of high- and low-pressure capnoperitoneum during laparoscopic cholecystectomy. Surg Endosc 13 (4):376–381
23. Chok KS, Yuen WK, Lau H, Fan ST (2006) Prospective randomized trial on low-pressure versus standard-pressure pneumoperitoneum in outpatient laparoscopic cholecystectomy. Surg Laparosc, Endosc Percutaneous Tech 16(6):383–386
24. Sarli L, Costi R, Sansebastiano G, Trivelli M, Roncoroni L (2000) Prospective randomized trial of low-pressure pneumoperitoneum for reduction of shoulder-tip pain following laparoscopy. Br J Surg 87(9):1161–1165
25. Wallace DH, Serpell MG, Baxter JN, O'Dwyer PJ (1997) Randomized trial of different insufflation pressures for laparoscopic cholecystectomy. Br J Surg 84(4):455–458
26. Vilos GA, Ternamian A, Dempster J, Laberge PY, The Society of Obstetricians and Gynaecologists of Canada (2007) Laparoscopic entry: a review of techniques, technologies, and complications. J Obstet Gynaecol Can 29(5):433–465
27. Agresta F, De SP, Ciardo LF, Bedin N (2004) Direct trocar insertion vs Veress needle in nonobese patients undergoing laparoscopic procedures: a randomized prospective single-center study. Surg Endosc 18(12):1778–1781
28. Bemelman WA, Dunker MS, Busch OR, Den Boer KT, de Wit LT, Gouma DJ (2000) Efficacy of establishment of pneumoperitoneum with the Veress needle, Hasson trocar, and modified blunt trocar (TrocDoc): a randomized study. J Laparoendosc Adv Surg Tech A 10(6):325–330
29. Borgatta L, Gruss L, Barad D, Kaali SG (1990) Direct trocar insertion vs. Verres needle use for laparoscopic sterilization. J Reprod Med 35(9):891–894
30. Byron JW, Markenson G, Miyazawa K (1993) A randomized comparison of Verres needle and direct trocar insertion for laparoscopy. Surg Gynecol Obstet 177(3):259–262
31. Gunec MZ, Yesildaglar N, Bingol B, Onalan G, Tabak S, Gokmen B (2005) The safety and efficacy of direct trocar insertion with elevation of the rectus sheath instead of the skin for pneumoperitoneum. Surg Laparosc, Endosc Percutaneous Tech 15(2):80–81
32. Tansatit T, Wisawasukmongchol W, Bunyavejchevin S (2006) A randomized, prospective study comparing the use of the missile trocar and the pyramidal trocar for laparoscopy access. J Med Assoc Thai 89(7):941–947
33. Melzer A, Riek S, Roth K, Buess G (1995) Endoscopically controlled trocar and cannula insertion. [Review] [25 refs]. Endosc Surg Allied Technol 3(1):63–68
34. Mettler L, Maher P (2000) Investigation of the effectiveness of the radially-expanding needle system, in contrast to the cutting trocar in enhancing patient recovery. Minim Invasive Ther Allied Technol 9(6):397–401

35. Turner DJ (1996) A new, radially expanding access system for laparoscopic procedures versus conventional cannulas. J Am Assoc Gynecol Laparosc 3(4):609–615
36. Ternamian AM (1997) Laparoscopy without trocars. Surg Endosc 11(8):815–818
37. Bhoyrul S, Payne J, Steffes B, Swanstrom L, Way LW (2000) A randomized prospective study of radially expanding trocars in laparoscopic surgery. J Gastrointest Surg 4(4):392–397
38. Feste JR, Bojahr B, Turner DJ (2000) Randomized trial comparing a radially expandable needle system with cutting trocars. JSLS 4 (1):11–15
39. O'Donovan PJ, McGurgan P (1999) Microlaparoscopy. Semin Laparosc Surg 6(2):51–57
40. Minervini A, Davenport K, Pefanis G, Keeley FX Jr, Timoney AG (2008) Prospective study comparing the bladeless optical access trocar versus Hasson open trocar for the establishment of pneumoperitoneum in laparoscopic renal procedures. Arch Ital Urol Androl 80(3):95–98
41. Audebert AJ, Gomel V (2000) Role of microlaparoscopy in the diagnosis of peritoneal and visceral adhesions and in the prevention of bowel injury associated with blind trocar insertion. Fertil Steril 73(3):631–635
42. Sutton CJG, Philips K (2008) Preventing entry-related gynaecological laparoscopic injuries. RCOG Green-top guideline
43. Hurd WW, Amesse LS, Gruber JS, Horowitz GM, Cha GM, Hurteau JA (2003) Visualization of the epigastric vessels and bladder before laparoscopic trocar placement. Fertil Steril 80(1):209–212
44. Halpern NB (1998) Laparoscopic cholecystectomy in pregnancy: a review of published experiences and clinical considerations. Semin Laparosc Surg 5(2):129–134
45. Levy BS (1997) Perforation of large vascular structures. Complications of Laparoscopy and Hysteroscopy: 2nd ed Oxford: Blackwell Science 26–9
46. Society of American Gastrointestinal and Endoscopic Surgeons (SAGES) (2007) Guidelines for Diagnosis, Treatment, and Use of Laparoscopy for Surgical Problems during Pregnancy. Practice/ Clinical Guidelines
47. Diamond MP, Corfman RS, DeCherney AH (1997) Insufflation of the obese patient. Complications of laparoscopy and hysteroscopy, 2nd edn. Blackwell Science, Oxford, pp 22–25

13

A multidisciplinary evidence-based guideline for minimally invasive surgery: Part 2 - laparoscopic port instruments, trocar site closure, and electrosurgical techniques

Claire F. la Chapelle · Willem A. Bemelman · Marlies Y. Bongers · Teus A. van Barneveld · Frank Willem Jansen · on behalf of the Dutch multidisciplinary guideline development group Minimally Invasive Surgery

Abstract Minimally invasive surgery (MIS) is practiced by different surgical disciplines applying similar basic techniques. In 2007, the Dutch Health Care inspectorate indicated the need for a guideline including multidisciplinary agreements for MIS aiming towards better patient care and safety. A multidisciplinary guideline development group was founded consisting of general surgeons, gynecologists, an anesthesiologist, and an urologist. All members were authorized by their scientific professional associations. Clinically important aspects were identified and discussed. The best available evidence on these aspects was gathered by systematic review. Recommendations for clinical practice were formulated based on the evidence and a consensus of expert opinion. The guideline was externally reviewed by members of the participating scientific associations and their feedback was integrated. Identified important topics were: laparoscopic entry techniques, intra-abdominal pressure, laparoscopic port instruments, electrosurgical techniques, prevention of trocar site herniation, patient positioning, anesthesiology, perioperative care, patient information, multidisciplinary user consultation, and complication registration. The text of each topic contains an introduction with an explanation of the problem and a summary of the current literature. The current available evidence on safety aspects in minimally invasive surgery is limited. Few conclusions could be deduced from evidence-based data. This underscores the need for larger studies with adequate design and methodology to define conclusions of importance. Above all, the development of this multidisciplinary guideline facilitated a rich discussion, which resulted in a very complete and implementable guideline. This is the second of three papers on the multidisciplinary guideline for minimally invasive surgery, in which we present our literature reviews, conclusions, and practical recommendations for the use of specific port instruments, port site closure, and electrosurgical and ultrasonic techniques.

Keywords Multidisciplinary guideline · Minimally invasive surgery · Laparoscopic ports · Trocars · Port-related complications · Electrosurgical techniques

C. F. la Chapelle (✉) · F. W. Jansen
Department of Gynecology, Leiden University Medical Center, K6 room 76, P.O. Box 9600, 2300 RC Leiden, the Netherlands
e-mail: c.f.la_chapelle@lumc.nl

W. A. Bemelman
Department of Surgery, Academic Medical Center, Amsterdam, the Netherlands

M. Y. Bongers
Department of Gynecology, Maxima Medical Center, Veldhoven, the Netherlands

T. A. van Barneveld
Department of Quality in Healthcare, Dutch Association of Medical Specialists, Utrecht, the Netherlands

Introduction and methods

Since the early 1990s, minimally invasive surgery (MIS) or laparoscopic surgery has been used extensively to diagnose and treat a variety of conditions. The advancing technology and methods of laparoscopic surgery offer increasing surgical possibilities. Laparoscopic surgery is practiced in different surgical disciplines, general surgery, gynecology, and urology, using relatively similar basic techniques. Despite these similarities, there is little cooperation between the different disciplines to assure and improve the quality of minimally invasive surgery. A number of monodisciplinary gynecological guidelines on laparoscopic entry techniques do exist, a well-known one is the guideline from the Royal College of Obstetricians and Gynaecologists [1]. Though, transcending the boundaries of monodisciplinary knowledge and skills and criticizing the differences between disciplines should result in multidisciplinary agreements to optimize patient safety. The Dutch Health Care Inspectorate encouraged the national scientific associations representing laparoscopically oriented surgeons to work together and develop a multidisciplinary guideline on MIS.

In our previous paper, we described the Evidence-Based Guideline Development (EBGD) methodology [2]. In short, the EBGD process includes the following steps: (1) problem analysis; (2) explicit formulation of the questions that the guideline is addressing (key questions); (3) defining eligibility criteria for evidence to be considered; (4) conducting a comprehensive search for evidence (search strategies are appended, see Appendix); (5) evaluating study quality; (6) summarizing the evidence and drawing scientific conclusions; (7) balancing the benefits and downsides of the alternative management strategies, discussing values and preferences (other considerations); (8) formulating recommendations based on evidence and consensus clinical opinion; (9) discussion about the draft guideline within working group; (10) setting up a final draft guideline; (11) external review by members of the participating scientific associations; (12) revision and finalization of the guideline; and finally, (13) authorization and (14) dissemination of the multidisciplinary guideline by the participating scientific professional associations.

In our first paper, we focused on primary entry techniques and the application of a pneumoperitoneum in laparoscopic surgery. The first technical step in laparoscopy is the primary entry: the introduction of a primary instrument (Veress needle or primary trocar) in the abdominal cavity, followed by the insufflation of carbon dioxide to create a pneumoperitoneum.

When the pneumoperitoneum is achieved, specific laparoscopic port instruments are introduced through the abdominal wall. Port instruments consist of several components: a central trocar, a corresponding peripheral cannula, a valve section, and a CO_2 stopcock. After insertion of this instrument, the central trocar is removed and the remaining cannula functions as an access port for laparoscopic instruments. The primary port, generally created in or near the umbilicus, is used for the introduction of the laparoscope. The creation of the primary laparoscopic port is called "primary entry." Secondary or ancillary ports are intended for the introduction of other laparoscopic instruments. The creation of secondary ports is called "secondary entry." The method of port creation, the port instruments' design, and the port location influence the risk of port-related complications.

Laparoscopic port instruments include a myriad of device designs, including over 100 brands from more than 20 manufacturers [3, 4]. Differences in diameter, shape, and material can result in an increased risk of laparoscopic port-related complications. An important postoperative port-related complication is port site herniation (PSH), a protrusion of intestine or omentum through a remaining defect at the laparoscopic port site. It is questionable whether closing the defect by suturing can prevent these herniations. In the initial problem analysis for this guideline, differences in the use of port instruments and port site closure were identified as important topics within laparoscopic surgery as well as electrosurgical and ultrasonic modalities. These modalities are very useful for coagulation and hemostasis in laparoscopic surgery but have been associated with serious complications. In this second paper on the multidisciplinary guideline on MIS, we discuss the evidence and consensus clinical opinion for the use of specific port instruments, port site closure, and electrosurgical and ultrasonic techniques.

Laparoscopic port instruments

Background

Laparoscopic port instruments are the most common device named in malpractice injury claims associated with laparoscopic procedures, representing one third of all claims [5]. The incidence is estimated to be 4.24 per 1,000 procedures [3]. Typical port-related complications are intra-abdominal vascular injury, visceral injury, port site bleeding, port site herniation, port site infection, and pain. In the last few decades, there has been continuous innovation of the instrument design aimed at reducing these complications.

Distinguishing primary from secondary port entry and different entry techniques

A distinction between primary and secondary entry needs to be made. Within the primary entry technique, it has to be taken into account whether the open/Hasson-, closed/Veress needle-, or non-insufflated/direct entry technique has been used. Less frequently used instruments for the primary entry are visual port systems and single port techniques. These different conditions may result in different outcomes. The type of primary port instrument depends on the applied primary entry technique where the type of secondary port instrument generally does not. In the Veress needle entry technique or the direct insertion technique, the insertion of the primary port instrument is a blind procedure while secondary port instruments are mandatorily inserted under direct laparoscopic vision.

Laparoscopic port instruments

A distinction can be made between reusable and disposable port instruments. Reusable instruments are composed of metal. The perforator tip can be completely blunt (cone shaped) or sharp with a conical, pyramidal, triflanged, or eccentric tip. Disposable instruments are usually made of plastic with bladed or bladeless tips. Shielded disposable port instruments are equipped with a retractable covering over the tip and were developed to protect against intra-abdominal vascular and visceral injury. These formerly called "safety trocars" are however also associated with major port-related complications [6]. The FDA does not allow anymore that the shielded port instruments are called safety trocars.

Radially expanding access (REA) systems represent yet another alternative in design. These port instruments are equipped with a radially expanding sleeve that can be dilated from 5 to 12 mm in diameter. The REA instrument is developed to minimize tissue trauma and, in theory, its use could result in fewer vascular injuries. The optical-access instruments are designed to decrease the risk of injury to the intra-abdominal structures by allowing the surgeon to visualize abdominal wall layers during placement [7]. A visual system that should be distinguished is the threaded visual cannula (TVC). The TVC enables body cavity access by applying a blunt cannula where a pointed or sharp central trocar is not required, linear penetration force is realigned to radial, and the cannula houses the laparoscope without an intervening pointed crystal that distorts visual layer enunciation [8]. The diameters of port instruments vary from 2 to 12 mm, depending upon the largest instrument needed for a particular port. For exceptional indications (for example extirpation of large cysts), larger or modified trocars are available [4].

Despite continuous innovation in the design of port instruments to enhance patient safety, port-related complications do still occur. The guideline development group indicated a need for advices on the use of specific laparoscopic port instruments to ensure patient safety.

Key question

1. What specific port instrument can be recommended to minimize the risks of port-related complications?

Summary of the literature

Major port-related complications

Major complications are mortality, visceral injury (such as perforation of the intestines or stomach, or injury of the bladder or liver), vascular injury (such as perforation of the aorta, vena cava, iliac artery, or iliac vein), and other injuries that required intensive care (IC) or intensive care unit (ICU) management or a subsequent surgical, endoscopic, or radiological intervention. In the recently updated Cochrane review from Ahmad et al., different laparoscopic port instruments were studied [9]. Eight RCTs were included comparing different port instrument designs. In four, REA instruments were compared with standard port instruments for primary port entry [10–13]. Two RCTs compared cutting and blunt port instruments for primary and secondary port entry [14, 15], and in two RCTs, the REA instrument was compared to a conventional instrument with cutting tip for secondary port entry [16, 17]. Trials that analyzed major complications with low incidences had too small sample sizes to identify any differences [10, 12, 15–17]. Meta-analyses demonstrated no significant differences for major complications (Table 1). Comparative prospective and retrospective studies on different laparoscopic port instruments did not evaluate major complications [18] or were underpowered [19].

Minor port-related complications

Minor port-related complications are port site herniation, port site bleeding or postoperative wound hematoma, port site infection, extraperitoneal insufflation and other injuries that did not require IC or ICU management or a subsequent surgical, and endoscopic or radiological intervention under general anesthesiology. In the meta-analyses of the Cochrane review, some differences were found for minor port-related complications. REA instruments compared to standard port instruments for primary entry were associated with a reduction of port site bleeding [OR 0.31 (95 % CI 0.15–0.62), three studies, 421 participants]. Comparing instruments with a cutting versus a blunt tip for primary port entry, no difference in port site bleeding [OR 0.33 (95 % CI 0.09–1.23), two studies, 195 participants] or wound infection [OR 7.76 (95 % CI 0.15–386.69), one study, 165 participants] was found. For secondary entry, radially expanding instruments were associated with lower rates of port site bleeding compared to conventional instruments with a cutting tip [OR 0.12 (95 %CI 0.02–0.92) one study, 68 participants]. No difference was found for port site infections after the use of REA instruments versus conventional instruments for secondary entry [OR 0.14 (95 % CI 0.01–2.21), one study, 61 participants].

A prospective cohort study comparing REA instruments to conventional sharp-shielded pyramidal instruments for secondary entry was probably underpowered to identify a difference in port site bleeding [OR 0.18 (95 % CI 0.01–4.00), 19 participants; 19]. A retrospective cohort study compared reusable steel cone-shaped non-cutting instruments to a historical group where disposable sharp cutting shielded instruments were used (n=600) for secondary entry [18]. A reduced risk was found for port site herniation [OR 0.09 (95 % CI 0.01–0.69)] and for port site bleeding [OR 0.27 (95 % CI 0.07–0.97)] when non-cutting instruments were used.

Port-related pain

No systematic reviews on pain related to laparoscopic port instruments were found. A total of seven RCTs evaluated

Table 1 Results from meta-analyses in Ahmad et al. for major port-related complications comparing different port instruments [9]

Radially expanding instruments versus standard instruments for primary port entry	
Vascular injury	OR 0.24 (95 % CI 0.05–1.21)
Visceral injury	OR 0.13 (95 % CI 0.00–6.37)
Solid organ injury	OR 1.05 (95 % CI 0.07–16.91)
Cutting instruments and blunt instruments for primary and secondary port entry	
Visceral injury	OR 7.67 (95 % CI 0.15–386.69)

OR odds ratio, 95 % CI 95 % confidence interval

postoperative pain after the use of REA instruments to standard port instruments for primary and/or secondary port entry. For primary and secondary ports, two RCTs found no differences (n=77 and n=56) [11, 15] and one was in favor of REA instruments (n=87) [12]. For primary ports specifically, one RCT found no difference (n=244) [10] whereas another RCT indicated less postoperative pain up to 12 h postoperative in patients where REA instruments were used (n=100) [13]. For secondary ports specifically, two RCTs reported less postoperative pain when REA instruments versus conventional instruments were used (n=68 and n=54) [16, 17]. Two RCTs found no differences for postoperative pain when blunt or cutting instruments were used [15, 20]. A prospective cohort study from Turner et al. (n=19) found less pain at secondary ports where REA instruments were used compared to conventionally cutting instruments [19].

There is substantial clinical and statistical heterogeneity between these trials. Within the studies, factors that could have influenced the results in these studies are fascial closure, manipulation at the port site, and postoperative analgesics. In most of the studies on pain regarding the use of different laparoscopic port instruments, no intention was made to identify any confounders neither to correct for confounders in the analysis.

Conclusions

Level 1	There is no evidence to suggest that any type of laparoscopic port instrument is more or less safe in terms of reducing severe complications either during primary or secondary entry. *Evidence level A1* [9]
Level 1	The use of radially expanding access instruments compared to standard (cutting) port instruments for primary and secondary port entry leads to fewer port site bleedings. *Evidence level A1* [9]
Level 3	The use of blunt port instruments compared to cutting port instruments for secondary port entry possibly leads to fewer port site bleedings and port site herniations. *Evidence level C* [18]
Level 1	REA instruments compared to conventional port instruments result in a decrease in postoperative pain. This reduction was not consistently found for primary entry. *Evidence level A1* [10–13, 16, 17, 19]
Level 2	It remains unclear whether the use of cutting or blunt port instruments has different postoperative pain scores. *Evidence level A2* [15, 20]

Considerations

In the preceding text, we described the best available data on different laparoscopic port instruments and specific port-related risks. The studies available to analyze are of very small numbers and basically no definite conclusions of importance can be deduced from their data. The expert's opinion in gynecology is that laparoscopic surgeons may continue to use their chosen technique for port creation [21].

Noticeably, the majority of trials compared REA instruments to conventionally cutting port instruments, even though they are not widely used in practice. A simple explanation could be encouragement by the pharmaceutical industry, though only two studies report that the REA instruments were supplied free of charge by the industry [15, 16]. REA instruments appear to have advantages in terms of less port site bleedings and postoperative pain. Reasons for their rare application probably are the higher cost price and a more complicated insertion technique of REA instruments compared to conventional instruments [15]. No appropriate cost–benefit analysis for REA instruments is available; therefore, one should be careful with the wide implementation of these systems.

Laparoscopic port instruments are either intended for single use (disposable instruments) or multiple uses (reusable instruments). Environmental concerns and spiraling health care costs generally encourage reusable instruments [22]. A disadvantage of reusable instrument is that their adequate function could diminish through repetitive use and sterilization. For example, reusable sharp instruments lose their sharpness through repetitive insertion; consequently, a relatively high puncture force for penetration through the abdominal wall is required, which could result in an abrupt and uncontrolled introduction of the laparoscopic port instrument leading to serious visceral and vascular injury [23]. No clinical trials comparing disposable to reusable laparoscopic port instruments were found. Multiple use of disposable port instruments is not recommended [24].

Another practical consideration that should not be overlooked is the use of port instruments with a smaller diameter (e.g., with 5 mm diameter compared to 10 mm) resulting in less postoperative pain and shorter convalescence [25].

A study revealed that blunt-tipped conical port instruments have a significantly greater fixity to the abdominal wall compared to cutting port instruments, resulting in significantly lower numbers of spontaneous port dislodgement during surgery [14]. Accordingly, the use of blunt-tipped instruments could reduce antecedent gas leak and loss of pneumoperitoneum and the need for port replacement with its associated increase in risk of trauma to the abdominal wall. On the other side, it appeared from animal studies that the entry force needed to perforate the abdominal wall is higher for conical blunt-tipped than pyramidal sharp port instruments [26]. The higher entry force could increase the risk of injuries to the intra- or retroperitoneal organs during insertion. The use of optical-access port instruments does not avoid serious injury despite having the ability to visualize tissue layers during insertion [7]. The TVC is a different system of which some experts consider it could be a less damaging approach [8]. We found insufficient evidence to formulate clear recommendations for safe and cost-effective use of laparoscopic port instruments. Larger comparative studies, with good methodological quality, are needed to clarify the important safety issues. The guideline development group supposes that the selection of a port instrument should, above all, be based on weighing the advantages against disadvantages of its characteristics and the experience of the surgeon with a safe application.

Recommendations

- The selection of a laparoscopic port instrument should be based on the benefits of its characteristics to the individual patient and the experience of the surgeon in a safe application of the particular instrument.
- The use of blunt-tipped instruments is preferred for laparoscopic ports with a 10–12 mm diameter.
- Whenever possible, it is recommended to use port instruments with small diameters.

Port site closure

Background

The introduction of a port instrument through the abdominal wall creates a fascial defect. The estimated prevalence of PSH is 0.5 % [27]. Closure of the fascial defect could reduce the risk of port site herniation. In clinical practice, there is a wide variety of suturing methods. No consensus exists regarding the closure of the fascial defect according to the port instrument diameter. Also, risk factors for PSH should be defined. Below, the available evidence on fascial closure of port sites is discussed.

Key questions

1. Does fascial closure of port sites prevent or reduce the risk of port site herniation?
2. What is the minimal port site diameter whereby fascial closure should be advised?
3. What fascial closure technique can be recommended?

Summary of the literature

No RCTs or prospective observational studies were found that investigated fascial closure as a measure to prevent PSH. In two retrospective cohort studies, the PSH prevalence among patients with or without fascial closure was compared [28, 29]. Mayol et al. observed that PSH in 10 mm umbilical ports occurred among patients with (3.3 %, n=151) or without (1.9 %, n=52) fascial closure [OR 1·8 (95 % CI 0·2 to 15)]. Kadar et al. neither identified a difference in prevalence of PSH in 12 mm extraumbilical ports when the fascia was closed or left open [8.0 %, n=25 versus 2.2 % n=136, OR 3.9 (95 % CI 0·6 to 24)]. The study does show that PSH could not completely be prevented by fascial closure: three hernias were found in 136 patients. Both studies were underpowered to detect statistically significant differences.

We then performed a search to identify the port site diameter from which the risk of herniation becomes significant. The majority of reported cases on PSH occurred at ≥10 mm ports [30, 31]; however, these studies did not compare this with the prevalence of PSH in ports with different diameters. Only one retrospective cohort study shows a relationship between port instrument size and PSH [28]. The prevalence of PSH was higher when instruments with a diameter of 12 mm compared to 10 mm were used [OR 13.7 (95 % CI 1.6–118.3)]. For 5 mm instruments compared to 10 mm trocars, no differences were found.

Closure technique

The standard closure technique for the fascia at the port site is a hand-sutured figure-of-eight. A variety of other methods have been described [32]. We found two comparative studies wherein different port closure techniques were compared with the standard technique [33, 34]. No PSHs were observed as the studies were underpowered to analyze for differences in prevalence of PSH.

More recently, cases of intrafascial incisional hernia were found in patients where 12 mm bladeless radially dilating instruments (without fascial closure) had been used [35]. In this type of hernia, also called partial wall hernia, bowel herniates through a defect in the transversal and internal oblique fasciae, but the external oblique fascia is intact. These patients present with symptoms of bowel obstruction but lack the typical signs of herniation during physical examination. This could be an argument for full-thickness closure of the port site, including all abdominal layers [27].

Conclusions

Level 3	It is unclear whether fascial closure of port sites reduces the risk of PSH. *Evidence level B* [28, 29]
Level 3	The prevalence of PSH is significantly increased in port sites where instruments with a diameter of 12 mm are used compared to sites where instruments with a diameter of 10 mm are used. *Evidence level B* [28, 29]
Level 4	It is unclear which fascial closure technique results in the least PSHs. *Evidence level D (opinion of guideline development group)*
Level 4	Full-thickness closure of port sites could reduce the risk of intrafascial herniation. *Evidence level D (opinion of the guideline development group)*

Considerations

From data obtained from current literature, it is generally recommended to close fascial defects ≥10 mm to reduce the risk of PSH [28, 31]. However, current information is inadequate and no evidence confirms that fascial closure reduces PSH. On the other hand, the risk of nerve injury, superficial vascular injury, and inadvertent injury of the bowel should be taken into account. Some suggested that risk factors for PSH are preexisting umbilical hernia [36] or a history of port site hernia, history of postoperative wound infection, poor wound healing (e.g., diabetes mellitus, wound infection, chemotherapy, steroid use, or poor nutrition), ascites, obesity, cachexia, asthma, connective tissue disorders, and manipulation of the port (e.g., to retrieve specimens) [31]. The extent in which these factors may pose a risk has been insufficiently researched.

In daily laparoscopic practice, some variety exists in the cutoff point of the port site diameter which should be closed; however, the fascia at port sites >10 mm are generally closed in all laparoscopic disciplines. In the literature, it appears that the risk of PSH is significantly increased in port site diameters ≥12 mm and it is supposed that fascial closure reduces the risk. The working group aligned their recommendation with current practice and recommends to close the fascia of port sites >10 mm diameter. The closure of smaller port site diameters should be considered, specifically when assumed risk factors are present.

As previously noted, the use of blunt trocars compared to cutting trocars for secondary port entry possibly leads to fewer TSHs. This is explained through the stretching and separating of tissues by blunt trocars rather than cutting through tissue layers by cutting trocars. This could be a reason for not closing a fascial defect with a diameter ≤12 mm, where a blunt trocar has been used.

It should be noted that single port surgery and robot-assisted surgery are not included in this guideline. It should be anticipated that in those techniques, a different port creation method is applied, probably increasing the occurrence of port site herniation and other port-related complications.

Recommendations

- Fascial closure is recommended for port sites with a diameter >10 mm. It could also be considered to close fascial defects of smaller ports, especially when assumed risk factors are present.
- When blunt port instruments of ≤12 mm diameter are applied, it is an option not to close the fascial defect.
- There are no recommendations for a specific fascial closure technique. Full-thickness closure of the port site could be considered, since it possibly reduces the risk of PSH.

Electrosurgical and ultrasonic energy techniques

Background

Electrosurgical and ultrasonic energy techniques have become indispensable in minimally invasive procedures. These techniques are used for coagulation, cutting, and hemostasis. The traditional modalities are monopolar and bipolar electrosurgery. Bipolar vessel sealing systems and ultrasonic technologies further improved the efficiency of operations and facilitated the surgical abilities to perform certain procedures. However, each of these energy sources can be associated with distressing complications. Compared to open surgery, a hazard in laparoscopic procedures is the visual field: the electrical current may damage adjacent structures outside the view of the laparoscope. Laparoscopic surgery presents additional hazards for electrosurgery, the primary ones being direct application, insulation failure, and direct- and capacitive coupling. Both electrosurgical instruments and ultrasonic instruments generate heat with the risk of thermal injury. It is important for users to have knowledge of the principles, applications, and safety aspects of the energy sources used in laparoscopy. We reviewed the literature concerning hazards of electrosurgical and ultrasonic energy sources in laparoscopy. Here we describe the specific complications and offer guidance to minimize the risks.

Monopolar electrosurgery

Monopolar electrosurgery is used for cutting, coagulation, and hemostasis. With monopolar electrosurgery, the active electrode is located at the surgical site while the return electrode (a dispersive pad) is attached elsewhere to the patient's body. The current flows from the active electrode, into the target tissue, through the patient, the dispersive pad, and subsequently returns to the generator. With the dispersive pad properly placed, the electrosurgical effects occur at the active electrode.

General surgeons rely more on monopolar than on bipolar electrosurgery because of its ease of use [37]. Monopolar electrosurgery provides a better penetration of the current density, which can be advantageous for hemostasis in certain tissues. A "blended cut" (blend of surgical effects) can be applied with a combined modus of cutting and coagulation. Additional capabilities are enhanced cutting, rapid dissection, and non-contact fulguration. With fulguration, a high-voltage electric current is used to destroy tissue; this may be useful to control diffuse bleedings.

Bipolar electrosurgery

With bipolar electrosurgery, both active and return electrodes are located close together within the tip of the surgical instrument. The current flows from one tip to the other; only the tissue between the two electrodes is exposed to the electric current. Tissue thermal energy can be localized more precisely and is effective at a lower voltage and power. This enables electrosurgical safety. Bipolar instruments cannot be used effectively for pure cutting, and for coagulating, the tissue should be gripped between the two electrodes. Because of lower power settings, bipolar coagulation of large areas and dense tissues requires more time. In addition, spray coagulation (fulguration) is not possible.

Vessel sealing

Vessel sealing technology is a type of bipolar electrosurgery developed to coagulate blood vessels from a diameter of 2–3 mm and with minimized collateral tissue damage. An electrothermal bipolar vessel sealer (EBVS) combines an advanced electrical current with mechanical pressure, in order to fuse the vessel walls and create a seal. The EBVS allows the secure sealing of vessels with a diameter of up to 7 mm [38, 39]. The seals obtained with EBVS have proven to be stronger compared to those obtained with traditional bipolar and ultrasonic technology [40, 41]. The available instruments have a diameter of either 5 or 10 mm [40]. EBVS rely on a computer-controlled tissue feedback system that senses tissue impedance or resistance and adjusts the current and output voltage: a consistent electrosurgical effect is obtained through all tissue types.

Ultrasonic technology

With ultrasonic technology, electrical energy is converted into vibration and heat. The combination of a vibrating blade together with the produced heat forms the mechanism by which the instrument cuts and coagulates tissue. The heat generated by ultrasonic instruments is typically less compared to mono- and bipolar electrosurgery, resulting in less thermal injury to surrounding tissues. This optimizes the histopathology assessment of surgical margins. An ultrasonic instrument ensues less smoke emission and probably less toxin production since tissue destruction is by vaporization and avoid charring [42]. As no electrical current is applied, there is no risk of direct coupling or capacitive coupling injuries. There are some disadvantages of ultrasonic technology: the formation of steam from tissues being treated can interfere with visualization through a laparoscope. After prolonged use, the vibrating blade may remain hot for a long period and create a risk of inadvertent thermal injury.

The ultrasonic technology enables the coagulation and sealing of blood vessels from 2 to 5 mm in diameter [43]. It has been shown that this modality can be used safely and effectively in different laparoscopic procedures such as myomectomy, hysterectomy, cholecystectomy, and colorectal laparoscopic surgery [43–46].

Key questions

1. What are the potential complications related to electrosurgery and what is the incidence of recognized injuries?
2. What measures can be taken to reduce the risk of electrosurgery-related complications?

Summary of the literature

Electrosurgery-related complications

Although electrosurgery-related complications are widely described, no systematic reviews, prospective or retrospective cohort studies, or case–control studies were identified that collected data on the incidence of electrosurgery-related complications in laparoscopy. Several studies retrospectively analyzed data on laparoscopic electrosurgery-related complications limited to specific procedures [47–49]. Consequently, a reliable incidence rate of electrosurgery-related complications is missing. The estimated incidence is 2 to 5 per 1,000 procedures [50]. One of the most serious complications is bowel perforation caused by an electrosurgical burn, frequently unrecognized at the time of occurrence. Symptoms of peritonitis are usually seen 4 to 10 days later and often lead to long-term complications.

Several RCTs comparing different electrosurgical and ultrasonic techniques were identified [41, 43, 45, 51–53]. There is considerable heterogeneity in the investigated surgical procedures between studies. In the majority of the trials, no difference in electrosurgery- and ultrasonic-related complications was found. However, the studies were generally underpowered to identify differences in complications. The use of distinct electrosurgical and ultrasonic instruments depends on the suitability of the instruments characteristics in the type of surgical procedure. Therefore, the following text is a delineated description of the electrosurgical mechanisms that may lead to complications and how to avoid potentially dangerous situations.

Hazards in monopolar electrosurgery

With monopolar electrosurgery, the patient forms a major part of the electrical circuit. This causes additional risks: stray currents, insulation failure, direct coupling, and capacitive coupling.

Stray currents through insulation failure

Insulation failure occurs when the insulation covering of the shaft of the active electrode is damaged. This allows the current to flow through alternative pathways and non-target-tissue. Breakdown of insulation can be caused by the use of high-voltage currents, repeated use, frequent re-sterilization, inappropriate use, or mechanical damage of instrumentation. The small and undetectable defects in the insulation are more dangerous, because this creates a higher current density.

Open circuit and detachment of the dispersive pad

hen the electrosurgical unit is activated without the active electrode in contact with the tissue (i.e., open circuit activation), a high-voltage level emerges at the active instrument. This may cause stray currents. Poor quality of contact between the dispersive pad and the patient's skin compromises a safe return of the current to the generator. The dispersive pad must be of low resistance with a large enough surface (>20 cm^2). When the dispersive pad is (partially) detached through bony prominences, adipose, excessive hair, scar tissue, presence of fluid or lotions, or dryness of the pad, the current exiting the body can have a high density. This may produce heat and unintended burns at the site of the dispersive pad. The use of a return electrode monitoring system averts these burns. This system inactivates the electrosurgical unit if the resistance between the patient's body and the dispersive pad is too high.

Direct coupling and capacitive coupling

Direct coupling occurs when the electrosurgical unit is accidentally activated while the active electrode is in close proximity to another secondary non-insulated instrument (e.g., a metal laparoscope). Electrical current flows from the active electrode to the secondary instrument and potentially damages adjacent structures.

Capacitive coupling occurs when current is transmitted from the active electrode through intact insulation and into adjacent materials without direct contact. Activation of the active electrode produces an alternating current inducing an electrostatic field between two "conductors" (conductive elements). When the net charge exceeds the insulator's capacity, the current is transferred from one conductor to the other. Hybrid cannulas are prone to induce capacitive coupling, since the plastic parts prevent the current dissipating from the metal part into the abdominal wall. This can result in electrical current passing through nearby structures. Longer instruments, thinner insulation, higher voltages, and narrow trocars increase the risk of injury [43, 50, 54].

Interference with (cardiac) implantable electronic device and prosthetics

Implantable devices that use electric current may be affected by the use of electrosurgery. In monopolar surgery, interaction of the current with a cardiac implantable electronic device (CIED) may have life-threatening consequences. Adverse effects include damage to the device, inability to deliver pacing or shocks, lead tissue interface damage, and electrical reset. The preoperative management of the CIED function should be guided by the cardiologist or anesthesiologist [42]. The risk of interference is low in procedures where the path between the active electrode and dispersive pad does not cross the CIED or its leads. There may be some diffusion of current and it is therefore safer to use bipolar electrosurgery or ultrasonic technology in patients with implantable electronic devices [55, 56]. Conductive prosthetics should as well be placed out of the direct path of the circuit since activation of the electrosurgical unit may cause heating of the prosthetic material.

Thermal injuries in electrosurgery and ultrasonic technology

Prolonged activation of both mono- and bipolar electrosurgical instruments as well ultrasonic instruments generate heat (up to 80–100 °C). The instrument can remain hot for some time after activation with the risk of thermal injury when it unintentionally touches surrounding tissue.

Conclusions

Level 4	Bowel perforation, biliary- and urinary tract injuries are among the most serious electrosurgical injuries. *Evidence level D (opinion of guideline development group)*
Level 2	There is insufficient evidence to define the differences in electrosurgery-versus ultrasonic-related complications. *Evidence level A2* [41, 44, 45, 51–53]

Level 4 Exact incidence rates of electrosurgery-related complications are unknown. The estimated incidence is 2 to 5 per 1,000 procedures.
Evidence level D (opinion of guideline development group)

Level 3 Additional risks of monopolar electrosurgery, compared to bipolar electrosurgery and ultrasonic technology, include: stray currents, insulation failure, direct coupling, and capacitive coupling.
Evidence level C [37, 43, 50, 54]

Level 4 Based on electrophysiology, the following factors increase the risk of electrosurgical injuries:
- The use of high-power and high-voltage settings
- Inadequate placement of the dispersive pad
- Hybrid cannulas
- The intermingling use of plastic and metal cannulas
- Long instruments and narrow cannulas
- Insulation failure
- Char of coagulated tissue on the instrument
- Prolonged activation of an electrosurgical instrument
- Activation of an electrosurgical instrument in an open circuit

Evidence level C [37, 42]

Level 4 When using electrosurgery, cardiac implantable electronic devices and conductive prosthetics are additional hazards.
Evidence level D [55, 56]

Considerations

The current available evidence on electrosurgical and ultrasonic energy techniques is inadequate to formulate definite evidence-based conclusions. Therefore, larger scale studies are needed. With the current information available, a safe application of these techniques can be achieved by adequate education of the surgical team and supporting staff. The team should be aware of the physics and hazards associated to the use of different energy sources used in MIS. Another obstacle in safety is that biomechanical engineers involved in the purchase of minimally invasive instruments are not routinely involved in the maintenance. Reusable trocars and instruments are often used until defects appear; this might represent a danger to the patient. Participation of biomechanical engineers in maintaining and testing instruments in use could possibly prevent those dangers. Instead of reusable instruments, disposable instruments could be used to prevent insulation failure through wear and tear. However, disposable instruments are often more expensive and not immune from insulation failures.

Finally, postoperative vigilance is required when a patient does not easily recover. The surgeon, physicians, and nurses on duty should be highly alert to the early manifestations of peritonitis. The warning signs may be insidious with atypical or mild symptoms such as slight abdominal discomfort, slight temperature increase, and inability to void. Symptoms of bowel perforation following electrothermal injury are usually seen 4 to 10 days after surgery, leading to a delay in diagnosis and treatment, with sometimes fatal consequences [54]. Laboratory results are often normal with a slight leukocytosis. Expedient evaluation and early intervention is demanded when a patient's recovery is below what should be expected [50].

Recommendations

- When using electrosurgical or ultrasonic techniques, one must have knowledge of electrophysiological functioning and effects.
- To reduce the risk of electrosurgical complications, the following precautions are recommended:
  - When both mono- and bipolar instruments are used, pedals and connections should be checked for accuracy before activating the electrosurgical units.
  - Instrument electrodes should be kept smooth and clean from char, to avoid disruption of current transfer.
  - To prevent capacitive coupling, an isolated position of metal trocars from the abdominal wall should be avoided. Use all-metal or all-plastic cannula systems; the use of metal–plastic hybrids is discouraged.
  - An instrument should be activated only when its electrode is fully visible and in contact with the target tissue. Do not activate in an open circuit.
  - Preferably use brief intermittent activation versus prolonged activation.
  - Use the lowest possible power setting and low-voltage waveform for the desired effect.
- Prior to each MIS procedure, monopolar instruments should be tested for insulation failure with a porosity detector at the central sterilization department.
- With monopolar electrosurgery, the dispersive pad should be applied to well-perfused, dry skin over a large muscle away from bony prominences and conductive prostheses. When disinfecting the skin, be cautious that there are no fluid leaks under the dispersive pad.
- In patients with conductive prosthesis, it is strongly recommended to place the prosthesis out of the direct path of the electrical circuit.
- For procedures in patients with a CIED, the use of bipolar over monopolar electrosurgery is preferred.
- Alertness for electrothermal injury is needed when a patient presents with mild symptoms such as slight abdominal discomfort or slight temperature increase.

Acknowledgments The authors would like to thank all members of the guideline development group Minimally Invasive Surgery for their critical contributions to the original guideline and this article. The Dutch Ministry of Health together with the Dutch Association of Medical Specialists supported the development of this guideline. We also thank Peggy de Vos van Steenwijk for the English correction of the manuscript.

Conflict of interest The authors report no conflicts of interest. The authors alone are responsible for the content and writing of the paper.

Appendix

Table 2 Literature searches

Subject	Data base	Search terms
Laparoscopic port instruments	Medline (OVID) 1950–March 2012	1. *Laparoscopy/
		2. (trocar* or troicar* or trocard*).ti.
		3. ((secondary adj trocar*) or (classical adj trocar*) or cannula or (disposable adj3 trocar*) or (radially adj expanding adj trocar*) or (STEP adj trocar*) or (visual adj entry) or systems or (conical adj trocar) or (pyramidal adj trocar*) or (reusable adj trocars*) or (disposable adj trocar*) or (single adj2 trocars) or optiview or endotip or visiport or (bladeless adj trocar*) or (sharp adj trocar*) or (trocar adj valve*)).ab,ti.
		4. 2 or 3
		5. *Surgical Instruments/
		6. "Equipment Design"/
		7. exp Gynecologic Surgical Procedures/is [Instrumentation]
		8. Laparoscopy/mt [Methods]
		9. or/5-9
		10. 1 and 4 and 9
		11. systematic reviews (filter)
		12. randomized controlled trials (filter)
		13. exp longitudinal studies/
	Embase (Elsevier) 1974–March 2012	14. 10 and 13 (trocar* OR troicar* OR trocard* OR 'secondary trocar' OR 'classical trocar' OR 'radially expanding trocar' OR 'step trocar' OR 'visual entry system' OR 'conical trocar' OR 'pyramidal trocar' OR 'reusable trocar' OR 'disposable trocar' OR 'single trocar' OR optiview OR endotip OR visiport OR 'bladeless trocar' OR 'sharp trocar' OR 'trocar valvë' OR 'secondary trocars' OR 'classical trocars' OR 'cannula'/exp OR 'radially expanding trocars' OR 'step trocars' OR 'visual entry systems' OR 'conical trocars' OR 'pyramidal trocars' OR 'reusable trocars' OR 'disposable trocars' OR 'single trocars' OR 'bladeless trocars' OR 'sharp trocars' OR 'trocar valves') AND 'surgical instrument'/exp/mj NOT [animals]/lim) AND ([dutch]/lim OR [english]/lim AND [embase]/lim
Port site closure	Medline (OVID) 1950–Nov 2009	1. exp *Laparoscopy/
		2. "laparascop*".m_titl.
		3. "minimal invasive*".m_titl.
		4. 1 or 2 or 3
		5. Surgical Wound Dehiscence/ Obesity/"obes*".m_titl./ Body Mass Index
		6. deep sheath closure*.mp. or Surgical Wound Infection/
		7. port closure*.mp.
		8. port site hernia*.mp.
		9. port infection*.mp.
		10. hernia/ or hernia, abdominal/
		11. herniation.mp.
		12. fascia defects.mp. or Hernia, Ventral/
		13. or/5-15
		14. exp *Sutures/
		15. exp *Suture Techniques/
		16. "suture*".m_titl.
		17. 17-19
		18. 4 and 16 and 20
		19. 9 or 10 or 11 or 12 or 14 or 15
		20. *Laparoscopy/ae [Adverse Effects]
		21. 22 and 23
		22. 21 or 24
		23. "ventral hernia repair*".m_titl.
		24. 25 not 26
		25. Roux-en-Y Gastric Bypass.m_titl.

Table 2 (continued)

Subject	Data base	Search terms
		26. (suture* or closure* or port*).m_titl.
		27. 27 and 29
		28. 30 not 28
	Embase (Elsevier) 1974–Nov 2009	(laparoscop*:ti OR 'laparoscopy'/exp/mj OR 'minimal invasive':ti AND ('deep sheath closure' OR 'port closure' OR 'port site hernia' OR 'port infection' OR 'herniation'/exp OR 'fascia defect' OR 'deep sheath closures' OR 'port closures' OR 'port site hernias' OR 'port infections' OR herniations OR 'fascia defects' OR 'wound dehiscence'/exp OR 'obesity'/exp OR 'body mass'/exp OR 'surgical infection'/exp OR 'abdominal wall hernia'/exp) AND ('suture'/exp/mj OR 'suture'/exp OR suture*:ti)) NOT ('roux en y' AND gastric AND bypass:ti)
		AND filter randomized controlled trials
Electrosurgical and ultrasonic techniques	Medline (OVID) 1950–Nov 2009	1. Laparoscopy/
		2. Laparoscopy.ti.
		3. 1 or 2
		4. Electrosurgery/
		5. Electrosurgery.ti.
		6. 4 or 5
		10. 3 and 6
		11. limit 10 to (dutch or english)
		12. limit 11 to (clinical trial, all or clinical trial or review or comparative study or consensus development conference or controlled clinical trial or evaluation studies or guideline or meta analysis or multicenter study or practice guideline or randomized controlled trial or research support, nih, extramural or research support, nih, intramural or research support, non us gov't or research support, us gov't, non phs or research support, us gov't, phs or technical report or validation studies)
		13. exp Epidemiologic Studies/
		14. 11 and 13
		15. systematic reviews (filter)
		43. randomized controlled trials (filter)
		68. 12 or 14
		69. 68 not (66 or 67)
	Embase (Elsevier) 1974–Nov 2009	'clinical study'/exp OR 'comparative study'/exp OR 'controlled study'/exp OR 'observational study'/exp AND ('electrosurgery'/exp/mj OR electrosurg*:ti) AND ('laparoscopy'/exp/mj OR laparoscop*:ti) NOT [animals]/lim) AND ([dutch]/lim OR [english]/lim AND [embase]/lim

Medline (OVID) and Embase were searched for relevant literature on the topics trocar use, trocar site closure and electrosurgical and ultrasonic techniques. The search was restricted to articles published in Dutch and English from 1966 to November 2009, with exception to the search for trocar use which we updated in March 2012. Additionally, the reference lists of all included studies and systematic reviews pertinent to this topic were screened. Methodological filters of the Scottish Intercollegiate Guidelines Network (http://www.sign.ac.uk/methodology/filters.html) were used to identify potential systematic reviews and randomized controlled trials

References

1. Sutton GJC (2009) Guideline on preventing entry-related gynaecological laparoscopic injuries: post-publication reflections of the senior author. Gynecol Surg 6:301–310
2. la Chapelle CF, Bemelman WA, Rademaker BMP, van Barneveld TA, Jansen FW (2012) A multidisciplinary evidence-based guideline for minimally invasive surgery. Part 1: entry techniques and the pneumoperitoneum. Gynecol Surg 9:271–282
3. Fuller J, Scott W, Ashar B, Corrado J (2003) Laparoscopic trocar injuries: a report from a U.S. Food and Drug Administration (FDA) Center for Devices and Radiological Health (CDRH) Systematic Technology Assessment of Medical Products (STAMP) Committee
4. Leibl BJ, Kraft K, Schmedt CG, Bittner R (2001) Access techniques for endoscopic surgery—types of trocars, ports and cannulae—an overview. Minim Invasive Ther Allied Technol 10(1):5–10
5. Fuller J, Ashar BS, Carey-Corrado J (2005) Trocar-associated injuries and fatalities: an analysis of 1399 reports to the FDA. J Minim Invasive Gynecol 12(4):302–307
6. Bhoyrul S, Vierra MA, Nezhat CR, Krummel TM, Way LW (2001) Trocar injuries in laparoscopic surgery. J Am Coll Surg 192 (6):677–683
7. Sharp HT, Dobson MK, Draper ML, Watts DA, Doucette RC, Hurd WW (2002) Complications associated with optical-access laparoscopic trocars. Obstet Gynecol 99:553–555
8. Ternamian AM, Vilos GA, Vilos AG, Abu-Rafea B, Tyrwhitt J, MacLeod NT (2010) Laparoscopic peritoneal entry with the reusable threaded visual cannula. J Minim Invasive Gynecol 17(4):461–467

9. Ahmad G, O'Flynn H, Duffy JM, Phillips K, Watson A (2012) Laparoscopic entry techniques. Cochrane Database Syst Rev 2: CD006583
10. Bhoyrul S, Payne J, Steffes B, Swanstrom L, Way LW (2000) A randomized prospective study of radially expanding trocars in laparoscopic surgery. J Gastrointest Surg 4(4):392–397
11. Bisgaard T, Jakobsen HL, Jacobsen B, Olsen SD, Rosenberg J (2007) Randomized clinical trial comparing radially expanding trocars with conventional cutting trocars for the effects on pain after laparoscopic cholecystectomy. Surg Endosc 21(11):2012–2016
12. Feste JR, Bojahr B, Turner DJ (2000) Randomized trial comparing a radially expandable needle system with cutting trocars. JSLS 4 (1):11–15
13. Mettler L, Maher P (2000) Investigation of the effectiveness of the radially-expanding needle system, in contrast to the cutting trocar in enhancing patient recovery. Minim Invasive Ther Allied Technol 9(6):397–401
14. Hamade AM, Issa ME, Haylett KR, Ammori BJ (2007) Fixity of ports to the abdominal wall during laparoscopic surgery: a randomized comparison of cutting versus blunt trocars. Surg Endosc 21(6):965–969
15. Venkatesh R, Sundaram CP, Figenshau RS, Yan Y, Andriole GL, Clayman RV et al (2007) Prospective randomized comparison of cutting and dilating disposable trocars for access during laparoscopic renal surgery. JSLS 11(2):198–203
16. Lam TY, Lee SW, So HS, Kwok SP (2000) Radially expanding trocar: a less painful alternative for laparoscopic surgery. J Laparoendosc Adv Surg Tech A 10(5):269–273
17. Yim SF, Yuen PM (2001) Randomized double-masked comparison of radially expanding access device and conventional cutting tip trocar in laparoscopy. Obstet Gynecol 97(3):435–438
18. Leibl BJ, Schmedt CG, Schwarz J, Kraft K, Bittner R (1999) Laparoscopic surgery complications associated with trocar tip design: review of literature and own results. J Laparoendosc Adv Surg Tech A 9(2):135–140
19. Turner DJ (1996) A new, radially expanding access system for laparoscopic procedures versus conventional cannulas. J Am Assoc Gynecol Laparosc 3(4):609–615
20. Stepanian AA, Winer WK, Isler CM, Lyons TL (2007) Comparative analysis of 5-mm trocars: dilating tip versus non-shielded bladed. J Minim Invasive Gynecol 14(2):176–183
21. Garry R (2009) Surgeons may continue to use their chosen entry technique. Gynecol Surg 6:87–92
22. Hurd WW, Diamond MP (1997) There's a hole in my bucket, the cost of disposable instruments. Fertil Steril 67:13–15
23. Tansatit T, Wisawasukmongchol W, Bunyavejchevin S (2006) A randomized, prospective study comparing the use of the missile trocar and the pyramidal trocar for laparoscopy access. J Med Assoc Thai 89(7):941–947
24. Chan ACW, Ip M, Koehler A, Crisp B, Tam JS, Chung SCS (2000) Is it safe to reuse disposable laparoscopic trocars. Surg Endosc 14:1042–1044
25. Matsuda T, Ogura K, Uchida J, Fujita I, Terachi T, Yoshida O (1995) Smaller ports result in shorter convalescence after laparoscopic varicocelectomy. J Urol 153(4):1175–1177
26. Bohm B, Knigge M, Kraft M, Grundel K, Boenick U (1998) Influence of different trocar tips on abdominal wall penetration during laparoscopy. Surg Endosc 12(12):1434–1438
27. Swank HA, Mulder IM, la Chapelle CF, Reitsma JB, Lange JF, Bemelman WA (2012) Systematic review of trocar-site hernia. Br J Surg 99(3):315–323
28. Kadar N, Reich H, Liu CY, Manko GF, Gimpelson R (1993) Incisional hernias after major laparoscopic gynecologic procedures. Am J Obstet Gynecol 168(5):1493–1495
29. Mayol J, Garcia-Aguilar J, Ortiz-Oshiro E, De-Diego Carmona JA, Fernandez-Represa JA (1997) Risks of the minimal access approach for laparoscopic surgery: multivariate analysis of morbidity related to umbilical trocar insertion. World J Surg 21(5):529–533
30. Montz FJ, Holschneider CH, Munro MG (1994) Incisional hernia following laparoscopy: a survey of the American Association of Gynecologic Laparoscopists. Obstet Gynecol 84(5):881–884
31. Tonouchi H, Ohmori Y, Kobayashi M, Kusunoki M (2004) Trocar site hernia. Arch Surg 139(11):1248–1256
32. Shaher Z (2007) Port closure techniques. Surg Endosc 21(8):1264–1274
33. Calik A, Yucel Y, Topaloglu S, Hos G, Aktas A, Piskin B (2008) Umbilical trocar site closure with Berci's needle after laparoscopic cholecystectomy. Hepato-Gastroenterology 55(88):1958–1961
34. Elashry OM, Nakada SY, Wolf JS Jr, Figenshau RS, McDougall EM, Clayman RV (1996) Comparative clinical study of port-closure techniques following laparoscopic surgery. J Am Coll Surg 183(4):335–344
35. Chiong E, Hegarty PK, Davis JW, Kamat AM, Pisters LL, Matin SF (2010) Port-site hernias occurring after the use of bladeless radially expanding trocars. Urology 75(3):574–580
36. Azurin DJ, Go LS, Arroyo LR, Kirkland ML (1995) Trocar site herniation following laparoscopic cholecystectomy and the significance of an incidental preexisting umbilical hernia. Am Surg 61 (8):718–720
37. Tucker RD (1995) Laparoscopic electrosurgical injuries: survey results and their implications. Surg Laparosc Endosc 5(4):311–317
38. Heniford BT, Matthews BD, Sing RF, Backus C, Pratt B, Greene FL (2001) Initial results with an electrothermal bipolar vessel sealer. Surg Endosc 15(8):799–801
39. Kossi J, Luostarinen M, Kontula I, Laato M (2007) Laparoscopic sigmoid and rectal resection using an electrothermal bipolar vessel sealing device. J Laparoendosc Adv Surg Tech Part A 17(6):719–722
40. Harold KL, Pollinger H, Matthews BD, Kercher KW, Sing RF, Heniford BT (2003) Comparison of ultrasonic energy, bipolar thermal energy, and vascular clips for the hemostasis of small-, medium-, and large-sized arteries. Surg Endosc 17 (8):1228–1230
41. Takada M, Ichihara T, Kuroda Y (2005) Comparative study of electrothermal bipolar vessel sealer and ultrasonic coagulating shears in laparoscopic colectomy. Surg Endosc 19(2):226–228
42. Harrell AG, Kercher KW, Heniford BT (2004) Energy sources in laparoscopy. Semin Laparosc Surg 11(3):201–209
43. Wang K, Advincula AP (2007) "Current thoughts" in electrosurgery. Int J Gynaecol Obstet 97(3):245–250
44. Litta P, Fantinato S, Calonaci F, Cosmi E, Filippeschi M, Zerbetto I et al (2010) A randomized controlled study comparing harmonic versus electrosurgery in laparoscopic myomectomy. Fertil Steril 94 (5):1882–1886
45. Rimonda R, Arezzo A, Garrone C, Allaix ME, Giraudo G, Morino M (2009) Electrothermal bipolar vessel sealing system vs. harmonic scalpel in colorectal laparoscopic surgery: a prospective, randomized study. Dis Colon Rectum 52(4):657–661
46. Tsimoyiannis EC, Jabarin M, Glantzounis G, Lekkas ET, Siakas P, Stefanaki NS (1998) Laparoscopic cholecystectomy using ultrasonically activated coagulating shears. Surg Laparosc Endosc 8:421–424
47. Fletcher DR, Hobbs MS, Tan P, Valinsky LJ, Hockey RL, Pikora TJ et al (1999) Complications of cholecystectomy: risks of the laparoscopic approach and protective effects of operative cholangiography: a population-based study. Ann Surg 229(4):449–457
48. Hulka JF, Levy BS, Parker WH, Phillips JM (1997) Laparoscopic-assisted vaginal hysterectomy: American Association of Gynecologic Laparoscopists' 1995 membership survey. J Am Assoc Gynecol Laparosc 4(2):167–171
49. Meikle SF, Nugent EW, Orleans M (1997) Complications and recovery from laparoscopy-assisted vaginal hysterectomy

compared with abdominal and vaginal hysterectomy. Obstet Gynecol 89(2):304–311

50. Wu MP, Ou CS, Chen SL, Yen EY, Rowbotham R (2000) Complications and recommended practices for electrosurgery in laparoscopy. Am J Surg 179(1):67–73
51. Holub Z, Jabor A, Kliment L, Lukac J, Voracek J (2002) Laparoscopic lymph node dissection using ultrasonically activated shears: comparison with electrosurgery. J Laparoendosc Adv Surg Tech Part A 12(3):175–180
52. Hubner M, Demartines N, Muller S, Dindo D, Clavien PA, Hahnloser D (2008) Prospective randomized study of monopolar scissors, bipolar vessel sealer and ultrasonic shears in laparoscopic colorectal surgery. Br J Surg 95(9):1098–1104
53. Morino M, Rimonda R, Allaix ME, Giraudo G, Garrone C (2005) Ultrasonic versus standard electric dissection in laparoscopic colorectal surgery: a prospective randomized clinical trial. Ann Surg 242(6):897–901
54. Jones CM, Pierre KB, Nicoud IB, Stain SC, Melvin WV III (2006) Electrosurgery. Curr Surg 63(6):458–463
55. Dawes JC, Mahabir RC, Hillier K, Cassidy M, de Haas W, Gillis AM (2006) Electrosurgery in patients with pacemakers/implanted cardioverter defibrillators. Ann Plast Surg 57(1):33–36
56. El-Gamal HM, Dufresne RG, Saddler K (2001) Electrosurgery, pacemakers and ICDs: a survey of precautions and complications experienced by cutaneous surgeons. Dermatol Surg 27 (4):385–390

Patients with adenomyosis are more likely to have deep endometriosis

Midgley Gonzales · Leandro Accardo de Matos · Manoel Orlando da Costa Gonçalves · Roberto Blasbalg · João Antônio Dias Junior · Sérgio Podgaec · Edmund Chada Baracat · Maurício Simões Abrão

Abstract This study seeks to analyze the association between adenomyosis diagnosed by magnetic resonance imaging (MRI) and endometriosis. This is a prospective study of consecutive patients. One hundred fifty-two patients with histologically confirmed endometriosis. Patients were submitted to MRI, then divided into Group A (with adenomyosis) and Group B (without adenomyosis). Thickness of the junctional zone and the presence of intramyometrial cysts were the principal criteria for diagnosis of adenomyosis. MRI data were correlated with clinical status, staging, sites affected, and histological classification of endometriosis. The prevalence of adenomyosis in endometriosis patients was 42.76 %. Patients with endometriosis and adenomyosis were more likely than those without adenomyosis to report severe or incapacitating dysmenorrhea (61.53 % in Group A; 44.83 % in Group B; $p=0.041$) and deep dyspareunia (64.61 % in Group A; 41.38 % in Group B; $p=0.005$), to have stage IV endometriosis (50.77 % in Group A; 33.34 % in Group B; $p=0.03$), to have endometriosis of the rectosigmoid (49.23 % in Group A; 32.18 % in Group B; $p=0.033$), and to have undifferentiated or mixed histological types of endometriosis (52.31 % in Group A; 34.48 % in Group B; $p=0.028$). A correlation was found between adenomyosis and deep endometriosis with poorer prognosis, particularly endometriosis of the rectosigmoid.

Keywords Endometriosis · Adenomyosis · Magnetic resonance imaging

Introduction

Adenomyosis is a gynecological disease characterized by the presence of endometrial glands and stroma in the myometrium, generally covered by smooth muscle hyperplasia [1–3]. Its prevalence is unclear, ranging from 15 % to 20 % [4–6] and reaching coefficients of up to 90 % when infertile patients are taken into consideration [7]. Classically, the diagnosis of adenomyosis was based on histology [1, 2]. Morphometric studies show that the myocytes of the subendometrial layer are characterized by a nuclear increase, a reduction in the extracellular matrix and in water volume compared with cells located in the external layer of the myometrium [8]. These cell differences observed in the subendometrial myocytes and around foci of adenomyosis permit identification of the junctional zone and poorly defined low density areas of the myometrium on T2-weighted magnetic resonance imaging (MRI) sequences [8].

The presence of endometrial components in the myometrium may be expressed by an increase in the thickness of the junctional zone on MRI [9]. Most authors agree that a junctional zone thickness ≥12 mm is indicative of a uterus with adenomyosis [5, 10, 11]. The presence of areas of low intensity and poorly defined borders surrounding points of

M. Gonzales · J. A. Dias Junior · S. Podgaec · E. C. Baracat · M. S. Abrão (✉)
Department of Obstetrics and Gynecology,
University of São Paulo Medical School,
Rua São Sebastião 550,
04708-001 São Paulo, São Paulo, Brazil
e-mail: msabrao@mac.com

L. A. de Matos · M. O. da Costa Gonçalves
Digimagem Diagnósticos,
São Paulo, Brazil

R. Blasbalg
Department of Radiology,
University of São Paulo Medical School,
São Paulo, Brazil

high signal intensity on T2-weighted sequences may represent a second criterion for diagnosis [5, 11–15], constituting what are referred to as intramyometrial cysts [5].

Transvaginal ultrasound is the natural first choice of image modality when investigating pelvic pain and endometriosis (including deep lesions) [16, 17]. MRI represents an accurate method for the detection of adenomyosis, sensitivity, and specificity varying from 86 % to 100 % [5, 14, 18–22], making this a highly effective tool for the diagnosis of this disease [14].

There is a multitude of theories with respect to the association between adenomyosis and endometriosis; however, other investigators consider them to be two distinct entities [23, 24]. No studies have yet been performed to correlate the two diseases from a diagnostic point of view, taking into consideration the relationship between the ectopic implantation of glands and endometrial stroma in the myometrium, and the sites of implantation and the severity of the foci of endometriosis. Therefore, the objective of the present study was to evaluate the prevalence of adenomyosis in patients with endometriosis and to verify the association of a diagnosis of adenomyosis according to MRI and the following parameters of endometriosis: clinical status, staging [25], the presence of undifferentiation according to histological classification [26] and the sites affected by the disease (peritoneum, ovary, or deep endometriosis).

Methods

A total of 170 patients consecutively attending the Endometriosis Clinic of the Teaching Hospital of the School of Medicine, University of São Paulo between February 2004 and October 2008 with an indication for videolaparoscopy based on clinical history, physical examination, pelvic echography, and MRI were evaluated according to the protocol used in cases of patients with a clinical suspicion of endometriosis.

In accordance with MRI, the patients were divided into two groups: Group A in which MRI findings were indicative of adenomyosis and Group B in which there were no signs indicative of adenomyosis.

Following surgery, 18 patients were excluded because they did not present endometriosis at laparoscopy and/or histological examination. According to the objectives of our study, to describe the MRI findings in patients with endometriosis, we decided to exclude these patients. The following inclusion criteria were applied to patients in Group A: age 20–45 years, histologically confirmed endometriosis, and MRI findings compatible with a diagnosis of adenomyosis. In addition, the patient should not have been in use of hormones in the 3 months preceding videolaparoscopy (including GnRH analogs, progestogens, and hormonal contraceptives) and should have no contraindications to undergoing MRI. For Group B, the same inclusion criteria were applied as for Group A; however, MRI findings for patients in this group had to indicate an absence of adenomyosis. The study was approved by the institution's Internal Review Board and all the patients read and signed an informed consent form.

With respect to the clinical status of endometriosis, the presence of acyclic pelvic pain, dysmenorrheal, and dyspareunia was recorded, as described by the patients with the use of a visual analog scale. Cyclic bowel and urinary abnormalities (during menstruation) and infertility status were also recorded.

In these patients, endometriosis was classified during laparoscopy as stages I to IV in accordance with the criteria defined by the American Society for Reproductive Medicine (ASRM), 1996 revision [25].

The most important site affected by endometriosis was defined in accordance with the severity of the disease in the affected organ. Three categories were established: peritoneal endometriosis, ovarian endometriosis, and deep endometriosis (lesions with a depth>5 mm), which included retrocervical and bowel lesions as well as lesions of the ureter, bladder, and vagina.

Tissue was analyzed histologically in accordance with the classification patterns proposed by Abrão et al. [26]: stromal, well-differentiated glandular, undifferentiated glandular, or mixed differentiation glandular (presence of epithelia with well-differentiated and undifferentiated patterns at the same site). To facilitate analysis, differential was defined as the presence or absence of endometriosis with an undifferentiated histological pattern, since this is the histological type with the poorest prognosis [26].

All pelvic MRI exams were performed using a 1.5 Tesla GE Signa scanner (General Electric Medical Systems, Milwaukee, WI) or a 1.5 Tesla Philips scanner with an 8-channel torso coil or cardiac coil for signal reception and transmission. All the patients had fasted for 4 h prior to the exam and were placed in the dorsal decubitus position with their arms raised above their heads. Vaginal gel was used when no contraindications were present. Gadolinium contrast medium (10–20 ml) was manually injected intravenously at a speed of approximately 2.0 ml/s.

Morphology of the junctional zone, a subendometrial region of low signal intensity, was evaluated on T1- (axial plane) and T2-weighted sequences (axial, sagittal and coronal planes). T1-weighted sequences were used to detect hemorrhagic foci in the junctional zone and in the myometrium. The other morphological alterations were observed in the T2-weighted sequences.

To determine a diagnosis of adenomyosis by pelvic MRI, the following criteria were taken into consideration [5, 9]: focal or diffuse thickening of the junctional zone ≥12 mm; the presence of intramyometrial cysts, which consists of a high signal area of the myometrium surrounded by an area of low intensity signal with poorly defined borders on T2-weighted sequences.

Categorical variables were analyzed using the chi-square test. Fisher's exact test was used whenever the distribution of the variable under analysis rendered the chi-square test inviable. The continuous quantitative variables were compared using Student's *t* test. All statistical analyses were performed using the SPSS statistical software program (SPSS Inc., USA), adopting a significance level of 5 %.

Results

A total of 152 women with endometriosis (diagnosed by histopathology following videolaparoscopy) were analyzed, 65 (42.8 %) of whom were found to have adenomyosis on pelvic MRI (Group A), while 87 (56.2 %) did not (Group B). The clinical and epidemiological characteristics of the study participants are shown in Table 1.

An association was found between a diagnosis of adenomyosis (Group A) and a greater likelihood of dysmenorrhea (severe or incapacitating) and deep dyspareunia. No differences were found between the two groups with respect to any of the other symptoms and there were no differences in findings detected at physical examination.

Table 1 Epidemiological and clinical characteristics of the patients in Group A (with adenomyosis) compared to the patients in Group B (without adenomyosis)

	Group A (N=65)	Group B (N=87)	p value
Skin color			
Yellow	4 (6.15 %)	8 (9.19 %)	
White	47 (72.30 %)	58 (66.67 %)	
Black	14 (21.55 %)	21 (24.14 %)	0.699
Pregnancies			
0	41 (63.10 %)	56 (64.37 %)	
1	20 (30.77 %)	26 (29.88 %)	
2	4 (6.15 %)	4 (4.60 %)	0.717
Mean age	33.43	32.82	0.474
Clinical data			
Dysmenorrhea	40 (61.53 %)	39 (44.83 %)	0.041*
Acyclic pelvic pain	22 (33.85 %)	19 (21.84 %)	0.099
Dyspareunia	42 (64.61 %)	36 (41.38 %)	0.005
Infertility	31 (47.69 %)	41 (47.13 %)	0.945
Cyclic bowel symptoms	32 (49.23 %)	32 (36.78 %)	0.124
Cyclic urinary symptoms	3 (4.61 %)	7 (8.04 %)	0.517

*p<0.05

When the staging of endometriosis obtained during videolaparoscopy in the 152 patients was compared between the two study groups, a relationship was found between adenomyosis and advanced stages of endometriosis (Table 2). This association was present when patients with stages III and IV were grouped together and became even more expressive when the presence of adenomyosis was investigated only in patients with stage IV endometriosis. Table 3 shows the distribution of the patients with and without adenomyosis according to the site most severely affected by pelvic endometriosis.

In the evaluation of the histological type of endometriosis (Table 4), the presence of undifferentiated or mixed histological patterns of endometriosis in the tissue studied was significantly more common in the patients with adenomyosis (Group A; p=0.028).

Discussion

Great advances have been made in the field of diagnosis and in the surgical treatment of deep endometriosis. In addition, new aspects are now beginning to be understood within the realm of etiopathogeny. Little is known about adenomyosis. There is an intuitive association with endometriosis. The tissues involved, the sites affected, the clinical status all connect these two diseases; however, a more objective confirmation of this association is required. Evaluating the characteristics of the two study groups, no differences were found between the two with respect to epidemiological parameters. There was a predominance of white patients, which is in agreement with data published by Arruda et al. [27]. The homogeneity found in the present study reinforces the power of this present analysis, since the only difference between the two groups was the variable under investigation: a diagnosis of adenomyosis on MRI.

The purpose of using imaging exams to diagnose adenomyosis is to study the disease in patients in whom hysterectomy is not indicated. This became feasible and MRI is

Table 2 Evaluation of the patients in Group A (with adenomyosis) compared with the patients in Group B (without adenomyosis), according to the stage of endometriosis (ASRM, 1996)

Stage	Group A (N=65)	Group B (N=87)	p value
I	9 (13.85 %)	26 (29.87 %)	0.020*
II	14 (21.54 %)	19 (21.84 %)	0.965
I/II	23 (35.38 %)	45 (51.72 %)	0.045*
III	9 (13.85 %)	13 (14.49 %)	0.849
IV	33 (50.77 %)	29 (33.34 %)	0.030*
III/IV	42 (64.61 %)	42 (48.27 %)	0.045*

*p<0.05

Table 3 Evaluation of the patients in Group A (with adenomyosis) in relation to the patients in Group B (without adenomyosis), according to the site of the endometriotic lesion

Site	Group A (N=65)	Group B (N=87)	p value
Peritoneal	26 (40 %)	49 (56.32 %)	0.046*
Ovarian	42 (64.61 %)	45 (51.72 %)	0.112
Deep			
Retrocervical	39 (60 %)	34 (39.08 %)	0.011*
Vagina	5 (7.69 %)	4 (4.60 %)	0.498
Bladder	6 (9.23 %)	8 (9.19 %)	0.994
Ureter	6 (9.23 %)	3 (3.45 %)	0.172
Rectosigmoid	32 (49.23 %)	28 (32.18 %)	0.033*

*p<0.05

currently considered to be a highly accurate tool for the diagnosis of this pathology [7, 11, 12, 14, 28]. The radiological criteria selected in the present study for the diagnosis of adenomyosis were those most generally accepted in the literature: thickness of the junctional zone ≥12 mm and the presence of intramyometrial cysts, regions of hyperintense signals surrounded by an area of low intensity signals and poorly defined borders on T2-weighted sequences [5, 14, 19–21]. In the 152 patients with a diagnosis of endometriosis in the present study, critical analysis of their MRI scans revealed that 65 patients (42.8 %) had a diagnosis of adenomyosis. The coefficient depends to a great extent on the characteristics, principally the clinical characteristics of the study population [1, 29].

The prevalence of adenomyosis in patients with endometriosis has been evaluated in few studies. Bazot et al. [30] reported a prevalence of adenomyosis of 27 % in patients with endometriosis. On the other hand, Kunz et al. [7] reported a prevalence of 79 %, which increased to 90 % when adenomyosis was diagnosed in patients with endometriosis and female infertility. Moreover, Larsen et al. [31] found that in 34.6 % of patients with endometriosis had adenomyosis compared to 19.4 % in the control patients. In a recent study published by Dai et al. [32], adenomyosis was diagnosed in 15.8 % of patients presenting deep endometriosis and it was significantly higher than in patients without deep endometriosis.

Table 4 Evaluation of the patients in Group A (with adenomyosis) in relation to the patients in Group B (without adenomyosis), according to the presence of undifferentiated histological pattern in the endometriotic lesion

Histology	Group A (N=65)	Group B (N=87)
Well-differentiated glandular or stromal disease	31 (47.69 %)	57 (65.52 %)
Undifferentiated glandular or mixed disease	34 (52.31 %)	30 (34.48 %)

p=0.028

Parker et al. [28] evaluated chronic pelvic pain in women with endometriosis and reported a prevalence of adenomyosis, as diagnosed by MRI, of 40 %. In the present study, the patients were symptomatic with respect to endometriosis, meeting the criteria for an indication for videolaparoscopy. Therefore, the 42.8 % prevalence of adenomyosis in endometriosis patients that was found in this study would appear to be compatible with the data in the literature considering the characteristics of the study population. Furthermore, there were statistically more cases of severe or incapacitating dysmenorrhea and deep dyspareunia in the group of patients with adenomyosis compared to the group with a diagnosis of endometriosis alone. It is comprehensible that dysmenorrhea would be more severe in this group bearing in mind the factors triggered by the combination of these two pathologies. Dyspareunia was more intense in patients of Group A, probably as a result of the associated deep endometriotic lesions, since the severity of symptoms is directly associated with the depth of the lesions [33–35]. Therefore, as has been shown in cases of endometriosis in which there is a significant correlation between deep dyspareunia and retrocervical endometriotic lesions [36], the severity of the symptoms in adenomyosis also correlates with the extension and depth of the myometrial invasion of the lesion [37, 38].

With respect to the endometriosis staging classification system proposed by the ASRM in 1985 and revised in 1996 [25], adenomyosis was found to be associated with more advanced stages of endometriosis, particularly stage IV of the disease. These data are in agreement with a study published by Kunz et al. [7] in which these authors correlated moderate and severe endometriosis with a junctional zone thickness of 12.4 mm (adenomyosis), with p=0.02. The stage IV was also found among women with severe endometriosis, 42.8 % had adenomyosis, with deeper wall invasion, compared to 29.4 % in the women with other stages of endometriosis [31].

Considering the site affected by endometriosis and its association with adenomyosis, a greater association was found between adenomyosis and cases of deep retrocervical endometriosis (60 %; p=0.01) and those in which endometriosis was affecting the rectosigmoid (49.2 %; p=0.03). Parker et al. [28] also suggested an association between adenomyosis and deep endometriosis; however, these authors emphasized that due to the small sample size in their study, it was impossible to correlate the data with the stage of endometriosis.

With respect to the histological classification of the disease [26], there was a significantly greater incidence of undifferentiated endometriosis, either in the pure or mixed form, in the group of patients with adenomyosis compared to the group of patients with endometriosis alone (p=0.028). These data are compatible with the finding that patients with undifferentiated endometriosis have more severe forms of endometriosis [26, 39].

These findings confirm previous data correlating adenomyosis with deep endometriosis (principally bowel endometriosis) and with advanced stages of the disease [25]. An association was therefore established between adenomyosis and cases of endometriosis with poor prognosis.

Despite the lack of studies in which patients with endometriosis were analyzed according to the present format, particularly correlating endometriosis with adenomyosis, it is worth mentioning the publication of Landi et al. [11], who reported poorer prognosis in patients with concurrent adenomyosis and endometriosis. However, they did not establish any satisfactory association with staging or the site of foci of endometriosis. Peritoneal lesions present as epithelial glands covered with endometrial-type stroma. This feature is absent in deep lesions that involve smooth muscle tissue [40, 41] similar to adenomyosis lesions. In the present study, an association was found between adenomyosis and deep endometriosis. It should be emphasized that it is the deep rather than the superficial endometriotic foci that resemble those found in adenomyosis [42].

When the three different forms of endometriosis, peritoneal, ovarian, and that affecting the rectovaginal septum were defined, Nisolle and Donnez [43] attributed different etiopathogenies to the peritoneal form of the disease (implants resulting from retrograde menstruation) and to the deep lesions, said to correspond to an adenomyotic nodule originating from Müllerian remnants by means of metaplasia [40, 41, 44]. These resemble an adenomyoma, an accumulation of smooth muscle tissue and endometrial glands with scarce stroma [40, 41, 44]. Well-grounded studies have shown that the nodules of deep retrocervical, and bowel endometriosis are not the result of deep infiltrative endometriosis but are similar to the nodules of adenomyosis that develop from Müllerian remnants by metaplasia [40, 41, 44].

As deep endometriosis, adenomyosis has also been explained [4, 45] as a condition originating from Müllerian remnants by metaplasia. These authors presume that there are transitional quiescent Müllerian elements between the endometrium and the myometrium that would have the capacity to develop by metaplasia.

The close association found in this study between adenomyosis and deep endometriosis, associated with advanced stages and pure or mixed undifferentiated histological patterns, permits some common theories to be expounded on the genesis of endometriosis and that of adenomyosis. According to the present findings, adenomyosis may be interpreted as a marker for deep endometriosis. Nevertheless, more studies need to be performed to supply further useful information and a better understanding of the association between these two diseases, providing greater knowledge on their etiopathogenies and developing new instruments for clinical practice.

Declaration of interest The authors report no conflicts of interest. The authors alone are responsible for the content and writing of the paper.

References

1. Bird CC, McElin TW, Manalo-Estrella P (1972) The elusive adenomyosis of the uterus—revisited. Am J Obstet Gynecol 112:583–593
2. Ferenczy A (1998) Pathophysiology of adenomyosis. Hum Reprod Update 4:312–322
3. Leyendecker G, Kunz G, Noe M et al (1998) Endometriosis: a dysfunction and disease of the archimetra. Hum Reprod Update 4:752–762
4. Racinet C, Morin X, Martin H (1987) Adenomyosis. Contrib Gynecol Obstet 16:183–191
5. Reinhold C, McCarthy S, Bret PM et al (1996) Diffuse adenomyosis: comparison of endovaginal US and MR imaging with histopathologic correlation. Radiology 199:151–158
6. Dueholm M, Lundorf E (2007) Transvaginal ultrasound or MRI for diagnosis of adenomyosis. Curr Opin Obstet Gynecol 19:505–512
7. Kunz G, Beil D, Huppert P et al (2005) Adenomyosis in endometriosis—prevalence and impact on fertility. Evidence from magnetic resonance imaging. Hum Reprod 20:2309–2316
8. Fusi L, Cloke B, Brosens JJ (2006) The uterine junctional zone. Best Pract Res Clin Obstet Gynaecol 20:479–491
9. Hricak H, Alpers C, Crooks LE et al (1983) Magnetic resonance imaging of the female pelvis: initial experience. AJR Am J Roentgenol 141:1119–1128
10. Bazot M, Cortez A, Darai E et al (2001) Ultrasonography compared with magnetic resonance imaging for the diagnosis of adenomyosis: correlation with histopathology. Hum Reprod 16:2427–2433
11. Landi S, Mereu L, Pontrelli G et al (2008) The influence of adenomyosis in patients laparoscopically treated for deep endometriosis. J Minim Invasive Gynecol 15:566–570
12. Reinhold C, Tafazoli F, Wang L (1998) Imaging features of adenomyosis. Hum Reprod Update 4:337–349
13. Stratton P, Winkel CA, Sinaii N et al (2002) Location, color, size, depth, and volume may predict endometriosis in lesions resected at surgery. Fertil Steril 78:743–749
14. Ascher SM, Arnold LL, Patt RH et al (1994) Adenomyosis: prospective comparison of MR imaging and transvaginal sonography. Radiology 190:803–806
15. Tamai K, Togashi K, Ito T, Morisawa N et al (2005) MR imaging findings of adenomyosis: correlation with histopathologic features and diagnostic pitfalls. Radiographics 25:21–40
16. Gonçalves MO, Podgaec S, Dias JA Jr et al (2010) Transvaginal ultrasonography with bowel preparation is able to predict the number of lesions and rectosigmoid layers affected in cases of deep endometriosis, defining surgical strategy. Hum Reprod 25:665–671
17. Gonçalves MO, Dias JA Jr, Podgaec S et al (2009) Transvaginal ultrasound for diagnosis of deeply infiltrating endometriosis. Int J Gynaecol Obstet 104:156–160
18. Mark AS, Hricak H, Heinrichs LW et al (1987) Adenomyosis and leiomyoma: differential diagnosis with MR imaging. Radiology 163:527–529

19. Togashi K, Nishimura K, Itoh K et al (1988) Adenomyosis: diagnosis with MR imaging. Radiology 166:111–114
20. Togashi K, Ozasa H, Konishi I et al (1989) Enlarged uterus: differentiation between adenomyosis and leiomyoma with MR imaging. Radiology 171:531–534
21. Hricak H, Finck S, Honda G et al (1992) MR imaging in the evaluation of benign uterine masses: value of gadopentetate dimeglumine-enhanced T1-weighted images. AJR Am J Roentgenol 158:1043–1050
22. Chamie LP, Blasbalg R, Gonçalves MO et al (2009) Accuracy of magnetic resonance imaging for diagnosis and preoperative assessment of deeply infiltrating andometriosis. Int J Gynaecol Obstet 106:198–201
23. Ridley JH (1968) The histogenesis of endometriosis. A review of facts and fancies. Obstet Gynecol Surv 23:1–35
24. Greaves P, White IN (2006) Experimental adenomyosis. Best Pract Res Clin Obstet Gynaecol 20:503–510
25. American Society for Reproductive Medicine (1997) Revised American Society for Reproductive Medicine classification of endometriosis: 1996. Fertil Steril 67:817–821
26. Abrão MS, Neme RM, Carvalho FM et al (2003) Histological classification of endometriosis as a predictor of response to treatment. Int J Gynaecol Obstet 82:31–40
27. Arruda MS, Petta CA, Abrão MS et al (2003) Time elapsed from onset of symptoms to diagnosis of endometriosis in a cohort study of Brazilian women. Hum Reprod 18:756–759
28. Parker JD, Leondires M, Sinaii N et al (2006) Persistence of dysmenorrhea and nonmenstrual pain after optimal endometriosis surgery may indicate adenomyosis. Fertil Steril 86:711–715
29. Atri M, Reinhold C, Mehio AR et al (2000) Adenomyosis: US features with histologic correlation in an in-vitro study. Radiology 215:783–790
30. Bazot M, Fiori O, Darai E (2006) Adenomyosis in endometriosis—prevalence and impact on fertility. Evidence from magnetic resonance imaging. Hum Reprod 21:1101–1102
31. Larsen SB, Lundorf E, Forman A et al (2011) Adenomyosis and junctional zone changes in patients with endometriosis. Eur J Obstet Gynecol Reprod Biol 157:206–211
32. Dai Y, Leng JH, Lang JH et al (2012) Anatomical distribution of pelvic deep infiltrating endometriosis and its relationship with pain symptoms. Chin Med J (Engl) 125:209–213
33. Koninckx PR, Meuleman C, Demeyere S et al (1991) Suggestive evidence that pelvic endometriosis is a progressive disease, whereas deeply infiltrating endometriosis is associated with pelvic pain. Fertil Steril 55:759–765
34. Porpora MG, Koninckx PR, Piazze J et al (1999) Correlation between endometriosis and pelvic pain. J Am Assoc Gynecol Laparosc 6:429–434
35. Chapron C, Fauconnier A, Dubuisson JB et al (2003) Deep infiltrating endometriosis: relation between severity of dysmenorrhea and extent of disease. Hum Reprod 18:760–766
36. Berbel BT, Podgaec S, Abrão MS (2008) Analysis of the association between symptoms referred by patients with endometriosis and the site of the disease. Rev Med (São Paulo) 87:195–200
37. Benson RC, Sneeden VD (1958) Adenomyosis: a reappraisal of symptomatology. Am J Obstet Gynecol 76:1044–1061
38. Nishida M (1991) Relationship between the onset of dysmenorrhea and histologic findings in adenomyosis. Am J Obstet Gynecol 165:229–231
39. Kamergorodsky G, Ribeiro PAA, Galvão MAL et al (2007) Avaliação da classificação histológica da endometriose observada em implantes de mulheres portadoras de endometriose pélvica superficial e profunda. RBGO 29:568–574
40. Nisolle M (1996) Peritoneal, ovarian and rectovaginal endometriosis are three distinct entities. Dissertation. Catholic University of Louvain
41. Nisolle M, Donnez J (1996) Peritoneal, ovarian and rectovaginal endometriosis: the identification of three separate diseases. Carnforth: Parthenon Publishing
42. Somigliana E, Infantino M, Candiani M et al (2004) Association rate between deep peritoneal endometriosis and other forms of the disease: pathogenetic implications. Hum Reprod 19:168–171
43. Nisolle M, Donnez J (1997) Peritoneal endometriosis, ovarian endometriosis, and adenomyotic nodules of the rectovaginal septum are three different entities. Fertil Steril 68:585–596
44. Donnez J, Nisolle M, Casanas-Roux F et al (1996) Stereometric evaluation of peritoneal endometriosis and endometriotic nodules of the rectovaginal septum. Hum Reprod 11:224–228
45. Minh HN, Smadja A, Orcel L (1986) An integrated histogenetic concept of internal and external endometriosis. J Gynecol Obstet Biol Reprod 15:29–35

15

Spontaneous intramyometrial pregnancy mimicking an intramural myoma: a diagnostic challenge

Maria-Laura Marotta · Jacques Donnez · Nathalie Michaux · Michaël Dupont · Monique Delos · Olivier Donnez

Abstract This study describes the diagnosis and treatment of a spontaneous intramyometrial pregnancy by a case report and review of the literature at a university hospital center. A 24-year-old woman presented with a spontaneous intramyometrial pregnancy without any previous uterine surgery. Successful laparoscopic resection and myometrial correction were performed. The presence of trophoblastic tissue was confirmed and the myometrium revealed complete healing at postoperative MRI. Intramyometrial pregnancy can occur without previous uterine surgery or uterine manipulation and may be difficult to diagnose. Conservative laparoscopic excision is possible without damage to myometrial integrity.

M.-L. Marotta (✉) · N. Michaux · O. Donnez
Department of Gynecology, CHU Mont-Godinne,
Université Catholique de Louvain,
Av. G. Thérasse, 1,
5530 Yvoir, Belgium
e-mail: maria-laura.marotta@uclouvain.be

J. Donnez
Pôle de Recherche en Gynécologie,
Institut de Recherche Expérimentale et Clinique (IREC),
Université Catholique de Louvain (UCL),
1200 Brussels, Belgium

J. Donnez
Department of Gynecology, Cliniques Universitaires Saint-Luc,
1200 Brussels, Belgium

M. Dupont
Department of Radiology, CHU Mont-Godinne,
Université Catholique de Louvain,
5530 Yvoir, Belgium

M. Delos
Department of Anatomopathology, CHU Mont-Godinne,
Université Catholique de Louvain,
5530 Yvoir, Belgium

Keywords Ectopic pregnancy · Intramyometrial · Myometrial pregnancy

Introduction

Intramyometrial pregnancy is a very rare type of ectopic pregnancy. This uncommon condition has been estimated to occur in less than 1 % of all ectopic gestations [1]. An intramyometrial pregnancy is located within the uterine wall, completely surrounded by myometrium, and separated from the uterine cavity and fallopian tubes [1], but confusion remains in the literature as to its physiopathology. Ong et al. explain intramyometrial ectopic pregnancy by increased lytic activity of the syncytiotrophoblast and defective decidualization, allowing the conceptus to penetrate the myometrium [1]. But, as described by Pijnenborg et al., in normal pregnancy, the decidua attracts the trophoblast and both intravascular and interstitial trophoblasts invade the inner myometrium [2]. Risk factors have been identified to explain the pathogenesis, including previous uterine trauma causing a sinus tract within the endometrium [1, 3, 4], implantation on a focus of intramural adenomyosis [5, 6], or difficult embryo transfer with a false passage [1, 7–9]. Others have described invasion of the uterine wall by placenta accreta and subsequent growth of the fetus deep within the myometrium [10].

Due to late and often difficult ultrasonographic diagnosis, the gestational sac can grow deep in the myometrium and cause the main complication, namely uterine rupture associated with life-threatening hemorrhage reported to occur between week 11 and week 30 of gestation [1]. To our knowledge, this is the first reported case of intramyometrial pregnancy to occur without any previous surgery or uterine manipulation.

Case report

A 24-year-old woman with a history of spontaneous abortion without dilatation–curettage was referred as an emergency case to our department with acute pelvic pain and suspected ectopic pregnancy. Vaginal examination provoked acute pain upon palpation of the right adnexa, while the uterus appeared to be of normal size. HCG was 102 IU/l, and vaginal ultrasound confirmed a normal-sized uterus, but containing a heterogeneous subserosal mass measuring 35× 30 mm and regularly circumscribed. An adenomyoma or necrotic uterine myoma was suspected. Both adnexa looked normal, but the Douglas pouch revealed the presence of blood. Because of acute pain at vaginal examination, low HCG level, and ultrasound status, ectopic pregnancy was suspected and diagnostic laparoscopy was performed.

At laparoscopy, the uterus showed a subserosal 3 cm mass located on the right side of the uterus below the right utero-ovarian ligament. Fifty milliliters of blood was found in the Douglas pouch. The fallopian tubes were both unremarkable, and no ectopic pregnancy was identified. The abdominal cavity was flushed with physiological serum. On day 1, the HCG level was 44 IU/l and the patient did not present with any abdominal pain. She was then discharged from the hospital, and monitoring of HCG levels was proposed. On day 10, her HCG was less than 1.2 IU/ml. One week after the first laparoscopy, vaginal examination revealed a 7-week-sized uterus, with tenderness on the right side.

Pelvic MRI was performed and confirmed the presence of a right lateral intramyometrial mass. Coronal and axial views of T2-weighted MRI images revealed a 35 mm heterogeneous mass at some distance from the uterine cavity (Fig. 1a, b). T1-weighted images (Fig. 1c, d) showed a discretely hyperintense mass. The right uterine horn was not distorted by the mass. The rest of the myometrium looked normal, as did both adnexa, and no uterine adenomyosis was found. A differential diagnosis was made between an intramural myoma in necrobiosis and intramyometrial pregnancy, but the T2-weighted signal was too heterogeneous.

Laparoscopic excision of the lesion was then proposed. Laparoscopic view of the right side of the uterus (Fig. 2a) confirmed a subserosal deformation of the myometrium below the right utero-ovarian ligament far from the right tube and uterine horn. To avoid bleeding after opening the myometrium, the right uterine artery was clipped at its origin (Fig. 2b). The uterine serosa and superficial layers of the myometrium were then opened using CO_2 laser (power 50 W) (Lumenis-Sharplan, Yokneam, Israel) at a safe distance from the right fallopian tube and right utero-ovarian ligament. The observed myometrial deformation corresponded to an intramyometrial cavity full of blood clots and fibrotic tissue (Fig. 2c). Intraoperative hysteroscopy was then performed and

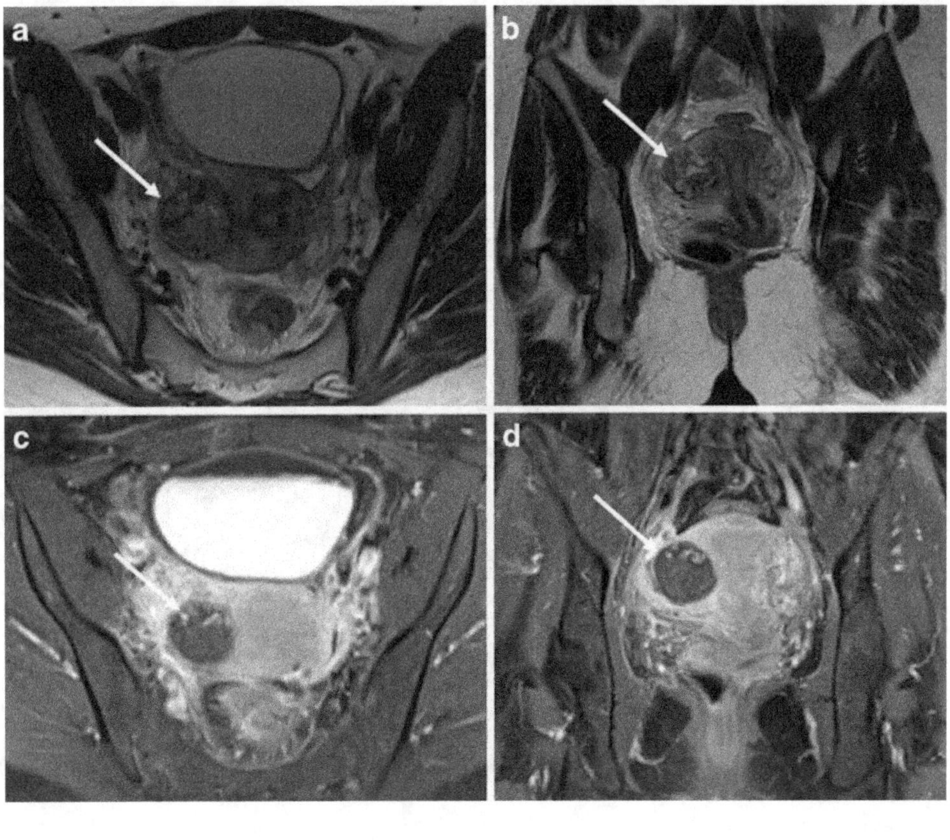

Fig. 1 **a** Axial T2-weighted image revealed a well-circumscribed heterogeneous mass (*white arrow*) subserously located far from the myometrial cavity. **b** Coronal view of a T2-weighted image showed the subserosal mass (*white arrow*) without any deformation of the right uterine horn. **c** Axial T1-weighted image with saturation of fatty tissue and injection of gadolinium into the slightly hypointense right uterine mass (*white arrow*), with hypocaptation of gadolinium. **d** Coronal T1-weighted image of the uterine mass (*white arrow*)

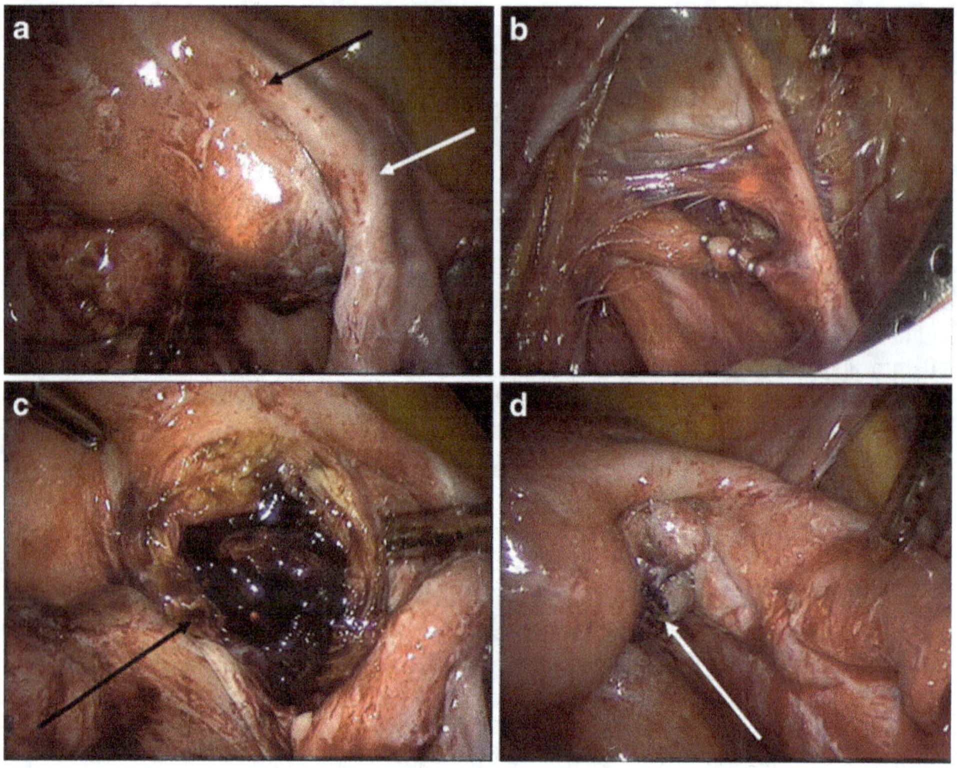

Fig. 2 **a** Laparoscopic view of the right side of the uterus with the subserosal mass located below the insertion of the right utero-ovarian ligament and tube (*white and black arrows*, respectively). **b** Laparoscopic view of the right uterine artery clipped at its origin (*white arrow*) to avoid intraoperative bleeding. **c** Laparoscopic view of the opened subserosal mass, revealing an intramyometrial cavity full of blood clots and fibrotic tissue (*black arrow*). **d** Final view of the two-layer running suture (*white arrow*)

revealed a normal uterine cavity and normal ostia. The endometrium covering the right side of the uterine cavity also looked unremarkable. There were no visible fistulas between the uterine cavity and intramyometrial cavity. After removing all the fibrotic tissue and washing the myometrial cavity, the myometrium was closed in two layers using a running suture of Quill™ SRS 0 (Angiotech, Reading, USA). The final result can be seen in Fig. 2d. In order to avoid more myometrial injury, no biopsy of the surrounding myometrium was performed. No drain was left in the peritoneal cavity, and the patient was discharged from hospital on day 1. Histologic examination of the excised tissue revealed degenerated villous tissue, proving the presence of a pregnancy inside the myometrium (Fig. 3a).

Pelvic MRI performed 3 months after surgery showed complete healing of the myometrium. No uterine scarring was visible (Fig. 3b). Clinical examination revealed a normal-sized uterus, and the patient did not experience any abdominal pain.

Discussion

Intramyometrial ectopic pregnancy is uncommon. Its etiology remains unclear, but most authors attribute it to a sinus tract within the endometrium caused by previous uterine surgery or manipulation [1, 3, 4], adenomyosis [5, 6], or a difficult embryo transfer [1, 7–9]. Leyder et al. described intramyometrial

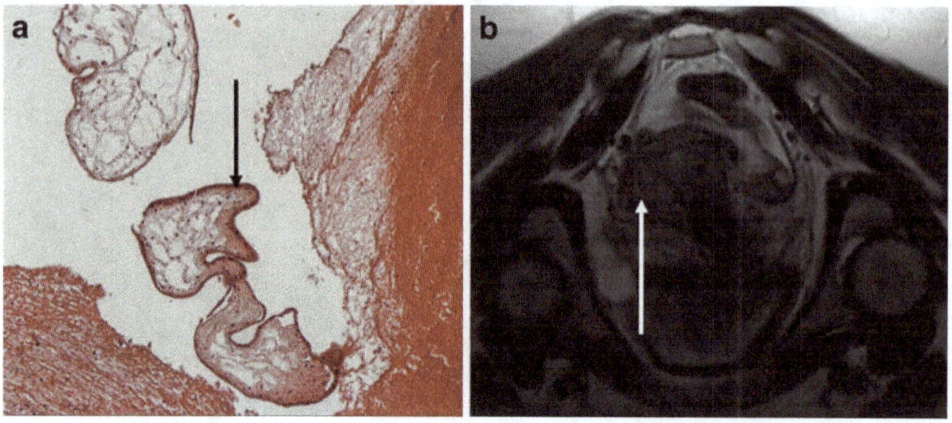

Fig. 3 **a** Histology (HES, ×10) confirmed the presence of blood clots with necrotic placental villi (*black arrow*). **b** T2-weighted MRI image performed 3 months after laparoscopy, showing complete healing of the right myometrial wall

Table 1 Therapies for intramyometrial pregnancies

	Number of patients	Past history	Diagnosis	Treatment	Outcome
Ginsburg et al. [5]	1	Adenomyosis	16 week pregnancy with hemoperitoneum and suspected uterine rupture	Laparotomic hysterectomy	–
Katano et al. [12]	1	1 D/C for a partial mole	US and MRI: GS with 22-mm CRL + FHB (−)	Laparoscopy: MTX injection into the GS + 2 US-guided injections of MTX	HCG (−) on 19th POD, HSG: pooling of contrast medium in the region of intramyometrial pregnancy
Bernstein et al. [10]	1	1 D/C + 1 spontaneous abortion	Transabdominal US: GS with a yolk sac Diagnostic laparoscopy	–	Spontaneous HCG (−) on 10th POD, HSG: small endometrial polyp with a moderately arcuate uterus
Lee et al. [15]	1	Right adnexectomy for torsion	US: GS with CRL and yolk sac	Laparotomic enucleation	–
Ko et al. [3]	1	5 D/C (last D/C 4 weeks before)	US and MRI: GS in the posterior wall	Alternating IM MTX and leucovorin for 8 days	HCG (−) after 8 weeks
Park et al. [4]	1	Myomectomy by laparotomy + transfer of 3 embryos	US: GS in subserosal region of the posterior wall with CRL and yolk sac	Laparoscopy: incision, aspiration, and interrupted sutures	HCG (−) on 14th POD, subsequent pregnancy after 4 frozen embryos transferred on 92nd POD + placental invasion of the myometrium
Ong et al. [1]	1	Bilateral endometriomas and adenomyosis	US: GS + CRL 3 mm + FHB (+)	US-guided intrafetal KCl and intra-amniotic MTX injections	HCG (−) on 82nd POD
Leyder et al. [9]	1	Uterine artery embolization for symptomatic uterine fibroids + transfer of 2 embryos	US and MRI	Systemic MTX injection	–
Glass et al. [11]	1	Tuberous sclerosis	US and MRI: GS without CRL, failure of US-guided curettage	Laparoscopy + laparotomic enucleation due to hemoperitoneum and size of the mass	–
Nabeshima et al. [14]	1	Left salpingectomy for ectopic tubal pregnancy and 1 C/S	US: GS + FHB (+)	Laparoscopy: myometrial injection of vasopression + section with Harmonic® scalpel + excision of surrounding myometrium + running suture + fibrin glue	HCG (−) on 14th POD, HSG: no change compared with before pregnancy
Present study	1	Spontaneous abortion without D/C	US and MRI Diagnostic laparoscopy	Laparoscopy: CO_2 laser section + no excision of myometrium + 2-layer running suture	Low HCG after first diagnostic laparoscopy, complete healing of the myometrium after second laparoscopy

D/C dilatation–curettage, *US* ultrasound, *GS* gestational sac, *CRL* crown-rump length, *FHB* fetal heartbeat, *MTX* methotrexate, *POD* postoperative day, *HSG* hysterosalpingography, *C/S* cesarean section, *KCl* potassium chloride pregnancy after an embryo transfer following uterine artery embolization [9], and Glass et al. described a case in a woman with tuberous sclerosis [11]. In our case, there was no previous uterine surgery or previous intrauterine manipulation and no sinus tract was found during hysteroscopy. This supports the theory of uterine wall invasion by placenta accreta and subsequent growth of the fetus deep in the myometrium, as described by Bernstein et al. [10].

Differential diagnosis based on 2D ultrasound remains difficult and may suggest a number of possibilities, including interstitial or cornual ectopic pregnancy, degenerating myoma, pregnancy in a congenitally abnormal uterus [1], sarcoma or molar pregnancy [11], or unruptured intramyometrial pregnancy.

The use of pelvic MRI allows visualization of multiple scan planes and helps to define the distance between the intramyometrial pregnancy and the uterine cavity [1, 3, 11, 12]. Ko et al. proposed MRI to distinguish an unruptured intramyometrial pregnancy, which looks like a homogeneous hyperintense mass on T2-weighted images, from a ruptured one, that shows a heterogeneous signal intensity on T2-weighted images. On the other hand, contrast-enhanced T1-weighted images show tree-like, solid components resulting from hemorrhages at various times [3]. In our case, T2-weighted views revealed a heterogeneous mass, but T1-weighted views showed a more homogeneous mass with only few remaining spots of contrast enhancement.

Treatment proposed in the literature differs and depends on the need to preserve future fertility. With enhancement by ultrasound and MRI, conservative medical treatment and conservative surgical treatment are options. All described therapies for intramyometrial pregnancies in the literature are summarized in Table 1.

Conservative medical management can be achieved using systemic intramuscular administration of methotrexate [13] or ultrasound-guided methotrexate injection into the chorionic cavity of patients with an intramyometrial pregnancy without a fetal heartbeat [12, 13]. Intra-amniotic injection of methotrexate can also be associated with intrafetal injection of potassium chloride in case of intramyometrial pregnancy with the presence of a fetal heartbeat [1].

Laparoscopic treatment with opening of the surrounding myometrium and suture by interrupted stitches was performed in a patient with an intramyometrial pregnancy in a myomectomy scar [4] and another who had undergone previous left salpingectomy [14]. Enucleation by laparotomy was also carried out for intramyometrial pregnancy after right adnexectomy [15] and due to massive hemoperitoneum [11].

Ginsburg et al. reported a case of suspected uterine rupture at 16 gestational weeks with hemoperitoneum. Hysterectomy was performed, and pathological examination showed the presence of an intramyometrial pregnancy [5].

In our case, despite a low HCG level, the patient still felt pain at vaginal examination. This led us to perform pelvic MRI, which was unable to differentiate between adenomyoma, necrotic leiomyoma, and intramyometrial pregnancy.

The low HCG level did not exclude uterine rupture. It can be compared to some ectopic pregnancies that occur with negative HCG levels. Ectopic pregnancy is due to growth of trophoblasts into the tubal mucosa that can cause erosion of tubal vessels, resulting in hematoma formation and tubal swelling. The persistence of ectopic pregnancy without rupture may lead, in some cases, to degeneration of trophoblasts and cessation of HCG production. Spontaneous abortion or repeated minor bleeding episodes in this type of chronic ectopic pregnancy can cause subsequent rupture associated with hemoperitoneum, with low or negative HCG levels [16]. Uterine conservative surgery was thus mandatory in our patient, with successful complete healing of the intramyometrial pregnancy site.

Conclusion

Intramyometrial ectopic pregnancy is a rare life-threatening entity. Our case suggests that spontaneous intramyometrial pregnancy can occur without any previous uterine surgery or intrauterine manipulation. Because of the paucity of cases described in the literature, diagnosis remains difficult and treatment tends to be conservative. Our case suggests that even in case of negative HCG levels, we cannot exclude ruptured intramyometrial pregnancy, and laparoscopic excision can be performed without damaging uterine wall integrity.

References

1. Ong C, Su LL, Chia D, Choolani M, Biswas A (2010) Sonographic diagnosis and successful medical management of an intramural ectopic pregnancy. J Clin Ultrasound 38(6):320–324
2. Pijnenborg R, Vercruysse L, Brosens I (2011) Deep placentation. Best Pract Res Clin Obstet Gynaecol 25(3):273–285
3. Ko HS, Lee Y, Lee HJ, Park IY, Chung DY, Kim SP, Park TC, Shin JC (2006) Sonographic and MR findings in 2 cases of intramural pregnancy treated conservatively. J Clin Ultrasound 34:356–360
4. Park WI, Jeon YM, Lee JY, Shin SY (2006) Subserosal pregnancy in a previous myomectomy site: a variant of intramural pregnancy. J Min Inv Gynecol 13:242–244
5. Ginsburg KA, Quereshi F, Thomas M, Snowman B (1989) Intramural ectopic pregnancy implanting in adenomyosis. Fertil Steril 51:354–356
6. Karakök M, Balat O, Sari I, Kocer NE, Erdogan R (2002) Early diagnosed intramural ectopic pregnancy associated with adenomyosis: report of an unusual case. Clin Exp Obstet Gynecol 29 (3):217–218

7. Hamilton CJ, Legarth J, Jaroudi KA (1992) Intramural pregnancy after in vitro fertilization and embryo transfer. Fertil Steril 57:215–217
8. Khalifa Y, Redgement CJ, Yazdani N, Taranissi M, Craft IL (1994) Intramural pregnancy following difficult embryo transfer. Hum Reprod 9:2427–2428
9. Leyder M, De Vos M, Popovic-Todorovic B, Dujardin M, Devroey P, Fatemi HM (2010) Intramyometrial ectopic pregnancy in an ICSI patient following uterine artery embolization. Reprod Biomed Online 20(6):831–835
10. Bernstein HB, Thrall MM, Clark WB (2001) Expectant management of intramural ectopic pregnancy. Obstet Gynecol 97:826–827
11. Glass T, Smith P, Hodges R, Holmes HJ (2010) Intramural pregnancy presenting in a patient with tuberous sclerosis. J Clin Ultrasound 38(7):393–396
12. Katano K, Ikuta K, Matsubara H, Oya N, Nishio M, Suzumori K (1999) A case of successful conservative chemotherapy for intramural pregnancy. Fertil Steril 72(4):744–746
13. Haimov-Kochman R, Sciaky-Tamir Y, Yanai N, Yagel S (2002) Conservative management of two ectopic pregnancies implanted in previous uterine scars. Ultrasound Obstet Gynecol 19(6):616–619
14. Nabeshima H, Nishimoto M, Utsunomiya H, Arai M, Ugajin T, Terada Y, Yaegashi N (2010) Total laparoscopic conservative surgery for an intramural ectopic pregnancy. Diagn Ther Endosc 2010:504062. Epub 2010 Oct 11
15. Lee GS, Hur SY, Kown I, Shin JC, Kim SP, Kim SJ (2005) Diagnosis of early intramural ectopic pregnancy. J Clin Ultrasound 33(4):190–192
16. Brennan DF, Kwatra S, Kelly M, Dunn M (2000) Chronic ectopic pregnancy—two cases of acute rupture despite negative beta HCG. J Emerg Med 19(3):249–254

16

Manual vacuum aspiration under local anaesthetic for early miscarriage: 2 years experience in a university teaching hospital in UK

Vinod Kumar · Jonathan Chester · Janesh Gupta · Manjeet Shehmar

Abstract Manual vacuum aspiration under local anaesthesia (MVA-LA) in an outpatient setting is an alternative to the standard surgical aspiration under general anaesthesia for miscarriage. We evaluate the feasibility, safety and clinical outcomes of MVA-LA in the management of miscarriage at less than 12 weeks of gestation in an outpatient setting. This prospective cohort study was conducted at the Birmingham Women's Hospital. One hundred and thirty-one women with ultrasound scan confirmed incomplete or missed miscarriage underwent MVA-LA between November 2010 and January 2013. A computer database was used to record relevant information. The mean gestation age was 8.3 weeks (±1.8). Successful evacuation was achieved in 100 % of cases. One hundred and fourteen (87 %) patients underwent the procedure with direct intracervical LA block and the remaining cases did not have LA. There were no reported complications in 96 % of procedures. Cervical injury and vasovagal symptoms noted in 3.8 % of cases. In all cases, vaginal bleeding was minimal or mild. The post-operative pain was controlled successfully with a combination of paracetamol and diclofenac in 82 % of patients. The MVA method was associated with high levels (93 %) of patient satisfaction and acceptability. MVA-LA in an outpatient setting is a safe and acceptable therapeutic option for women diagnosed with early missed or incomplete miscarriage.

Keywords Vacuum curettage/methods · Early pregnancy loss · Manual vacuum aspiration · Early miscarriage management · Surgical evacuation

Background

In 2009, over 45,000 of 900,000 pregnancies ended with miscarriage in England and Wales [1, 2]. In the UK, current guidelines provide several options for the management of miscarriage; expectantly by awaiting spontaneous expulsion of the remaining products, medically with misoprostol or surgically by evacuation of the uterus [3, 4]. Expectant and medical management have good efficacy rates of 70–80 % [5] although these methods are proved to be less acceptable to women [6, 7]; 88 % of women are managed through surgical methods, mainly electric vacuum aspiration (EVA) under general anaesthesia (GA) [8, 9]. However, an alternative method now exists, in the form of manual vacuum aspiration (MVA).

Unlike EVA, MVA is a light-weight, quiet, inexpensive syringe which can be used under local anaesthetic in a clinic or ward environment and does not require electricity, which makes it especially useful in emergencies. Many studies have shown MVA to be comparable to EVA in efficacy and rates of complications, such as uterine bleeding and perforation [10–14]. Data from a cost analysis study has shown that MVA performed in the ambulatory setting is significantly less expensive than EVA performed under GA [15]. Despite the proven benefits, MVA under local anaesthesia (LA) is still underused in the United Kingdom [14, 16, 17].

Given the current economic climate and the benefits shown in previous studies, a service was set up in November

V Kumar and J Chester have contributed equally to this research.

V. Kumar (✉)
University Hospitals Birmingham NHS Foundation Trust, Birmingham, UK
e-mail: vinodkumar1@nhs.net

J. Chester
Good Hope Hospital, Birmingham, UK

J. Gupta · M. Shehmar
Birmingham Women's NHS Foundation Trust, Birmingham, UK

2010 at Birmingham Women's Hospital. MVA under LA was offered in the outpatient setting to women following an incomplete or early miscarriage within the first 12 weeks of gestation. The aim of this study was to assess the feasibility, safety and clinical outcomes of MVA under LA in the outpatient setting.

Methods

This prospective cohort study was carried out between November 2010 and January 2013. All women, with ultrasound scan (USS) confirmed incomplete or early missed miscarriage at less than 12 weeks of gestation, were offered the MVA procedure under LA as an option for the management of miscarriage. Exclusion criteria included suspected septic miscarriage, known uterine anomalies, molar pregnancy, multiple pregnancy and previous cervical knife cone treatment.

Written consent was obtained by the operating surgeon on the gynaecological ward prior to the procedure. All patients were given the option of further intra-operative analgesia or Entonox® (50 % nitrous oxide and 50 % oxygen; BOC Healthcare, Manchester, UK) should they require it.

As the procedure was performed under local anaesthetic, there was no need to fast beforehand. Therefore, all elective patients were encouraged to eat and drink before the procedure to reduce the incidence of hypoglycaemia and vasovagal episodes [18]. As per protocol, all women were administered 800 μg of vaginal misoprostol (Pharmacia Ltd. Milton Keynes, UK) for cervical priming at least 2 h before the procedure. All patients had a full blood count and group and save measured before the procedure except in emergency cases.

The procedure was mostly performed electively in the outpatient setting by two hospital consultants in the early pregnancy assessment unit (EPAU). However, in emergency situations of heavy haemorrhage with cardiovascular compromise, the procedure was carried out in the gynaecology ward treatment room, accident and emergency (A&E) or in an operating theatre. Pre-procedure vaginal misoprostol was not administered in emergency situations.

During the MVA, every effort was made to keep the procedure room a relaxed and comfortable environment. One dedicated registered nurse and one health care assistant (HCA) were present to support the clinician performing the procedure. The patient was positioned on a couch in a lithotomy position and a HCA stood beside her to offer psychological support (Vocal Local) and Entonox if required.

The clinician visualised the cervix, cleaned it with antiseptic solution (Unisept®) and applied a single tooth volsellum to stabilise the anterior lip of cervix. The LA consisted of a direct intracervical block using 6.6 ml 3 % mepivacaine hydrochloride (Scandonest, Septodont ltd.) infiltration deep at the cervical isthmus level at 12, 3, 5, 6, 7, and 9 o'clock positions using dental needle (Solo Supra). The cervix was dilated to a minimum of 7 mm and the MVA curette of 6 to 9 mm was introduced into the uterine cavity to commence the aspiration using a 60-ml self-locking syringe (Ipas MVA Plus® aspirator). Typically, the MVA procedure consisted of no more than three separate suction events, initially rotating the syringe and then finishing with an in and out motion, lasting in total between 60 s to 2 min. The products retrieved were sent to pathology for histopathology evaluation.

Immediately, post-procedure, 50–100 mg diclofenac and 1 g paracetamol were given rectally for pain relief. When patients could not be prescribed diclofenac due to contraindications then co-dydramol two tablets or Tramadol 100 mg was given orally. In all emergency cases, IV morphine was given in a titrated 5-mg bolus dose up to a maximum of 20-mg dose with Entonox®.

Anti-D prophylaxis was administered to all Rhesus negative women. Oxygen saturation monitoring was carried out for at least 2 h prior to discharge in women who underwent emergency MVA and had IV morphine. Patients were usually discharged within 2 h of the procedure. All women were advised to rest for the remainder of the day and were advised to return to work usually within 24–48 h.

On discharge, the patient was given the ward's contact number, in case of problems, and analgesia in the form of diclofenac or co-dydramol. The patient was instructed to do a urine pregnancy test 2 weeks after the procedure. No follow-up was specifically arranged. The patient was instructed to get in contact if experiencing heavy bleeding, pyrexia, severe abdominal pain, abnormal vaginal discharge or had a positive pregnancy test.

A computer database was used to record relevant information relating to the procedure. Data was collected immediately post-procedure and updated once the patient was discharged. Recorded data included any post procedural complications and analgesia requirements by the operating clinician. Patient experience was evaluated in a sample of patients using an anonymous questionnaire survey on the gynaecology ward by the staff nurses over a 2-month period (n=28). This included questions on acceptability, anxiety and pain before and after the procedure and free comments. The collected data was then analysed using SPSS (version 16, IBM SPSS Statistics).

Findings

A total of 131 women with USS confirmed early miscarriage at less than 12 weeks of completed gestation or incomplete miscarriage underwent the MVA procedure. The majority of procedures were carried out in a dedicated outpatient setting in EPAU (82 %) whilst a minority in the gynaecology ward

(13.0 %), theatre (4.6 %) whilst piloting the service, and A&E (0.8 %) for emergency procedures.

The mean gestation age was 8.3 weeks (±1.8 weeks) (Table 1). The seven patients that had MVA at gestation greater than 12 weeks were patients with an incomplete miscarriage.

The majority of patients (87.0 %) required an LA cervical block for the procedure. Most patients were managed immediately post operatively with diclofenac and/or paracetamol combination (81.7 %). Only four patients required the use of anti-emetics immediately post-procedure.

Vaginal misoprostol for cervical priming was administered in all elective missed miscarriage patients. Of the 127 patients with results recorded, 71 (54.2 %) had an open cervical os at the time of procedure and only 16 (22.5 %) required further cervical dilation.

All women had a successful evacuation of the uterus. Only five (3.8 %) cases had intra-operative complications; two with vasovagal symptoms, two with cervical injury and one with suspected uterine perforation which was managed with a short course of antibiotics and no further intervention was required. There were no major, life threatening or fatal complications. All patients reported minimal or mild vaginal bleeding after the procedure. None of the patients required a blood transfusion. All patients were managed as a day case.

Data about procedure acceptability and experience are shown in Table 2. The majority (82 %) reported that procedure duration was shorter or as expected; 68 % said they would recommend this option to a friend, and 61 % stated that they would choose this method again. Level of pain during the procedure was satisfactory with only 11 % reported unbearable pain which settled after the procedure.

Table 1 Results of women managed with MVA-LA in an outpatient setting for early miscarriage, $n=131$ (*n percentage*)

Indication for MVA	
Missed miscarriage	112 (85 %)
Incomplete miscarriage	19 (15 %)
Mean gestation age by USS (weeks)	
<9	91 (70 %)
9–12	33 (25 %)
>12	7 (5 %)
Intra-operative analgesia (some patients required multiple analgesics)	
Cervical block LA	114 (87 %)
None	21 (16 %)
Morphine	12 (9 %)
Entonox®	6 (5 %)
Cervical dilatation required	
Yes	72 (55 %)
No	55 (42 %)
Not recorded	4 (3 %)
Intra-operative complications	
None	126 (96 %)
Uterine perforation (suspected)	1 (1 %)
Severe haemorrhage	0 (0 %)
Cervical injury	2 (2 %)
Vasovagal	2 (2 %)
Post-operative analgesia (some patients required multiple drugs)	
Diclofenac and paracetamol	107 (82 %)
Codeine	4 (3 %)
Morphine/pethidine	8 (6 %)
Entonox®	18 (14 %)
None	10 (8 %)
Post-operative complications	
None reported	129 (98 %)
RPOC	1 (1 %)
USS to confirm complete evacuation	1 (1 %)

MVA-LA manual vacuum aspiration under local anaesthesia, *USS* ultrasound scan, *RPOC* retained products of conception

Table 2 Post procedure responses to questionnaire about acceptability and experience with MVA under LA, $n=28$ (data showed in percentage (number of patients))

Overall experience (as compared to what was expected)			
Much better	61 %		
A bit better	14 %		
As expected	18 %		
Worse	0 %		
No reply	7 %		
Procedure duration?			
As expected	82 %		
Longer	14 %		
No answer	4 %		
Happy to recommend?			
Yes	68 %		
No	21 %		
Don't know	11 %		
Choose the method again?			
Yes	61 %		
No	11 %		
Don't know	29 %		
	During procedure	At 1 h	At discharge
Patients with anxiety (%)			
None	14 %	46 %	54 %
Moderate	61 %	50 %	39 %
Severe	25 %	4 %	0 %
No reply	0 %	0 %	7 %
Patients with pain (%)			
None	18 %	18 %	39 %
Moderate	68 %	79 %	54 %
Severe	11 %	4 %	0 %
No reply	3 %	0 %	7 %

Table 3 Characteristics of studies investigating the use of MVA in the management of early pregnancy loss

Study	Study period	Study design	Participants	Setting	Interventions	Comparison	Conclusions
Blumenthal and Remsburg [15]	1990–1992	Open, serial, quasi-experimental	35 women with first trimester incomplete abortions	OT, ER or LW, USA	Outpatient MVA under sedation using Fentanyl or Midazolam	Electrical suction curettage in OT	Significant reduction in both procedure time (42 %) and costs (41 %) with MVA
Egziabher et al. [22]	1997	Double blind RCT	142 women with incomplete miscarriage	Health Centre, Nairobi	MVA under paracervical block with 1 % lignocaine (LA)	MVA under paracervical block with sterile water	LA significantly reduced pain during MVA
Gazvani et al. [14]	1998–2000	Prospective	57 women with first trimester miscarriage	OT, UK	MVA under systemic analgesia using IV Alfentanil or Midazolam	MVA under patient controlled sedation	No significant differences in MVA success and acceptability rates (100 %) between the anaesthetic techniques
Edwards et al. [10]	2002–2004	RCT, multicenter, non inferiority	157 women with first trimester miscarriage	OT, ER USA	MVA under LA	EVA under GA or spinal anaesthesia	MVA success rate 97 % vs. EVA 95.2 %, MVA acceptability 70 % vs. EVA 77 %
Milingos et al. [17]	2003–2005	Retrospective observational study	245 women with first trimester miscarriage	EPAU, UK	MVA under LA	None	MVA success rate 94.7 %
Tasnim et al. [23]	2007–2008	RCT	176 women with early pregnancy failure	OT, Pakistan	MVA under paracervical block	EVA under GA	MVA success rate 90 % vs. EVA 91 %, Significant less blood loss, shorter hospital stay and reduced cost with MVA
Kinariwala et al. [24]	2011–2012	Retrospective case series	9 women with early pregnancy failure	A&E, USA	MVA under paracervical 1 % lidocaine, IV and oral analgesia	None	MVA success rate 100 %

MVA manual vacuum aspiration, *OT* operation theatres, *ER* outpatient emergency or procedure room, *LW* labour ward, *RCT* randomised controlled trial, *LA* local anaesthetic, *IV* intravenous, *EVA* electric vacuum aspiration, *GA* general anaesthesia, *EPAU* early pregnancy assessment unit, *A&E* accident and emergency

Discussion

The data from our study suggest that MVA under LA can be successfully used for the management of confirmed early missed or incomplete miscarriages in an outpatient setting.

The procedure was introduced in our hospital with the aim of providing a safe, effective and value-for-money alternative to other methods of surgical management, which increased convenience and reduced recovery time. Milingos et al. [17], in a retrospective observational study, showed that the procedure was effective in 95 % cases with no major complications and our experiences from the first 2 years of its use support these findings. The procedure was completed successfully in all cases and there were no major complications in our cohort.

Cervical priming with vaginal misoprostol before MVA has shown to significantly reduce the need for cervical dilation and improve the efficacy of the procedure [19]. For many of the elective patients in the study, the use of misoprostol alone before procedure was enough to ensure that the cervix was dilated, allowing safer evacuation by minimising cervical trauma related to instrumental dilation and reducing the discomfort of cervical dilation.

MVA is a procedure in which most of the patients experience a moderate level of pain [20]; however, local anaesthesia in the form of a cervical block provides effective pain control ensuring MVA is a quick, inexpensive and the preferred alternative to other surgical methods requiring GA [20]. For many patients in our study, vaginal misoprostol and LA to the cervix (if required) was adequate to complete the procedure. It is important, however, to ensure that the level of pain relief can be increased if required during the evacuation and this can be achieved with the use of Entonox® and/or IV morphine.

Although further research is needed to examine acceptability of MVA among users, findings of our survey indicate that women's perceptions and experiences with MVA are favourable. Women often feel nervous about undergoing uterine evacuation under LA, and their anxiety aggravates their perception of pain. Conversely, women who feel less anxious are less likely to perceive pain. Therefore the role of a nurse or HCA to psychologically support the patient cannot be undermined as it is important that the patient's attention is diverted during the procedure (Vocal Local). We are currently studying patients' acceptability of MVA in a trial involving patient questionnaire and interviews of their experience.

Although women were not followed up after their discharge, all women were given the ward's contact number in case of any problems and were advised to contact on a 24-h basis. However, there is a possibility that a few patients may have seen their local GPs with minor problems and these would have been missed in the data analysis.

The World Health Organization (WHO) has listed MVA as an effective and safe method of surgical management of miscarriage [21], however it remains underused in the UK [14, 16, 17] (Table 3).

The unfamiliarity of this method and lack of confidence among clinicians when counselling women about options of surgical evacuation may be the contributing factor of its infrequent use in the UK. Given the current economic climate and the benefits shown by our study, it is an option that requires further consideration as a more efficient alternative method of surgical evacuation. MVA-LA for evacuation of early miscarriage is an ideal procedure to be taken into the ambulatory outpatient setting. Although the procedure was mostly performed by two hospital consultants in our study, this simple and mostly complication-free procedure can be easily performed by trainees under direct or indirect supervision as the learning curve for this is a simple procedure.

Our data suggest that MVA-LA can be a feasible and effective therapeutic alternative to conventional suction curettage options in the management of first trimester pregnancy losses. It may result in considerable improvements in patient care and patient choices who do not wish for a general anaesthesia or prolonged conservative/medical treatment, and substantial savings for health service. However, these findings now need to be assessed in the context of randomised trials comparing MVA-LA with other conventional suction curettage methods for managing early pregnancy loss.

Conclusions

The outcome data of MVA under LA for early pregnancy loss are consistent with previously published studies. The results are favourable and MVA-LA for early pregnancy loss could be a safe, efficient and acceptable alternative to surgical management methods under GA. However, a well-designed randomised controlled trial is required to confirm these findings. This easily performed procedure can be undertaken in a variety of outpatient settings. Moreover, it is efficient, safe, provides better patient experience and increases patient's choice, making it suitable to respond to current healthcare needs.

Conflict of interest On behalf of all authors, the corresponding author states that there is no conflict of interest.

References

1. Office of National Statistics (2011) Conception in England and Wales 2009. Office of National Statistics [Online]. Available at http://www.ons.gov.uk/ons/rel/vsob1/conception-statistics–england-and-wales/2009/index.html. Accessed 11 March 2013

2. Hospital Episode Statitistics (2010) Total deliveries, miscarriages and ectopic pregnancies per 100 deliveries, 1997–98 to 2009–10. Hospital Episode Statistics [Online]. Available at http://www.hesonline.nhs.uk/Ease/servlet/ContentServer?siteID=1937&categoryID=1064. Accessed 11 March 2013
3. Trinder J, Brocklehurst P, Porter R et al (2006) Management of miscarriage: expectant, medical, or surgical? Results of randomised controlled trial (miscarriage treatment (MIST) trial). BMJ 332(7552):1235–1240
4. Ankum WM, Wieringa-De Waard M, Bindels PJ (2001) Management of spontaneous miscarriage in the first trimester: an example of putting informed shared decision making into practice. BMJ 322(7298):1343–1346
5. Shelley JM, Healy D, Grover S (2005) A randomised trial of surgical, medical and expectant management of first trimester spontaneous miscarriage. Aust N Z J Obstet Gynaecol 45(2):122–127
6. Petrou S, McIntosh E (2009) Women's preferences for attributes of first-trimester miscarriage management: a stated preference discrete-choice experiment. Value Health 12(4):551–559
7. Ryan M, Hughes J (1997) Using conjoint analysis to assess women's preferences for miscarriage management. Health Econ 6:261–273
8. Kulier R, Fekih A, Hofmeyr GJ et al (2001) Surgical methods for first trimester termination of pregnancy. Cochrane Database Syst Rev 4(CD002900)
9. Bradley E, Hamilton-Fairley D (1998) Managing miscarriage in early pregnancy assessment units. Hosp Med 59:451–456
10. Edwards S, Tureck R, Fredrick M et al (2007) Patient acceptability of manual versus electric vacuum aspiration for early pregnancy loss. J Womens Health (Larchmt) 16(10):1429–1436
11. Wen J, Cai QY, Deng F, Li YP (2008) Manual versus electric vacuum aspiration for first-trimester abortion: a systematic review. BJOG 115(1):5–13
12. Bird ST, Harvey SM, Beckman LJ et al (2003) Similarities in women's perceptions and acceptability of manual vacuum aspiration and electric vacuum aspiration for first trimester abortion. Contraception 67(3):207–212
13. Westfall JM, Sophocles A, Burggraf H et al (1998) Manual vacuum aspiration for first-trimester abortion. Arch Fam Med 7(6):559–562
14. Gazvani R, Honey E, MacLennan FM et al (2004) Manual vacuum aspiration (MVA) in the management of first trimester pregnancy loss. European Journal of Obstetrics & Gynecology and Reproductive Biology 112(2):197–200
15. Blumenthal PD, Remsburg RE (1994) A time and cost analysis of the management of incomplete abortion with manual vacuum aspiration. Int J Gynaecol Obstet 45(3):261–267
16. Dean G, Cardenas L, Darney P et al (2003) Acceptability of manual versus electric aspiration for first trimester abortion: a randomized trial. Contraception 67(3):201–206
17. Milingos DS, Mathur M, Smith NT et al (2009) Manual vacuum aspiration: a safe alternative for the surgical management of early pregnancy loss. BJOG 116(9):1268–1271
18. Clark TJ, Gupta JK (2005) Handbook of outpatient hysteroscopy: a complete guide to diagnosis and therapy. Hodder Arnold, London
19. Mittal S, Sehgal R, Aggarwal S et al (2011) Cervical priming with misoprostol before manual vacuum aspiration versus electric vacuum aspiration for first-trimester surgical abortion. Int J Gynaecol Obstet 112(1):34–39
20. López JC, Vigil-De Gracia P, Vega-Malek JC et al (2007) A randomized comparison of different methods of analgesia in abortion using manual vacuum aspiration. Int J Gynaecol Obstet 99(2):91–94
21. World Health Organization (1991) Essential elements of obstetric care at first referral level. Geneva: WHO. Available at http://whqlibdoc.who.int/publications/1991/9241544244.pdf. Accessed 11 March 2013
22. Egziabher TG, Ruminjo JK, Sekadde-Kigondu C (2002) Pain relief using paracervical block in patients undergoing manual vacuum aspiration of uterus. East Afr Med J 79(10):530–534
23. Tasnim N, Mahmud G, Fatima S et al (2011) Manual vacuum aspiration: a safe and cost-effective substitute of electric vacuum aspiration for the surgical management of early pregnancy loss. J Pak Med Assoc 61(2):149–153
24. Kinariwala M, Quinley KE, Datner EM et al (2013) Manual vacuum aspiration in the emergency department for management of early pregnancy failure. Am J Emerg Med 31(1):244–247

17

Transvaginal cystocele repair using tension-free polypropylene mesh at the time of sacrospinous colpopexy for advanced uterovaginal prolapse

Ayman Qatawneh · Fawaz Al-Kazaleh · Shawqi Saleh · Fida Thekrallah · Majed Bata · Issa Sumreen · Mahmoud Al-Mustafa

Abstract The management of an advanced multi-compartment prolapse requires a combination of techniques. The objective of this study was to report the anatomical outcomes of a prospective randomised trial comparing tension-free polypropylene mesh-reinforced anterior vaginal prolapse with anterior colporrhaphy at the time sacrospinous colpopexy and posterior fascial plication for the management of massive uterovaginal prolapse. A total of 116 patients with a stage III or IV (Pelvic Organ Prolapse Quantification System/International Continence Society) uterovaginal prolapse were randomised into two groups. The mesh group includes transvaginal cystocele repair using a tension-free polypropylene mesh, while the non-mesh group includes anterior colporrhaphy. All patients in the two groups underwent a sacrospinous colpopexy and posterior fascial plication. The primary outcome was objective success < stage 2 prolapse. The secondary outcomes were reoperation for recurrent prolapse, subjective success rates, patient satisfaction with the surgery and complications. The overall objective success rates (in all compartments) were 79 % (42/53) in the mesh group and 62 % (39/63) in the non-mesh group (p=0.043). The objective success rates in the anterior compartment were 85 % (45/53) in the mesh group and 62 % (39/63) in the non-mesh group (p=0.006). Three (6 %) patients in the mesh group and 12 (19 %) in the non-mesh group underwent repeat surgery for recurrent pelvic organ prolapse (p=0.03). The subjective success rates were 89 % (47/53) in the mesh group and 76 % (48/63) in the non-mesh group (p value=0.08). The mean patient satisfaction rates with the surgery were 84 % in the mesh group and 76 % in the non-mesh group (p=0.08). The development of a urinary tract infection, right-sided buttock pain (temporary sciatic neuralgia) and new-onset stress urinary incontinence were not significantly different between the two groups. The mesh exposure rate was 8 %. Transvaginal cystocele repair using tension-free polypropylene mesh at the time of sacrospinous colpopexy and posterior fascial plication offers lower anatomic recurrence and less need for further prolapse surgery to correct recurrent pelvic floor defects than anterior colporrhaphy, sacrospinous colpopexy and posterior fascial plication.

Keywords Uterovaginal prolapse · Sacrospinous ligament fixation · Cystocele · Anterior vaginal wall repair · Mesh · Polypropylene

Background

The management of multi-compartment advanced pelvic organ prolapse (POP) remains a major challenge for gynaecologists. It is estimated that a woman has an 11 % lifetime risk of undergoing a surgical procedure for the correction of pelvic floor dysfunction with almost one third of such women requiring a repeat operation either due to the failure of the first operation or due to the prolapse of another compartment [1]. Transvaginal sacrospinous ligament fixation is a widely used procedure for massive uterovaginal prolapse that is usually performed concomitantly with a

A. Qatawneh (✉) · F. Al-Kazaleh · S. Saleh · F. Thekrallah · M. Bata · I. Sumreen
Department of Obstetrics and Gynaecology, Faculty of Medicine, The University of Jordan,
PO Box 13046, Amman 11942, Jordan
e-mail: aymenfida@yahoo.com

M. Al-Mustafa
Department of Anaesthesia, Faculty of Medicine, The University of Jordan,
Amman, Jordan

vaginal hysterectomy [2]. The procedure has a variable success rate but is known to lead to anterior vaginal wall prolapse [3].

Recent randomised controlled trials have demonstrated that the use of synthetic mesh at the anterior compartment is superior to anterior colporrhaphy in reducing the risk of recurrent anterior vaginal wall prolapse [4, 5]. de Tayrac et al. reported a low recurrence rate of anterior vaginal wall prolapse with the use of tension-free polypropylene mesh after 5 years of follow-up [6].

The combined use of anterior trans-obturator mesh (Perigee®, AMS) and sacrospinous ligament fixation for apical support and fascial repairs for posterior compartments in treating massive urogenital prolapse has been shown to effectively restore the anatomy and achieve favourable pelvic function 30 months postoperatively [7]. A combination of anterior vaginal mesh (Gynecare Prolift™), sacrospinous hysteropexy and posterior fascial plication has also been reported to effectively restore the anatomy and achieve favourable bladder, bowel and sexual function in a prospective study with a 12-month follow-up for women with anterior compartment-dominated uterovaginal prolapse [8].

To our knowledge, no prospective randomised trials have compared the use of native tissue repair versus the use of anterior vaginal wall tension-free polypropylene monofilament mesh at the time of sacrospinous colpopexy and posterior fascial placation to treat massive uterovaginal prolapse. The purpose of this study, therefore, was to evaluate the anatomical outcomes and reoperation rates following anterior vaginal wall mesh (Gynemesh™, PS) augmentation versus traditional anterior repair using native tissues with concomitant sacrospinous ligament fixation and posterior fascial plication in cases of massive uterovaginal prolapse.

Subjects and methods

The study group included women attending the Department of Obstetrics and Gynaecology at Jordan University Hospital (JUH), Amman, Jordan, for symptomatic uterovaginal prolapse or vaginal vault prolapse between January 2005 and January 2010.

All women with severe symptomatic pelvic organ prolapse (i.e. uterine or vaginal vault prolapse of stages III and IV according to the International Continence Society (ICS) grading system on maximum Valsalva manoeuvre) were eligible to take part in the study [9]. Women who had less than a stage III prolapse of any compartment or previous procedures with implants as a part of pelvic reconstructive surgery were excluded from the study. Other exclusion criteria included a known coagulation disorder, previous pelvic irradiation and women who wished to preserve their uterus. The study protocol was explained to the patients, and a written consent form was signed by all women before taking part in the study. Ethical approval was obtained from the local Ethics Committee at the JUH.

Prior to surgery, the pelvis was evaluated according to the recommendation of the ICS using the ordinal stages of pelvic organ prolapse (POP quantification (POP-Q)) system (grades 0–IV) as has been described [9]. A computer-generated randomisation list was made, and the patients were divided into two groups (mesh vs. non-mesh) as shown in Fig. 1.

Surgical technique

A midline longitudinal incision was made in the vaginal epithelium from the vaginal apex to 2.5 cm from the urethral meatus. This incision was preceded by a vaginal hysterectomy in patients with a uterine prolapse. In women who had previously undergone a hysterectomy, the procedure began with a transverse incision through the vaginal epithelium distal to the cuff. The anterior vaginal wall was sharply dissected from the underlying pubocervical fascia. The dissection was continued laterally in each direction to the pelvic side wall and distally to the level of the urethrovesical junction.

In the non-mesh group, the underlying pubocervical fascia was plicated in the midline with a delayed absorbable 2-0 polydioxanone suture (Ethicon, Somerville, NJ, USA). In the mesh group, the retropubic space was widened using sharp and blunt dissection before plication of the pubocervical fascia as mentioned, and a monofilament polypropylene Gynemesh™ PS (Gynecare, Ethicon Inc., Somerville, NJ, USA) was designed and tailored, leaving two tabs on each side. The mesh used was usually 15 cm long and 3 cm wide and was positioned by placing the tabs into the retropubic space in a tension-free fashion without sutures. The central part of the mesh was drawn down to the lowermost

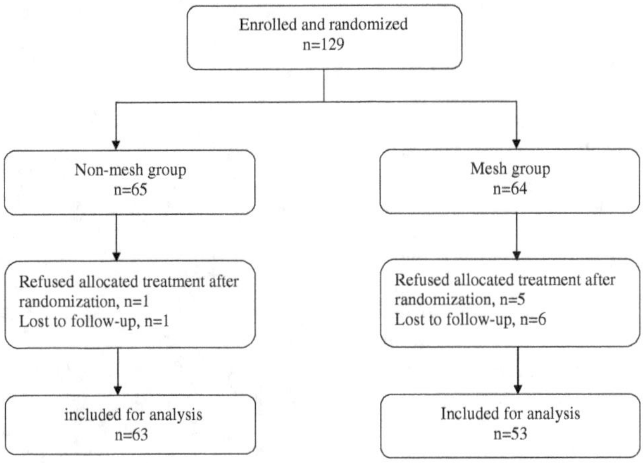

Fig. 1 Patient enrolment, randomisation and analysis

portion of the cystocele; excessive inlaying mesh was trimmed. The mesh was adjusted to avoid any folding and loosely fixed at four points using a 3-0 polyglactin absorbable suture (Vicryl; Ethicon, Somerville, NJ, USA) [10]. The vaginal incision was closed with a continuous 0 polyglactin absorbable suture (Vicryl; Ethicon, Somerville, NJ, USA) as shown in Fig. 2.

In both groups, a sacrospinous colpopexy was performed as previously described [11]. Briefly, a midline incision was performed in the posterior vaginal wall starting from the hymenal ring to the vault to expose the rectovaginal space. The vaginal skin was dissected laterally to expose the pararectal fat. Using the index finger, a window was created between the rectovaginal space and the ischial spine through the right rectal pillar to expose the sacrospinous ligament. A Miya hook ligature carrier was used to insert a triple No. 0 delayed absorbable polydioxanone suture (Ethicon, Somerville, NJ, USA) into the right sacrospinous ligament 2 cm medial to the ischial spine. The rectum was retracted medially using a Breisky–Navratil vaginal retractor, and the sutures were retrieved using a nerve hook. Pulley sutures were created using a no. 4 Mayo needle to ensure good contact between the vaginal skin and the sacrospinous ligament when the sutures were tied. The rectovaginal fascia was plicated in continuity with the perineum, and the vaginal incision was closed as previously described [12]. The PDS sutures were tied, pulling the vault to the sacrospinous ligament. A concomitant TVT-O™ (Ethicon, Somerville, NJ, USA) procedure was performed using a separate incision for patients with urodynamic stress urinary incontinence. Postoperatively, a vaginal pack was placed for 24 h, and a Foley catheter was kept in situ for 24 h. All participants received a preoperative intravenous antibiotic (cefuroxime 1 g) and low-molecular weight heparin as antithrombotic prophylaxis which we routinely give to all patients who underwent pelvic surgery according to the guidelines in our hospital. All procedures were performed under regional or general anaesthesia.

The patient demographics, previous surgeries, preoperative pelvic organ prolapse quantification (POP-Q) and perioperative information including operating time, blood loss, in-hospital stay, length of catheter use, time to return to activities of daily living and complications were collected. A postoperative evaluation occurred at 6 weeks and every 6 months thereafter and included a pelvic examination using the POP-Q grading system performed by an independent investigator. Patient satisfaction was recorded on a 0 to 100 visual analogue scale.

The primary outcome measure of this study was the objective success rate, defined as less than a stage II prolapse at the anterior vaginal wall and in all compartments. The secondary outcome measures included the need for repeat surgery to correct a recurrent prolapse, the subjective success rate (defined as no prolapse sensation), patient satisfaction and complication rates.

Statistical analysis was performed using Statistical Package for the Social Sciences (SPSS) version 15 (SPSS Inc., Chicago, IL, USA). Descriptive statistics were used for the patient demographics and peri-operative data. The continuous variables were compared with the paired t test, and the categorical variables were compared with the $\chi 2$ or McNemar test. A p value <0.05 was considered statistically significant for all comparisons.

The number of patients was calculated by a power analysis using the G-power programme, assuming the type I error to be 5 % and the power to be 80 %. The assumed rates of recurrent prolapse were estimated to be 10 % in the mesh group [6] and 35 % in the non-mesh group [15]. The effect size was estimated to be 0.25, and the dropout rate was estimated to be 10 %. Therefore, it was assumed that 57 patients were needed in each arm of the study.

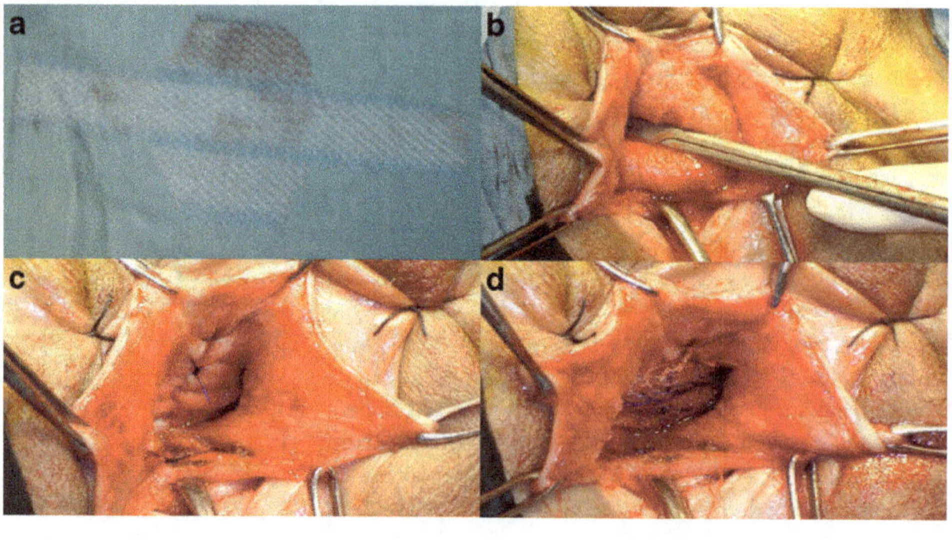

Fig. 2 Transvaginal cystocele repair using a tension-free polypropylene mesh. **a** A monofilament polypropylene mesh was designed and tailored, leaving two tabs on each side. **b** The retropubic space was widened using sharp and blunt dissection. **c** The underlying pubocervical fascia was plicated in the midline with a delayed absorbable 2-0 polydioxanone suture. **d** The mesh was positioned by placing the tabs into the retropubic space in a tension-free fashion

Findings

Overall, 129 patients were recruited into the study, and six dropped out on the day of surgery. Complete pre- and postoperative data were obtained for 116 patients. Seven patients were lost to follow-up. The clinical and demographic characteristics were similar in the two study groups (Table 1).

Overall, a stage II recurrence occurred in 19 % (10/53) of patients in the mesh group and in 24 % (15/63) of patients in the non-mesh group. Only one patient (2 %) developed a stage III prolapse in the mesh group, but 14 % (9/63) of patients developed a stage III prolapse in the non-mesh group. There were no stage IV recurrences in any group. The overall objective success rates (in all compartments) were 79 % (42/53) in the mesh group and 62 % (39/63) in the non-mesh group (p=0.043). A stage II anterior vaginal wall recurrence occurred in 13 % (7/53) of patients in the mesh group and in 24 % (15/63) of patients in the non-mesh group. Only one patient (2 %) in the mesh group developed a stage III anterior vaginal wall recurrence compared to 14 % (9/63) of patients in the non-mesh group. No stage IV anterior vaginal wall recurrences were noted in any of the two groups. The overall objective success rate in the anterior compartment was 85 % (45/53) in the mesh group and 62 % (39/63) in the non-mesh group (p=0.006). The postoperative POP-Q stages for all compartments are summarised in Table 2.

The preoperative POP-Q values were similar in both groups. The preoperative values for the anterior, vaginal cuff and posterior vaginal wall (point Ba, C and Bp) improved significantly after surgery in both groups. Between the study groups, the points Ba and C were significantly shifted proximally in the mesh group (Table 3).

The subjective success rates were 89 % (47/53) in the mesh group and 76 % (48/63) in the non-mesh group (p value=0.08). The mean patient satisfaction with the surgery was 84 % in the mesh group and 76 % in the non-mesh group (p=0.08).

The need for repeat surgery to correct a recurrent prolapse in any compartment during the follow-up period was significantly higher in the non-mesh group (Table 4). Only three (6 %) patients in the mesh group underwent repeat surgery for recurrent pelvic organ prolapse; two involved the anterior and apical compartments, and one involved an isolated rectocele. Conversely, 12 (19 %) patients in the non-mesh group underwent repeat surgery for the anterior and apical compartments; two of the patients also underwent rectocele repair (p=0.03).

The occurrence of a postoperative urinary tract infection and right-sided buttock pain (temporary sciatic neuralgia) which was resolved spontaneously after 2–3 weeks in all cases was not significantly different between the two groups (Table 4).

Mesh exposure was identified in four (8 %) patients and in all cases measured 1 cm or less in diameter and was asymptomatic. All mesh exposures were located under the suture line in the distal anterior vaginal wall. The initial management included topical oestrogen therapy and the

Table 1 Baseline demographic and clinical data of the two study groups

	No-mesh group (n=63)	Mesh group (n=53)	p value
Mean age ± SD (years)	56±10	57±7	0.58
Median (range) parity	6 (1–15)	6 (3–14)	0.69
Mean BMI ± SD (kg/m^2)	30±4	30±3	0.95
Postmenopausal	39 (62)	36 (68)	0.50
Postmenopausal with HRT	6 (10)	6 (11)	0.24
Prior pelvic surgery			
Abdominal hysterectomy	9 (14)	4 (8)	0.50
Vaginal hysterectomy	0 (0)	1 (2)	
Vaginal repair	11 (18)	12 (22)	
Vaginal repair > once	1 (2)	2 (4)	
Overall vaginal POP-Q stage			
Stage III	49 (78)	39 (74)	0.49
Stage IV	14 (22)	14 (26)	
Urodynamic stress urinary incontinence	10 (16)	9 (17)	0.87
Mean operating time ± SD (min)	89±26	88±19	0.85
Mean estimated blood loss ± SD (ml)	267±222	257±205	0.81
Median (range) hospitalisation length (days)	4 (2–9)	4 (2–9)	0.37
Median (range) catheter use (days)	2 (1–8)	2 (1–7)	0.15
Median (range) return to ADL (weeks)	6 (3–10)	6 (3–10)	0.14
Median (range) period of follow-up (months)	29 (6–60)	28 (10–60)	0.58

Data are n (%) unless otherwise specified

SD standard deviation, *BMI* body mass index, *HRT* hormone replacement therapy, *ADL* activities of daily living, *POP-Q* pelvic organ prolapse quantification

Table 2 Overall and compartment-specific pelvic organ prolapse quantification stages at the last follow-up in the two study groups

POP-Q stage	Non-mesh group (n=63)	Mesh group (n=53)	p value
Overall			0.043
Stage 0–I	39 (62)	42 (79)	
Stage II	15 (24)	10 (19)	
Stage II	9 (14)	1 (2)	
Anterior			0.006
Stage 0–I	39 (62)	45 (85)	
Stage II	15 (24)	7 (13)	
Stage III	9 (14)	1 (2)	
Vaginal vault			0.11
Stage 0–I	52 (82)	49 (92)	
Stage II	8 (13)	3 (6)	
Stage III	3 (5)	1 (2)	
Posterior			0.51
Stage 0–I	56 (89)	49 (92)	
Stage II	6 (9)	4 (8)	
Stage III	1 (2)	0 (0)	

Data are number (n) and percentage (%)

mobilisation and excision of the exposed mesh with oversewing of the vaginal epithelium.

Stress urinary incontinence was cured in all patients in the two groups who underwent a TVT-O™ (Ethicon, Somerville, NJ, USA) procedure as a part of the surgery. Postoperative de novo stress urinary incontinence occurred in 5 % (2/44) of patients in the mesh group and in 4 % (2/53) of patients in the non-mesh group (Table 4).

Conclusion

We reported the results of two approaches for the management of multi-compartment vaginal prolapse with or without the use of mesh to support the anterior vaginal wall. To our knowledge, this study is unique in that it compared the outcome of two different techniques for the support of the anterior vaginal wall in conjunction with sacrospinous fixation; posterior fascial placation and vaginal hysterectomy were indicated. Our results suggest that the use of mesh is associated with a higher objective success rate on the anterior wall and in all compartments compared to native tissue repair (85 and 79 % with mesh and 62 and 62 % with native repair, respectively). This is not surprising given that the use of grafts has grown in pelvic reconstructive surgery under the rationale that a POP is similar to a hernia in its aetiology [13] and that reinforcement would most likely lower the recurrence rates, whereas putting stitches in already weakened tissue would not be the best way to achieve a long-lasting correction. A multi-compartment prolapse is more challenging to treat and achieve a favourable outcome than a single compartment prolapse, especially if an apical defect is involved.

Feiner et al. [8] reported a 1-year success rate of 87 % in the anterior compartment and a 75 % success rate in all compartments after the combination of anterior mesh repair (Gynecare Prolift™, Ethicon, Somerville, NJ, USA), sacrospinous hysteropexy and posterior fascial placation. Our results using mesh revealed a similar success rate, albeit with a longer follow-up period.

Previously, an objective cure rate of 91.8 % and an anterior compartment cure rate of 100 % were reported at

Table 4 Reoperation rates and postoperative complications in the two study groups

Complication	Non-mesh group (n=63)	Mesh group (n=53)	p value
Repeat surgery for recurrent prolapse	12 (19)	3 (6)	0.03
Temporary sciatic neuralgia	7 (11)	8 (15)	0.52
Urinary tract infection	9 (14)	11 (20)	0.35
Mesh exposure	NA	4 (8)	
New-onset stress urinary incontinence	2 (3)	2 (4)	0.86

Data are number (n) and percentage (%)

Table 3 POP-Q values at baseline and at the last follow-up in patients in the two study groups

POP-Q measurements (cm)	No-mesh group (n=63)			Mesh group (n=53)			p value
	Baseline	Follow-up	Difference	Baseline	Follow-up	Difference	
Point Ba	4.0±2.2	−1.0±1.9	−5.0±2.6	4.0±2.0	−2.2±1.3	−6.2±2.1	0.004
Point C	4.7±2.5	−4.8±2.8	−9.5±3.5	4.9±2.2	−6.0±2.2	−10.9±3.3	0.024
Point Bp	3.9±2.2	−1.8±1.1	−5.7±2.3	3.7±2.3	−2.4±0.6	−6.1±2.4	0.322

Data are mean ± SD. The POP-Q measurements are as recommended [9]. Point Ba is the anterior wall, most-dependent part (in centimetres); point C, cervix or vaginal cuff (in centimetres); point Bp, posterior wall, most-dependent part (in centimetres)

POP-Q pelvic organ prolapse quantification

a median follow-up of 30 months using a different technique of combined anterior vaginal wall mesh (Perigee® AMS) and conventional vaginal pelvic reconstructive surgery using sacrospinous ligament fixation [7].

An objective cure rate of 89 % was reported by de Tayrac et al. [6] in his study of transvaginal cystocele repair using tension-free polypropylene mesh at a mean follow-up of 37 months. We performed a similar technique to de Tayrac, but our procedure was performed at the time of a sacrospinous colpopexy and posterior fascial plication for massive uterovaginal prolapse.

Nguyen [4] evaluated the outcome after anterior vaginal prolapse repair in a randomised controlled trial and demonstrated 55 % optimal and satisfactory anterior vaginal support after anterior colporrhaphy and 87 % optimal and satisfactory anterior vaginal support after anterior vaginal prolapse repair with polypropylene mesh reinforcement. In our control group, we observed a 38 % rate of recurrent anterior and apical prolapse, which is similar to the results of Maher's and Paraiso's trials. Maher reported a cumulative anterior and vault prolapse recurrence of 45 % at the time of sacrospinous colpopexy, and Paraiso reported a 37 % cystocele rate after sacrospinous colpopexy [14, 15].

In our study, only two patients (4 %) in the mesh group required surgical correction of a prolapse at the anterior and apical compartments during the follow-up period. In the control group, the need for surgical correction of a recurrent prolapse was required in 12 patients (19 %); all included apical and anterior vaginal wall defects. Cervigni et al. [16] reported a 24 % recurrence rate after 38 months of follow-up after repair using polypropylene mesh and only a 5 % occurrence of repeat surgery. The risk for a recurrent anterior vaginal wall prolapse using tension-free polypropylene mesh seems to increase over time, but no repeat procedures were required from 6 to 79 months of follow-up [17].

The concomitant sacrospinous suspension and the surgical technique we chose for (tension-free) mesh insertion may explain the number of cystocele recurrences (15 %) in the mesh group because of the lack of both lateral and apical support. The few cases of repeat surgery (6 %) may be explained by the elevated subjective success rate and higher patient satisfaction in the mesh group. However, these did not reach statistical significance, most likely due to the high number of withdrawals and the patients that were lost to follow-up in the mesh group.

The high cure rate in all patients with stress urinary incontinence can be attributed to the TVT-O™ procedure. New-onset stress urinary incontinence is low and similar in the two groups. The effect of anterior vaginal wall mesh on urinary incontinence is somewhat controversial, but our results show that mesh placement does not increase the risk of postoperative urinary incontinence, similar to the results reported by Nieminen et al. [5] and in accordance with results reported after trans-obturator mesh placement [7].

We reported 8 % asymptomatic mesh exposure during the follow-up period. Vaginal mesh exposure is the complication of greatest concern, and the rate of exposure using Gynemesh™ PS ranges from 3.8 to 20 % [6, 18–20], although the definition of exposure in these reports was usually absent or confusing. The avoidance of thinning of the vaginal epithelium, pre- and posttreatment with local oestrogen, placement of the mesh in a tension-free fashion and intraoperative coverage with antibiotics significantly reduce the serious exposure rates.

Urinary tract infection was the most common postoperative complication in both groups, and all cases responded to antibiotic therapy. This could be explained by the long catheter use time (2 days), which increases the risk of a urinary tract infection, but there was no difference between the two study groups. The relationship between urinary tract infection and vaginal mesh reconstructive surgery is not well reported in the literature.

We reported a 13 % occurrence of right-sided buttock pain with no difference between the two study groups; the pain was mild and disappeared after 2–3 weeks. Postoperative sciatic neuralgia was induced by the traction of the suture in the sacrospinous ligament. The incidence varied between 1 and 30 % [21–25], and the resulting pain was mild and could be controlled by simple analgesics with no need for suture removal.

The main limitation of this study was the lack of validated quality of life questionnaires as none are available in the Arabic language. Additionally, this was a single-centre study, and the sample size was not sufficient to assess complications.

In conclusion, anterior vaginal wall repair reinforced with tension-free polypropylene mesh with concomitant sacrospinous colpopexy and posterior fascial plication has significantly higher objective cure rates and less need for reoperation compared to pubocervical fascial plication with sacrospinous colpopexy and posterior fascial plication for women with massive uterovaginal prolapse at a median follow-up of 28 months with acceptable complication rates.

Declaration of interest The authors report no conflicts of interest. The authors alone are responsible for the content and writing of the paper.

References

1. Olsen AL, Smith VJ, Bergstrom JO, Colling JC, Clark AL (1997) Epidemiology of surgically managed pelvic organ prolapse and urinary incontinence. Obstet Gynecol 89:501–506

2. Hoffman MS, Harris MS, Bouis PJ (1996) Sacrospinous colpopexy in the management of uterovaginal prolapse. J Reprod Med 41:299–303
3. Morgan DM, Rogers MAM, Huebner M, Wei JT, DeLancey JO (2007) Heterogeneity in anatomic outcome of sacrospinous ligament fixation for prolapse. Obstet Gynecol 109:1424–1433
4. Nguyen JN, Burchette RJ (2008) Outcome after anterior vaginal prolapse repair: a randomized controlled trial. Obstet Gynecol 111:891–898
5. Nieminen K, Hiltunen R, Takala T, Heiskanen E, Merikari M, Niemi K, Heinonen PK (2010) Outcomes after anterior vaginal wall repair with mesh: a randomized, controlled trial with a 3 year follow-up. Am J Obstet Gynecol 203(235):e1–e8
6. de Tayrac R, Deffieux X, Gervaise A, Chauveaud-Lambling A, Fernandez H (2006) Long term anatomical and functional assessment of trans-vaginal cystocele repair using a tension-free polypropylene mesh. Int Urogynecol J 17:483–488
7. Lo T-S, Ashok K (2011) Combined anterior trans-obturator mesh and sacrospinous ligament fixation in women with severe prolapse —a case series of 30 months follow-up. Int Urogynecol J Pelvic Floor Dysfunct 22:299–306
8. Feiner B, Gietelink L, Maher C (2010) Anterior vaginal mesh sacrospinous hysteropexy and posterior fascial placation for anterior compartment dominated uterovaginal prolapse. Int Urogynecol J Pelvic Floor Dysfunct 21:203–208
9. Bump RC, Mattiasson A, Bø K et al (1996) The standardization of terminology of female pelvic organ prolapse and pelvic floor dysfunction. Am J Obstet Gynecol 175(1):10–17
10. de Tayrac R, Gervaise A, Chauveaud A, Fernandez H (2005) Tension-free polypropylene mesh for vaginal repair of anterior vaginal wall prolapse. J Reprod Med 50(2):75–80
11. Hefni M (2002) Place of sacrospinous colpopexy at vaginal hysterectomy. In: Sheth S, Studd J (eds) Vaginal hysterectomy, 1st edn. Taylor and Francis, London, pp 249–261
12. Maher CF, Qatawneh AM, Baessler K, Schluter PJ (2004) Midline rectovaginal fascial plication for repair of rectocele and obstructed defecation. Obstet Gynecol 104:685–689
13. Shull BL (1999) Pelvic organ prolapse: anterior, superior and posterior vaginal segment defects. Am J Obstet Gynecol 181:6–11
14. Maher CF, Qatawneh AM, Dwyer PL, Carey MP, Cornish A, Schluter PJ (2004) Abdominal sacral colpopexy or vaginal sacrospinous colpopexy for vaginal vault prolapse: a prospective randomized study. Am J Obstet Gynecol 190:20–26
15. Paraiso MF, Ballard LA, Walters MD, Lee JC, Mitchinson AR (1996) Pelvic support defects and visceral and sexual function in women treated with sacrospinous ligament suspension and pelvic reconstruction. Am J Obstet Gynecol 175:1423–1430
16. Cervigni M, Natale F, La Penna C, Panei M, Mako A (2008) Transvaginal cystocele repair with polypropylene mesh using a tension free technique. Int Urogynecol J Pelvic Floor Dysfunct 19:489–496
17. Letouzey V, Deffieux X, Gervaise A, Mercier G, Fernandez H, de Tayrac R (2010) Trans-vaginal cystocele repair using a tension-free polypropylene mesh: more than 5 years of follow-up. Eur J Obstet Gynecol Reprod Biol 151(1):101–105
18. Adhoute F, Soyeur L, Pariente JL, Le Guillou M, Ferriere JM (2004) Use of trans-vaginal polypropylene mesh (Gynemesh) for the treatment of pelvic floor disorders in women. Prospective study in 52 patients. Prog Urol 14:192–196
19. Hardiman P, Oyawoye S, Browning J (2000) Cystocele repair using polypropylene mesh. Br J Obstet Gynaecol 107:825–826
20. Deffieux X, de Tayrac R, Huel C, Bottero J, Gervaise A, Bonnet K et al (2007) Vaginal mesh erosion after trans-vaginal repair of cystocele using Gynemesh or Gynemesh-Soft in 138 women: a comparative study. Int Urogynecol J Pelvic Floor Dysfunct 18:73–79
21. Lovatsis D, Drutz HP (2002) Safety and efficacy of sacrospinous vault suspension. Int Urogynecol J Pelvic Floor Dysfunct 13:308–313
22. Nichols DH (1982) Sacrospinous fixation for massive eversion of the vagina. Am J Obstet Gynecol 142:901–904
23. Cruikshank SH, Cox DW (1990) Sacrospinous ligament fixation at the time of vaginal hysterectomy. Am J Obstet Gynecol 162:1611–1619
24. Baker MH (1992) Success with sacrospinous suspension of the prolapsed vaginal vault. Surg Gynecol Obstet 175:419–420
25. Carey MP, Slack MC (1994) Vaginal vault prolapse. Br J Hosp Med 51:417–420

18

A meta-analysis of the use of 4 % icodextrin solution to prevent adhesion formation after gynaecological surgery

Fiona L. Mackie · Sofia Dias · Andrew Watson · Gaity Ahmad

Abstract Post-surgical adhesions are common and can cause substantial co-morbidity. The aim of this review was to investigate the efficacy of 4 % icodextrin solution, a widely used adhesion prevention agent, in gynaecological surgery. Randomised-controlled trials comparing the use of 4 % icodextrin solution vs. Ringer's-lactated saline (control) in women of any age undergoing fertility-conserving surgery either by laparoscopy or laparotomy were searched and meta-analysis performed. Compared to Ringer's-lactated saline, there was no significant difference in the number of patients free from de novo adhesions at second-look laparoscopy (SLL) (odds ratio, 1.21 [0.76, 1.93]), the adhesion score reduction at SLL (mean difference (MD), 0.71 [−0.66, 2.08]), the percentage reduction in adhesion extent (MD, 5.47 [−4.18, 15.12]) or severity (MD, 13.49 [−23.78, 50.75]). The included studies reported the effect of 4 % icodextrin in different ways thus limiting meta-analysis. This is the first meta-analysis of icodextrin and the lack of evidence found to support the use of icodextrin suggests further research is required which should be presented in a uniform manner.

Keywords Adhesions · Gynaecological · Icodextrin · Adept · Meta-analysis

F. L. Mackie
Education and Research Centre, Pennine Acute Trust,
Royal Oldham Hospital,
Rochdale Road,
Oldham OL12JH, UK

S. Dias
School of Social and Community Medicine,
University of Bristol,
Canynge Hall, 39 Whatley Road,
Bristol BS8 2PS, UK

A. Watson
FRCOG, Department of Obstetrics and Gynaecology,
Tameside General Hospital,
Fountain Street, Ashton Under Lyne,
Lancashire OL6 9RW, UK

G. Ahmad (✉)
MRCOG, Department of Obstetrics and Gynaecology,
Pennine Acute Trust, Royal Oldham Hospital,
Rochdale Road,
Oldham OL12JH, UK
e-mail: Gaity.ahmad@pat.nhs.uk

Background

Adhesions are fibrin bands which develop due to aberrant healing of the peritoneum [3]. Damage to the peritoneum results in an inflammatory response which activates the coagulation cascade and a fibrin plug then forms over the damaged mesothelial tissue. Normally, the fibrin plug is broken down, revealing regenerated peritoneum. However, in adhesion formation, less fibrinolysis occurs and a fibrin matrix develops. The presence of adhesions may have no consequence but can cause infertility, pain, bowel obstruction and their presence is associated with increased risks of complications from further surgery.

Pelvic adhesions are the commonest complication of gynaecological surgery and form in 50–100 % of women who undergo gynaecological surgery [2]. Other causes of adhesions include: infection, particularly pelvic inflammatory disease, endometriosis, and ischaemia [2]. Five percent of patients are re-admitted with problems related to adhesions [2]. These consequences can have a negative impact on a patient's quality of life and may necessitate further surgery.

Adhesions also have considerable public health and financial implications. It is estimated that the direct cost of readmissions related to adhesions in the first year after lower abdominal surgery is £24.2million, which increases to £95.2million 10 years after the initial surgery [6].

Adhesiolysis although accepted in clinical practice is still controversial [2]. Thus, the focus of adhesion management is prevention. There are a variety of adhesion prevention agents available which can be divided into solid mechanical barriers and fluid agents. Icodextrin (4 %) solution (Adept, Baxter, Berkshire, UK) is widely used as an adhesion prevention agent as it is easy to use and store, and is relatively cheap compared to other adhesion prevention agents. It is a non-viscous, iso-osmotic fluid which contains icodextrin—a glucose polymer (molecular weight, ~16,500 Da) [3]. The agent is said to act by hydroflotation over several days, thus preventing contact between organs and traumatised tissue and thus adhesions are unable to form [3].

The aim of this review was to evaluate the efficacy of 4 % icodextrin solution in the prevention of adhesion formation after fertility-conserving gynaecological surgery.

Methods

MEDLINE, EMBASE, CINAHL, PsychINFO and the Cochrane Menstrual Disorders and Subfertility Group Specialised Register of controlled trials were searched using the keywords: adhesion(s), adhesion barrier(s), adhesion prevention, gynaecological, pelvic, adept, and icodextrin. The reference lists of published papers were cross-checked. Studies published up to February 2012 were considered for inclusion. Randomised controlled trials (RCTs) which investigated the efficacy of 4 % icodextrin solution as an anti-adhesion agent in gynaecological surgery were included. The surgery was fertility-conserving and may have either been performed by laparoscopy or laparotomy, on women of any age. Studies involving non-gynaecological surgery were excluded. There was no restriction on language. Two authors (FM and GA) independently assessed the suitability of the trials for inclusion. Any disagreements

Table 1 Characteristics of the included randomised controlled trials on the efficacy of 4 % icodextrin solution on the prevention of adhesion formation in gynaecological surgery

Study	Brown et al. [1]	diZerega et al. [3]	Trew et al. [5]
Patients analysed (*n*)	402	53	330
Indication for surgery	Planned laparoscopic gynaecological surgery which included adhesiolysis	Planned laparoscopic gynaecological surgery for pelvic pain and/or infertility problems	Planned laparoscopic gynaecological surgery for primary removal of myomas or endometriotic cysts. (≤4 myomas and largest myoma 2–8 cm in diameter, endometriotic cysts 3–7 cm in diameter)
Inclusion criteria	All participants were ≥18 years old, in good general health and undergoing laparoscopic gynaecological surgery only. SLL performed 4–16 weeks after initial procedure		
Exclusion criteria (common)	Pregnancy, active pelvic/abdominal infection, known allergy to study materials, non-gynaecological procedures to be performed during surgery, cancer, and concomitant use of steroids/antineoplastics/radiation		
Exclusion criteria (unique)	<3 available anatomical study sites with adhesions, or <3 sites lysed.	More than half available anatomical study sites contained adhesions.	Conversion to laparotomy, mAFS adhesion score moderate or severe, AFS endometriosis class III or IV (excluding cysts), or adhesions which required lysing
Time of SLL after initial procedure (weeks)	4–8	6–12	4–16
Timing of randomisation	Intraoperatively	Recruitment	24 h prior to surgery
Method of randomisation	Computer generated	Envelope used, no more information given	Telephone randomisation
Single or multicentre (*n*)	Multicentre (16)	Multicentre (not known)	Multicentre (25)
Presence of blinding	Double-blinded (patient and assessor)	Single-blinded (surgeon)	Double-blinded (patient and assessor)
Use of independent blinded assessor	Yes	Yes	Yes
Presence of power calculation	No	No	Yes
Was analysis intention to treat?	Yes	Yes	Yes
Timing and location of trial	July 2001-March 2004 USA	Not known USA	September 2003-August 2005 Europe
Sources of funding	Innovata Ltd, Vectura Group	No sources of funding stated	Shire Pharmaceutical Development Ltd, Baxter BioSurgery

SLL second-look laparoscopy, *mAFS* modified American Fertility Society, *AFS* American Fertility Society were settled by consensus with a third author (AW). The outcomes of the review were all related to the adhesions found at second-look laparoscopy (SLL). Specifically, these were: changes in severity of pelvic pain, pregnancy rate, incidence of adhesions, number of patients free from de novo adhesions, adhesion score, adhesion score reduction at SLL compared with initial laparoscopy, mean percentage reduction in the extent of adhesions, mean percentage reduction in the severity of adhesions and improvement or worsening in adhesion score.

The quality of the studies was evaluated, including: the timing and method of randomisation, whether it was a single or multicentre trial, the presence of blinding, the number of patients who were analysed, the presence of a power calculation, whether analysis was by intention to treat, the timing and location of the trial, and any sources of funding.

Data were input and analysed using Metaview of Review Manager (RevMan; RevMan version 5.2 Copenhagen: The Nordic Cochrane Centre, The Cochrane Collaboration, 2011). Dichotomous data (e.g. the number of patients free from de novo adhesions, and improvement or worsening of adhesion score) were expressed as an odds ratio (OR) with 95 % confidence intervals (CIs). Continuous data (e.g. adhesion score at SLL, mean adhesion score reduction, mean percentage reduction in extent and severity) were presented as the mean difference (MD) with 95 % CIs. The mean adhesion score reduction in DiZerega et al. [3] was calculated by subtracting the mean baseline adhesion score from the mean adhesion score at SLL, the standard deviation was calculated by assuming a within-patient correlation of 0.5 to calculate the variance of the mean reduction. It has been suggested that plausible values for the within-patient correlation could be in the range of 0.5–0.7 [4]. Sensitivity to the assumed correlation was checked and the conclusions were unchanged. Meta-analysis was performed assuming a random effects model (DerSimonian–Laird). Results were considered statistically significant when $p<0.05$.

Findings

The initial search revealed 45 studies, three of which were eligible for inclusion, with a total of 785 participants [1, 3, 5] (see Table 1). All three studies compared 4 % icodextrin solution with Ringer's lactated saline (RLS) as the control. The administration of the agent was the same in the three studies: the abdomen was irrigated with >100 ml of agent every 30 min and 1,000 ml instilled at the end, although DiZerega et al. instilled 400–1,000 ml of RLS at the end of the procedure. The modified American Fertility Society (mAFS) adhesion scoring system was used by all the studies

Table 2 Efficacy of 4 % icodextrin solution on the prevention of adhesion formation in gynaecological surgery

Study	Adhesions at SLL
Brown et al. [1]	Number of patients free from de novo adhesions: OR 1.49 [1.01, 2.21]
	Adhesion score at SLL: outcome not analysed
	Adhesion score reduction at SLL: MD 1.51 [0.32 2.70]
	Mean % reduction in extent of adhesions: MD 5.10 [−4.67, 14.87]
	Mean % reduction in severity of adhesions: MD 2.70 [−5.73, 11.13]
	Improvement in adhesion score: outcome not analysed
	Worsening in adhesion score: outcome not analysed
diZerega et al. [3]	Number of patients free from de novo adhesions: outcome not analysed
	Adhesion score at SLL: outcome not analysed
	Adhesion score reduction at SLL[a]: MD 0.10 [−0.50, 0.70]
	Mean % reduction in extent of adhesions: MD 21.00 [−42.36, 84.36]
	Mean % reduction in severity of adhesions: MD 47.00 [−15.76, 109.76]
	Improvement in adhesion score: OR 3.24 [0.86, 12.12]
	Worsening in adhesion score: OR 0.28 [0.07, 1.21]
Trew et al. [5]	Number of patients free from de novo adhesions: OR 0.92 [0.55, 1.54]
	Adhesion score at SLL: MD −0.29 [−2.97, 2.39]
	Adhesion score reduction at SLL: outcome not analysed
	Mean % reduction in extent of adhesions: outcome not analysed
	Mean % reduction in severity of adhesions: outcome not analysed
	Improvement in adhesion score: outcome not analysed
	Worsening in adhesion score: outcome not analysed

SLL second-look laparoscopy, *OR* odds ratio, *MD* mean difference, *SD* standard deviation

[a] Calculated by subtracting the mean score at SLL from the mean baseline score. SD calculated by assuming a within-patient correlation of 0.5 for the sensitivity analysis

a Number of patients free of de novo adhesions

Study	4% icodextrin		Ringer's-Lactated Saline (RLS)		Weight (%)	Odds Ratio
	Patients free of de novo adhesions	Total number of patients	Patients free of de novo adhesions	Total number of patients		M-H, Random, 95% CI
Brown 2007	108	203	86	199	56.1	1.49 [1.01, 2.21]
Trew 2011	38	170	38	160	43.9	0.92 [0.55, 1.54]
Total (95% CI)		**373**		**359**	**100.0**	**1.21 [0.76, 1.93]**

Heterogeneity: Tau² = 0.06; Chi² = 2.12, df = 1 (P = 0.15); I² = 53%
Test for overall effect: Z = 0.80 (P = 0.42)

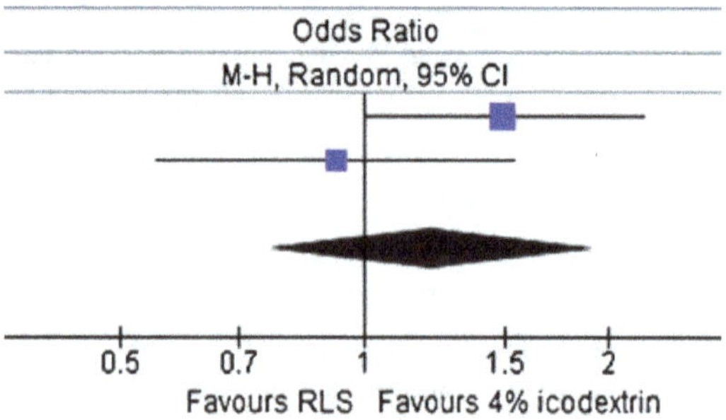

b Mean reduction in mAFS score per patient – 0.5 variance

Study	4% icodextrin		Ringer's-Lactated Saline (RLS)		Weight (%)	Mean difference
	Mean (SD)	Total number of patients	Mean (SD)	Total number of patients		IV, Random, 95% CI
Brown 2007	2.7 (6.18)	203	1.19 (5.98)	199	43.1	1.51 [0.32, 2.70]
diZerega 2002	0.19 (1.27)	23	0.09 (0.69)	19	56.9	0.10 [-0.50, 0.70]
Total (95% CI)		**226**		**218**	**100.0**	**0.71 [-0.66, 2.08]**

Heterogeneity: Tau² = 0.76; Chi² = 4.29, df = 1 (P = 0.04); I² = 77%
Test for overall effect: Z = 1.01 (P = 0.31)

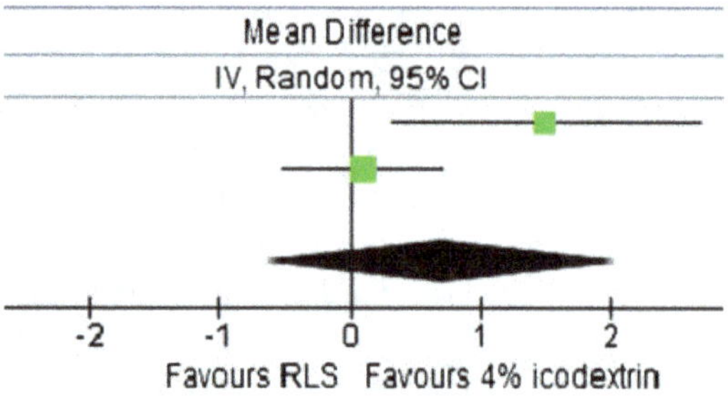

Fig. 1 Meta-analyses of adhesions at second-look laparoscopy. **a** Number of patients free from de novo adhesions. **b** Mean reduction in mAFS score per patient, 0.5 variance. **c** Mean percent reduction in extent of adhesions per patient. **d** Mean percent reduction in severity of adhesions per patient. *mAFS* modified American Fertility Society, *SD* standard deviation, *CI* confidence interval

which assesses the incidence, extent and severity of adhesions at 23 specified anatomical sites. None of the included studies provided data on the outcomes of the pregnancy rate, or the incidence of adhesions at SLL. Brown et al. found that in the patients with a primary diagnosis of pelvic pain, 118/152 (83 %) patients treated with 4 % icodextrin solution demonstrated a clinically significant decrease in pelvic pain, compared to 108/134 (82 %) of patients who received RLS. None of the outcomes were reported by all three studies (see Table 2).

c Mean % reduction in extent of adhesions per patient

Study	4% icodextrin		Ringer's-Lactated Saline (RLS)		Weight (%)	Mean difference
	Mean (SD)	Total number of patients	Mean (SD)	Total number of patients		IV, Random, 95% CI
Brown 2007	26.9 (51.4)	203	21.8 (48.5)	199	97.7	5.10 [-4.67, 14.87]
diZerega 2002	4 (88)	23	-17 (116)	19	2.3	21.00 [-42.36, 84.36]
Total (95% CI)		**226**		**218**	**100.0**	**5.47 [-4.18, 15.12]**

Heterogeneity: $Tau^2 = 0.00$; $Chi^2 = 0.24$, df = 1 (P = 0.63); $I^2 = 0\%$
Test for overall effect: Z = 1.11 (P = 0.27)

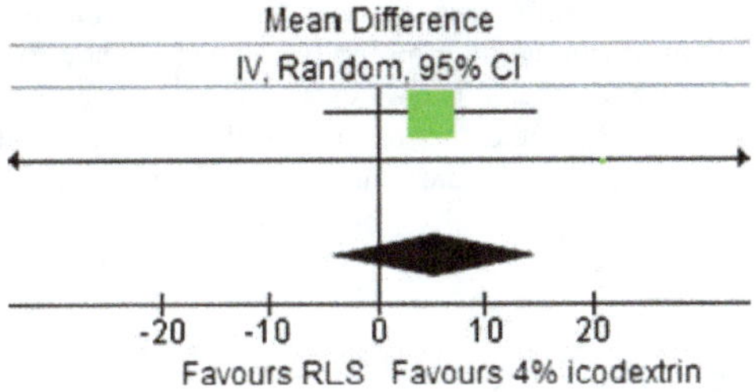

d Mean % reduction in severity of adhesions per patient

Study	4% icodextrin		Ringer's-Lactated Saline (RLS)		Weight (%)	Mean difference
	Mean (SD)	Total number of patients	Mean (SD)	Total number of patients		IV, Random, 95% CI
Brown 2007	24.2 (45.2)	203	21.5 (41)	199	75.6	2.70 [-5.73, 11.13]
diZerega 2002	21 (82)	23	-26 (118)	19	24.4	47.00 [-15.76, 109.76]
Total (95% CI)		**226**		**218**	**100.0**	**13.49 [-23.78, 50.75]**

Heterogeneity: $Tau^2 = 459.39$; $Chi^2 = 1.88$, df = 1 (P = 0.17); $I^2 = 47\%$
Test for overall effect: Z =0.71 (P = 0.48)

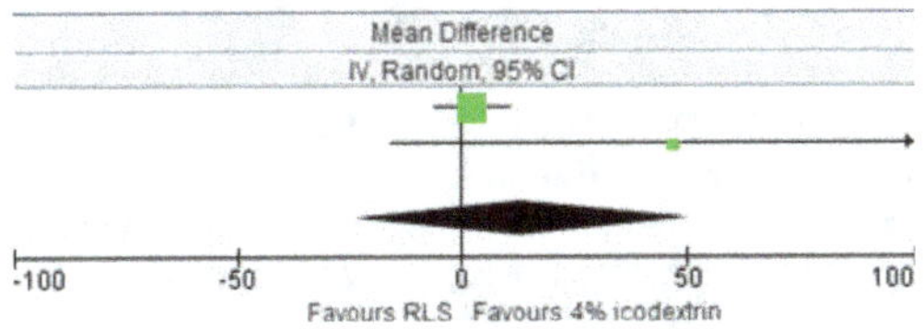

Fig. 1 (continued)

Meta-analysis of Brown et al. and Trew et al. showed a non-statistically significant reduction in the number of patients free from de novo adhesions with 4 % icodextrin when compared to patients who received RLS (OR 1.21 [0.76, 1.93]) (see Figure 1). The mean adhesion score reduction per patient at SLL which was reported by Brown et al. and diZerega et al. was not statistically significant (MD 0.71 [−0.66, 2.08]). Nor was the meta-analysis of the mean percentage reduction in the extent of adhesions (MD 5.47 [−4.18, 15.12]), or the severity of adhesions (MD 13.49 [−23.78, 50.75]) which were both investigated by Brown et al. and diZerega et al. The remainder of the outcomes, i.e. the adhesion score at SLL and improvement or worsening in adhesion score between first-look laparoscopy and SLL, were explored by individual studies, which found no significant difference between 4 % icodextrin solution and RLS (see Table 2).

Conclusions

This review failed to demonstrate the effectiveness of 4 % icodextrin in preventing adhesions after pelvic surgery. The three studies included presented data relating to the adhesion score at SLL, but they all used different actual outcomes. Because of this no meta-analysis used data from more than two studies.

One issue this review has raised is the low number of RCTs which have been conducted on 4 % icodextrin solution in gynaecological surgery, despite its widespread use. Another issue was the different ways the authors reported the effect of 4 % icodextrin solution on adhesions. Out of the eight different measurements of adhesions at SLL which were analysed, none were reported by all three studies. Although the three studies used the mAFS adhesion score, often different aspects were reported. For example, it was not possible to analyse the incidence of adhesions at SLL as Brown et al. stated the reduction in the number of sites of adhesions at SLL but did not provide the number of adhesion sites at baseline, whereas DiZerega et al. reported the incidence of adhesions in patients with at least one adhesion at baseline, and Trew et al. reported only the incidence of de novo adhesions. There was also no long-term follow-up with contact terminating after SLL and the longest time between the initial laparoscopy and the SLL being 16 weeks. It would be interesting to see if there was any difference in the safety/adverse events such as bowel obstruction with further follow up.

This is the first meta-analysis of the efficacy of 4 % icodextrin solution as an adhesion prevention agent in gynaecological surgery to the authors' knowledge. It has demonstrated that there is a dearth of evidence regarding the use of 4 % icodextrin solution. The findings suggest that currently, there is insufficient evidence to support that 4 % icodextrin solution is effective at preventing adhesions in gynaecological surgery compared to RLS. Although 4 % icodextrin solution is cheaper and easier toapply than other commercial adhesion-prevention agents, if it does not prevent adhesions it is neither in the patient's best interest, or cost-effective to continue using it. The American Society for Reproductive Medicine recommends that the mAFS score should be used when evaluating adhesion prevention agents; however in addition to this, data should be published in complete and in a way which allows for comparison with other studies. Alternative adhesion prevention agents should continue to be considered for gynaecological surgery.

This review does not support the use of 4 % icodextrin solution as an anti-adhesion agent in gynaecological surgery. More research is required into adhesion prevention agents, the results of which should be reported in a uniform manner to enable comparison.

Acknowledgments The Cochrane Menstrual Disorders and Subfertility Group, Department of Obstetrics and Gynaecology, University of Auckland, Auckland, New Zealand who helped with the search for relevant studies, particularly Marian Showell.

Declaration of interest Dr. Watson received consultancy and lecture fees in 2003 from Shire Pharmaceuticals. Dr. Watson has received lecture fees from Gynaecare, Shire and Baxter all of whom distributed adhesion prevention modalities when the lecture on adhesion prevention was given. In addition he received a consultancy fee from Shire when the use of icodextrin to prevent adhesions was first being promoted. The other authors report no conflicts of interest. The authors alone are responsible for the content and writing of the paper.

Reference list

1. Brown C, Luciano A, Martin D, Peers E, Scrimgeour A, DiZerega G (2007) Adept (icodextrin 4% solution) reduces adhesions after laparoscopic surgery for adhesiolysis: a double-blind, randomized, controlled study. Fertil Steril 88:1413–1426
2. Diamond M, Freeman M (2001) Clinical implications of postsurgical adhesions. Hum Reprod Update 7:567–576
3. diZerega G, Verco S, Young P, Kettel M, Kobak W, Martin D et al (2002) A randomized, controlled pilot study of the safety and efficacy of 4% icodextrin solution in the reduction of adhesions following laparoscopic gynaecological surgery. Human Reprod 17:1031–1038
4. Frison L, Pocock S (1992) Repeated measures in clinical trials: analysis using mean summary statistics and its implications for design. Stat Med 11:1685–1704
5. Trew G, Pistofidis G, Pados G, Lower AM, Mettler L, Wallwiener D et al (2011) Gynaecological endoscopic evaluation of 4% icodextrin solution: a European, multicentre, double-blind, randomized study of the efficacy and safety in the reduction of *de novo* adhesions after laparoscopic gynaecological surgery. Human Reprod 26:2015–2027
6. Wilson M, Menzies D, Knight A, Crowe A (2002) Demonstrating the clinical and cost effectiveness of adhesion reduction strategies. Colorec Dis 4:355–360

19

Classification of intra-abdominal adhesions after cesarean delivery

Togas Tulandi · Deirdre J. Lyell

Abstract The objective of the study was to develop a standard classification for adhesions after cesarean delivery. We searched the Medline, Pubmed, EMBASE, and the Cochrane database of systematic reviews from 1996 through 2011 for all articles pertaining to adhesion scoring after a cesarean delivery. We performed the search using the keywords "cesarean, adhesions, repeat cesarean, intra-abdominal adhesions, adhesion scoring system, and adhesion classification." Most published adhesion scoring systems were non-site-specific or unclearly described. The most comprehensive adhesion scoring systems were described in three prospective studies that came from two institutions. The scoring systems were similar, site-specific, involving over four sites, and assessing the severity and consistency of adhesions. We combined the two scoring systems to develop a standardized classification of adhesions after cesarean delivery. To date, there are no uniform classifications of intra-abdominal adhesions after cesarean delivery. We hereby outline the first standardized classification of adhesions after cesarean delivery.

Keywords Adhesion · Cesarean · Classification · Scoring system

Background

Cesarean delivery is one of the most common operations performed on women, and its rate keeps increasing. The rates of cesarean in the USA in 1996 and 2009 were 20.7 and 32.9 % respectively, an increase of over 50 % [1, 2]. In the states of Louisiana and New Jersey, the rates were close to 40 %. The increasing rate of cesarean deliveries can be attributed to many factors including an increased repeat cesarean delivery rate. The repeat cesarean delivery rate among all live births was 6.7 % in 1996 and 14.8 % in 2001, representing an increase of over 120 %. [3]. Martin et al. reported that the repeat cesarean delivery rate increased from 69.8 in 1996 to 88.7 in 2003 per 100 births among low-risk women with a previous cesarean [2].

Adhesions develop frequently following cesarean delivery, with estimates of adhesions following the first cesarean ranging from 24.4 % overall [4] to 73 % when the parietal peritoneum is left open [5]. Several studies have demonstrated that adhesions develop more frequently and with greater density with each repeat cesarean and are associated with increasing maternal morbidity [4, 6–8].

In studies of post-cesarean adhesions, however, each institution has used a different adhesion-grading system and approach, which may explain the significant variation in reporting. In the field of infertility, the classification of adnexal adhesions of the American Society for Reproductive Medicine has been widely used clinically and for research purposes [9]. Yet, to date, there has been no standardization of adhesions after cesarean delivery. Indeed, there is a paucity of information about adhesions in obstetric settings, and its consequences have been underappreciated [10].

The purpose of our literature review is to develop a standard classification for adhesions after cesarean delivery.

Materials and methods

We searched Medline, EMBASE, Pubmed, and the Cochrane database of systematic reviews from 1996 through 2011for all articles pertaining to adhesion scoring after a

T. Tulandi (✉)
Department of Obstetrics and Gynecology, McGill University,
687 Pine Ave. West,
Montreal, Quebec H3A 1A1, Canada
e-mail: togas.tulandi@mcgill.ca

D. J. Lyell
Department of Obstetrics and Gynecology, Stanford University,
Stanford, CA, USA

cesarean delivery. We performed the search using the keywords "cesarean, adhesions, repeat cesarean, intra-abdominal adhesions, adhesion scoring system, and adhesion classification". We reviewed reference lists from any identified article including reviews to find other publications.

Study selection

We examined all articles that studied adhesions after cesarean deliveries and the outcome. Those with adhesion scoring systems or classifications of adhesions were evaluated for whether scoring was performed prospectively and whether it was site-specific. We included studies where the adhesions were evaluated prospectively with site-specific adhesion scoring systems (Table 1) [5, 11, 12]. Studies with unclear evaluation of adhesions (Table 2) [13–18] and retrospective studies (Tables 3 and 4) [19–25] were excluded.

Findings

Besides studies listed on Table 1, all adhesion scoring systems were non-site-specific or unclearly described [13–18]. There were three randomized studies (Table 2). Roset et al. evaluated a subgroup of patients involved in a previous randomized trial; adhesions were evaluated retrospectively [13]. Weerawetwat et al. used an adhesion scoring system (no adhesions, mild, moderate, and severe adhesions) based on the width of the adhesion bands and described whether the adhesions involved the uterus, bladder, omentum, or abdominal wall [14]. The study lacks detailed description of site-specific adhesions. Another randomized study [18] used a different grading of adhesions based on the ease of removal of adhesion bands between the uterus and omentum or rectus muscle. The study involved a small number of cases.

Of three prospective non-randomized studies, Salim et al. used a site-specific adhesion scoring system, and severity of adhesions was divided into light filmy or dense vascular adhesions [16]. However, detailed description of site-specific adhesions was not provided. Komoto et al. evaluated the frequency of adhesions but not the severity [15]. Malvasi et al. evaluated adhesions in limited locations, primarily between the bladder and the uterus, and severity of adhesions was graded as none, mild, or severe [17].

The most comprehensive adhesion scoring systems were described in three prospective studies (Table 1). Although they came from two institutions, the scoring systems were similar, site-specific involving over four sites, and assessed the severity and consistency of adhesions. The validity of the two scoring systems was evaluated by each institution, with inter-rater reliability of 0.85 and 0.84, respectively. As a result, we combined the two scoring systems (Table 5). In this new classification, we use a point system, and the scores from multiple sites are additive. The area of incision covered by adhesions is divided into <3 cm, 3–6 cm, and >6 cm. This is based on the estimate that in general, the length of incision for cesarean delivery is approximately 10 cm. Three centimeters is about one third of the incision length and 6 cm is approximately two third of the length.

Comment

There have been many studies evaluating adhesion formation after cesarean delivery, mainly comparing the effects of peritoneal closure and non-closure. Due to the increasing number of repeat cesarean deliveries, several authors have started to examine the effects of repeated cesareans on adhesion formation.

To date, there has never been a uniform classification of intra-abdominal adhesions after cesarean delivery. Previous studies have used either no adhesion scoring system or a non-site-specific scoring system [19–25]. For example, Chapa et al. graded the adhesions as no adhesions (grade 0), minimal or filmy adhesions (grade 1), moderate/thick adhesions (grade 2), and absence of free space between the uterus and anterior abdominal wall/viscera [25]. The system does not

Table 1 Prospective studies with site-specific adhesion scoring system

Authors	Type of study	Main outcome measures	Number of patients analyzed	Number of adhesion sites	Results
Lyell et al. [5]	Prospective cohort	Effect of parietal peritoneal closure	173	Over 4 sites	Parietal peritoneal closure is associated with reduced adhesion formation
Tulandi et al. [11]	Prospective cohort	Prevalence of adhesions with or without keloids	429	Over 4 sites	Women with keloids have increased adhesions between the uterus and the bladder or the abdominal wall
Tulandi et al. [12]	Prospective cohort	Prevalence and extent of adhesions after repeated cesareans	1,026	Over 4 sites	Adhesion are mainly between the uterus and the bladder or the anterior abdominal wall

Table 2 Randomized and prospective studies with unclear evaluation of adhesions

Authors	Type of study	Main outcome measures	Number of patients analyzed	Results	Comments
Roset et al. [13]	Randomized clinical trial	Effect of combined parietal and visceral peritoneum closure	29	No difference in long-term morbidity between closure and non-closure of peritoneum	Outcomes were evaluated by patient report
Weerawetwat et al. [14]	Randomized clinical trial	Effect of parietal and visceral peritoneum closure	65	No difference in adhesion formation between closure and non-closure of peritoneum	Adhesion score (no, mild, moderate and severe) based on the width of the adhesion bands; lack of detailed description of site-specific adhesions
Komoto et al. [15]	Prospective cohort	Effect of combined parietal and visceral peritoneum closure	50	Increased adhesion formation with parietal and visceral peritoneum closure	Frequency of adhesions was evaluated, and severity was based on whether adhesiolysis was performed
Salim et al. [16]	Prospective cohort	Relationship between abdominal scar characteristics and adhesions	107	Depressed previous scar is associated with increased adhesions.	Adhesion severity: light filmy or dense vascular
Malvasi et al. [17]	Prospective cohort	Effect of visceral peritoneum closure	112	Increased adhesions with visceral peritoneum closure	Evaluation of mainly adhesions between the bladder and the uterus. Severity of adhesions was graded using the American Fertility Society classification for adnexal adhesions
Zareian et al. [18]	Randomized clinical trial	Effect of combined parietal and visceral peritoneum closure	31	Parietal and visceral peritoneum closure may decrease adhesion formation	Adhesion score based on the ease of removal of adhesion bands between the uterus and omentum or rectus muscle. Small number of cases

indicate which viscera are involved in most of the adhesions. Others used the Bristow and Montz scoring system [26], a non-site-specific scoring system that has been used to evaluate adhesions after oncologic surgery as well as in an animal model. It consists of no adhesions (0 point), avascular adhesions (1 point), vascular adhesions (3 points), and thick adhesions (5 points). Some studies have not reported overall adhesions; rather, they stratified adhesions into minor or dense adhesions.

The need for a standardized adhesion classification is obvious. It will allow investigators and readers to evaluate and compare results from different studies. Routine use of a standardized adhesion classification might also enable future investigators to conduct more reproducible retrospective studies. More importantly, knowledge of the presence and severity of adhesions will prepare the obstetrician for future repeat cesarean deliveries. We and others found that rates of dense adhesion after one cesarean was greater than 20 % and after two cesareans, greater than 40 % [4, 27].

We propose a classification of intra-abdominal adhesions after cesarean delivery. Our proposed classification is based on our previous prospective studies of adhesions after cesareans, site-specific, and assessed the severity and consistency of adhesions. We also use a point system (Table 5). Because vascularity especially at the time of repeat cesarean delivery is difficult to evaluate, we did not include it in our classification system. The application and results of using this classification system remain to be seen.

Table 3 Retrospective studies with site-specific adhesion scoring system

Authors	Type of study	Main outcome measures	Number of patients analyzed	Results
Morales et al. [6]	Retrospective cohort	Prevalence of adhesions after cesareans	542	Cesareans result in adhesion formation. Site-specific locations available only if described in operative notes
Tulandi et al. [4]	Retrospective cohort	Prevalence of adhesion after repeat cesareans	1,283	Increased adhesion with each subsequent cesarean. Site-specific locations available only if described in operative notes. Scores assigned based on severity of adhesion

Table 4 Retrospective studies with no or unclear description of site-specific adhesions

Authors	Type of study	Main outcome measures	Number of patients analyzed	Results
Myers and Bennett [19]	Retrospective study	Effect of combined parietal and visceral peritoneum closure	191	Combined parietal and visceral peritoneum closure was associated with decreased adhesion formation
Phipps et al. [20]	Case control study	Identification of risk factor of bladder injury	126	Adhesions from prior cesarean is a risk factor for bladder injury at repeat cesarean
Zhu et al. [21]	Retrospective cohort	Effect of parietal peritoneum closure	612	Non-closure of parietal peritoneum is associated with increased visceral adhesions
Nisenblat et al. [22]	Retrospective cohort	Complications after repeated cesareans	768	Increased complications and dense adhesion with cesarean number. Dense adhesions were defined as multiple adhesions between the uterus and surrounding organs
Hamel [23]	Retrospective cohort	Incidence and severity of adhesions	62	Decreased adhesions with closure of the rectus muscle or the parietal peritoneum.
Fatusic and Hudic [24]	Retrospective study	Prevalence of adhesions	400	Decreased adhesions after MisgavLadach cesarean. Adhesion scores based on Bristow and Montz scoring system
Chapa et al. [25]	Retrospective cohort	Effect of adhesion barriers at cesarean	112	An adhesion barrier and parietal peritoneum closure reduced adhesion formation

The characteristics of the previous incision scar might provide an idea about the severity of intra-abdominal adhesions [11, 28]. In a study, the authors reported that elevated scars are associated with increased dense adhesions [28]. In another study, women with keloids on the cesarean scar have increased adhesions between the uterus and the bladder, and between the uterus and the abdominal wall [11]. A uniform reporting of adhesions at the time of previous cesareans will be very useful.

Indeed, adhesions after a cesarean delivery are common, and their extent and density increase with repeated cesarean deliveries. The presence of adhesions increases time to delivery of the fetus and time of the procedure [4, 11, 29]. Greenberg et al. reported that the mean interval of incision to delivery in women with severe adhesions (19.8 min) was significantly longer than in those with less severe adhesions (15.6 min). In addition, more women with severe adhesions remained undelivered at 30 min after incision [29]. Maternal morbidities can also increase with each subsequent cesarean delivery. This includes increased bowel and bladder injury, uterine and wound dehiscence, hysterectomy, post-partum hemorrhage, and pulmonary emboli [4, 30, 31].

Conclusion

We hereby outlined the first standardized classification of adhesions after cesarean delivery. It is site-specific and evaluates the prevalence and severity of adhesions. We encourage clinicians and investigators to adopt this classification into a standard practice.

Table 5 Proposed classification of intra-abdominal adhesions after cesarean delivery

Adhesions	Consistency of the adhesions	<3 cm	3–6 cm	>6 cm
Between uterus and bladder	Filmy	1	2	4
	Dense	4	8	16
Between uterus and abdominal fascia	Filmy	1	2	4
	Dense	4	8	16
Between uterus and omentum	Filmy	1	2	4
	Dense	4	8	16
Between omentum and abdominal fascia	Filmy		2	
	Dense		8	
Adhesions to other pelvic structure that interfere with the delivery	Filmy		4	
	Dense		8	

Acknowledgments Togas Tulandi received a travel grant as advisor for Genzyme for adhesion related research.

References

1. Hamilton BE, Ventura SJ, Osterman MJK, Kirmeyer S, Mathews TJ, Wilson E (2011) Births: final data for 2009. Nat Vital Stat Rep 60:1–35
2. Martin JA, Hamilton BE, Ventura SJ et al. Births: Final data for 2003. National vital statistics reports; vol 54 no 2. Hyattsville, MD. National Center for Health Statistics. 2005. http://www.cdc.gov/nchs/births.htm
3. Barber EL, Lundsberg LS, Belanger K, Pettker CM, Funai EF, Illuzzi JL (2011) Indications contributing to the increasing cesarean delivery rate. Obstet Gynecol 118:29–38
4. Tulandi T, Agdi M, Zarei A, Miner L, Sikirica V (2009) Adhesion formation and morbidity after repeat cesarean delivery. Am J Obstet Gynecol 201:56.e.1–56.e.16
5. Lyell DJ, Caughey AB, Hu E, Daniels K (2005) Peritoneal closure at primary cesarean delivery and adhesions. Obstet Gynecol 106:275–280
6. Morales KJ, Gordon MC, Bates GW Jr (2007) Postcesarean delivery adhesions associated with delayed delivery of infant. Am J Obstet Gynecol 196:461.e1–461.e16.8
7. Nisenblat V, Barak S, Griness OB, Degani S, Ohel G, Gonen R (2006) Maternal complications associated with multiple cesarean deliveries. Obstet Gynecol 108:21–26
8. Makoha FW, Felimban HM, Fathuddien MA, Roomi F, Ghabra T (2004) Multiple cesarean section morbidity. Int J Gynecol Obstet 87:227–232
9. American Fertility Society (1988) The American Fertility Society classifications of adnexal adhesions, distal tubal occlusion, tubal occlusion secondary to tubal ligation, tubal pregnancies, müllerian anomalies and intrauterine adhesions. Fertil Steril 49:944–955
10. Diamond MP (2011) Postoperative adhesions: an underappreciated complication of cesarean deliveries. Am J Obstet Gynecol 205(6 Suppl):S1
11. Tulandi T, Al-Sannan B, Akbar G, Ziegler C, Miner L (2011) Prospective study of intraabdominal adhesions among women of different races with or without keloids. Am J Obstet Gynecol 204:132.e1–132.e14
12. Tulandi T, Al-Sannan B, Akbar G, Miner L, Ziegler C, Sikirica V (2011) Clinical Relevance of intra-abdominal adhesions in cesarean delivery. Gynecol Surg 8(4):399–403
13. Roset E, Boulvain M, Irion O (2003) Nonclosure of the peritoneum during caesarean section: long-term follow-up of a randomised controlled trial. Eur J Obstet Gynecol Reprod Biol 108:40–44
14. Weerawetwat W, Buranawanich S, Kanawong M (2004) Closure vs. non-closure of the visceral and parietal peritoneum at cesarean delivery: 16 year study. J Med Assoc Thail 87:1007–1011
15. Komoto Y, Shimoya K, Shimizu T, Kimura T, Hayashi S, Temma-Asano K, Kanagawa T, Fukuda H, Murata Y (2006) Prospective study of non-closure or closure of the peritoneum at cesarean delivery in 124 women: impact of prior peritoneal closure at primary cesarean on the interval time between first cesarean section and the next pregnancy and significant adhesion at second cesarean. J Obstet Gynaecol Res 32:396–402
16. Salim R, Kadan Y, Nachum Z, Edelstein S, Shalev E (2008) Abdominal scar characteristics as a predictor of intra-abdominal adhesions at repeat cesarean delivery. Fertil Steril 90:2324–2327
17. Malvasi A, Tinelli A, Farine D, Rahimi S, Cavallotti C, Vergara D, Martignago R, Stark M (2009) Effects of visceral peritoneal closure on scar formation at cesarean delivery. Int J Gynaecol Obstet 105:131–135
18. Zareian Z, Zareian P (2006) Non-closure versus closure of peritoneum during cesarean section: a randomized study. Eur J Obstet Gynecol Reprod Biol 128:267–269
19. Myers SA, Bennett TL (2005) Incidence of significant adhesions at repeat cesarean section and the relationship to method of prior peritoneal closure. J Reprod Med 50:659–662
20. Phipps MG, Watabe B, Clemons JL, Weitzen S, Myers DL (2005) Risk factors for bladder injury during cesarean delivery. Obstet Gynecol 105:156–160
21. Zhu Y, Cai Q, Wu W (2006) Closure vs. nonclosure of the peritoneum at cesarean delivery. Int J Gynaecol Obstet 94:103–107
22. Nisenblat V, Barak S, Griness OB, Degani S, Ohel G, Gonen R (2006) Maternal complications associated with multiple cesarean deliveries. Obstet Gynecol 108:21–26
23. Hamel KJ (2007) Incidence of adhesions at repeat cesarean delivery. Am J Obstet Gynecol 196:e31–e32
24. Fatusic Z, Hudic I (2009) Incidence of post-operative adhesions following Misgav-Ladach cesarean section—a comparative study. J Matern Fetal Neonatal Med 22:157–160
25. Chapa HO, Venegas G, Vanduyne CP, Antonetti AG, Sandate JP, Silver L (2011) Peritoneal adhesion prevention at cesarean section: an analysis of the effectiveness of an absorbable adhesion barrier. J Reprod Med 56:103–109
26. Bristow RE, Montz FJ (2005) Prevention of adhesions formation after radical oophorectomy using a sodium hyaluronate-carboxymethylcellulose (HA-CMC) barrier. Gynecol Oncol 99:301–308
27. Soltan MH (1996) Al Nuaim L, Khashoggi T, Chowdhury N, Kangave D, Adelusi B. Sequelae of repeat cesarean sections. Int J Gynaecol Obstet 52:127–132
28. Dogan NU, Haktankacmaz SA, Dogan S, Ozkan O, Celik H, Eryilmaz OG, Doganay M, Gulerman C (2011) A reliable way to predict intraabdominal adhesions at repeat cesarean delivery: scar characteristics. Acta Obstet Gynecol Scand 90:531–534
29. Greenberg MB, Daniels K, Blumenfeld YJ, Caughey AB, Lyell DJ (2011) Do adhesions at repeat cesarean delay delivery of the newborn? Am J Obstet Gynecol 205:380.e1–380.e15
30. Silver RM, Landon MB, Rouse DJ, Leveno KJ, Spong CY, Thom EA, Moawad AH (2006) Caritiset al. Maternal morbidity associated with multiple repeat cesarean deliveries. Obstet Gynecol 107:1226–1232
31. Andolf E, Thorsell M, Kallen K (2010) Cesarean delivery and risk for postoperative adhesions and intestinal obstruction: a nested case–control study of the Swedish Medical Birth Registry. Am J Obstet Gynecol 203:406.e1–406.e16

20

Outcome of conservative surgical treatment of deep infiltrating endometriosis

Sylvie Gordts · Patrick Puttemans · Rudi Campo · Marion Valkenburg · Stephan Gordts

Abstract Deep infiltrating endometriosis, which is frequently associated with pain, is diagnosed at clinical examination and with indirect imaging techniques like ultrasound and MRI. The aim of this study was to evaluate complications and recurrence rate after laparoscopic resection of deep infiltrating endometriosis by shaving technique. Between January 2004 and December 2010, 74 procedures for deep infiltrating endometriosis were performed in patients with pain and/or infertility. The endometriotic plaques were resected laparoscopically using scissors and bipolar and/or unipolar current. If rectosigmoidal invasion was present, a shaving was performed. Mean age was 31.7 years (SD ± 4.4). The vaginal nodule was a solitary lesion in 4 % of the patients without involvement of the ovaries, rectum or bladder. In 86 % of the cases, the rectosigmoid was involved as well. Mean follow-up was 776 days (SD= 465). One patient developed postoperatively a severe complication with intestinal perforation secondary to thermal necrosis (1.4 %). In four patients recurrence of symptoms was noted (8 %). Conservative surgery for deep infiltrating endometriosis resulted in the relief of pain, with a low postoperative complication rate (1.4 %). This shaving technique also resulted in a limited risk of recurrence of the symptoms (8 %).

Keywords Deep endometriosis · Surgery · Outcome

S. Gordts (✉) · P. Puttemans · R. Campo · M. Valkenburg · S. Gordts
LIFE,
Tiensevest 168,
Leuven 3000, Belgium
e-mail: Sylvie.Gordts@lifeleuven.be

Background

Endometriosis is characterized by the presence of endometrial glands and stroma outside the uterine cavity. It primarily affects women of fertile age, and represents a relevant clinical issue as it causes pain [1, 2] and infertility [2, 3]. Rectovaginal endometriosis (RVE) consists of an endometriotic nodule within the connective tissue between the anterior rectal wall and the vagina. The incidence of bowel infiltration among women with endometriosis varies between 6 and 12 % [4]. Deep endometriosis involving the bowel is most frequently localised in the rectovaginal septum [4, 5] and less in the sigmoid. Other bowel localisations are relatively rare [6].

Surgery is the best therapeutic option for symptomatic rectovaginal endometriosis. Several surgical techniques have been proposed with no consensus existing. Different procedures have been described in terms of parameters such as the size of the nodule and the affected bowel circumference, depth of lesions on the rectal wall, presence of other endometriotic foci and experience of the surgeon [7–9]. The most common surgical procedures used in the treatment of RVE are the following: superficial thickness excision (shaving), resection of the nodule with excision of the anterior side of the rectum (discoid resection) and colorectal segmental resection. At present, some surgeons prefer colorectal resection, as they are convinced that this is the treatment of choice to improve pain and to avoid relapses [10–13]. Other groups prefer the excision of the endometriotic nodule, since the rate of morbidity is lower and the recurrence of pain is similar [14, 15]. The choice for colorectal resection is supported by studies showing that microscopic endometriotic lesions usually exist around the main rectal nodule [16, 17]. But the clinical implication of leaving microscopic foci of endometriosis on the digestive tract remains unknown [18]. The aim of this study was to evaluate complications and recurrence rate after laparoscopic resection of deep infiltrating endometriosis by the shaving technique.

Materials and methods

Between January 2004 and December 2010, 74 procedures for deep infiltrating endometriosis were performed in patients with pain and/or infertility. Fifteen patients presented with pain symptoms, without fertility problems; 57 patients presented with pain and fertility problems, while two patients had only fertility problems and no pain (Table 1). These procedures were retrospectively reviewed for complications and relapse of symptoms.

Examination with a speculum revealed either a normal vaginal mucosa or a protruded blue nodule in the posterior fornix. By palpation, the diameter of the lesion could be evaluated. Palpation is often painful, and the presence of a nodule accounts for symptoms such as deep dyspareunia and dysmenorrhea. Preoperatively, a full bowel preparation was performed in all patients.

The endometriotic nodules were resected laparoscopically. In all cases a 5-mm laparoscope, in the umbilical position, and three 5-mm trocars were used. First, an adhesiolysis was performed. When ovarian endometriotic cysts were present, these were treated in the first step by opening the cyst and coagulation of the inner endometriotic wall using a BICAP probe (Storz). Resection of the nodule was performed using scissors and bipolar and/or unipolar current. Excision was guided visually and by tactile feedback of the indurations during the endoscopic excision.

Dissection was started by freeing the anterior rectum until the loose tissue of the rectovaginal space was reached. If rectosigmoidal invasion was present, a shaving was performed. With this technique as much as possible of the endometriotic tissue is removed without opening the intestine. This technique was performed independently of the size and depth of the lesion. A careful sharp dissection was performed until the rectum was completely free and identifiable below the lesion. Excision of the fibrotic tissue on the side of the rectum was performed after the rectal dissection was complete. The rectal muscle defects could be closed with suture. The lesions extending totally through the vagina were treated with *en bloc* laparoscopic resection of the lesion with the vaginal mucosa. In these cases the fornix posterior was opened. After complete resection of the nodule, the posterior vaginal wall was closed laparoscopically.

In order to exclude unnoticed rectum perforations, at the end of the operation, the pouch of Douglas was filled with irrigation fluid and subsequently, air was brought into the rectum. If the endometriotic nodule or fibrosis included ureter involvement, intra-operative ureter stents were used. The women were normally kept in the hospital for 36 h after surgery.

Table 1 Number of patients with respective sites of endometriosis lesions according to symptoms

Site of endometriosis	Pain[a]	Infertility[b]	Infertility + pain	Total
Ovarian endometriosis	4	2	31	37
Rectosigmoid	13	0	51	64
Bladder	1	1	8	10
Total	15	2	57	74

[a] Pain symptoms without infertility

[b] Infertility without any symptoms of pain

Findings

The mean age of the patients was 31.7 years (SD ± 4.4). The mean size of the rectovaginal nodule was 1.9 cm. The size of the nodule was estimated by clinical examination and inspection during surgical resection of the nodule. By excision of the nodule, the posterior fornix of the vagina was opened in 42 % of the cases.

The vaginal nodule was a solitary lesion in 4 % of the patients without involvement of ovaries, rectum or bladder. In most cases the endometriosis was a complex disease involving different structures (sacrouterine ligaments, rectosigmoid, ureter and ovaries). In 37 cases one or both ovaries had an endometriotic cyst. In 86 % (n=64) of the cases, the bowel was involved. In 14 % of the patients, bladder endometriosis was present (Table 1). Thirteen patients had been operated for endometriosis in the past in other centres.

In 91 % (n=58) of the patients with bowel involvement, shaving was performed. During the shaving, opening of the bowel mucosa was performed in five patients (8 %). Only on one patient a discoid resection was performed. In two patients when the appendix was involved, appendectomy was carried out. In four patients no treatment of the bowel involvement was performed since they had no bowel symptoms. In these patients only a resection of the vaginal part of the nodule was performed. In one of these four patients, a second laparoscopy with bowel shaving is performed 2 years later because of bowel symptoms.

One patient developed postoperatively a complication with intestinal perforation secondary to thermal necrosis (1.4 %). This patient presented with pain and fever 10 days postoperatively. An urgent laparoscopy was performed showing bowel perforation with necrosis. A partial bowel resection was performed. Other complications like ureteral damage, urinary retention or fistulas were not noted.

Only two patients received preoperatively GnRH analogues because of pain and waiting period before the

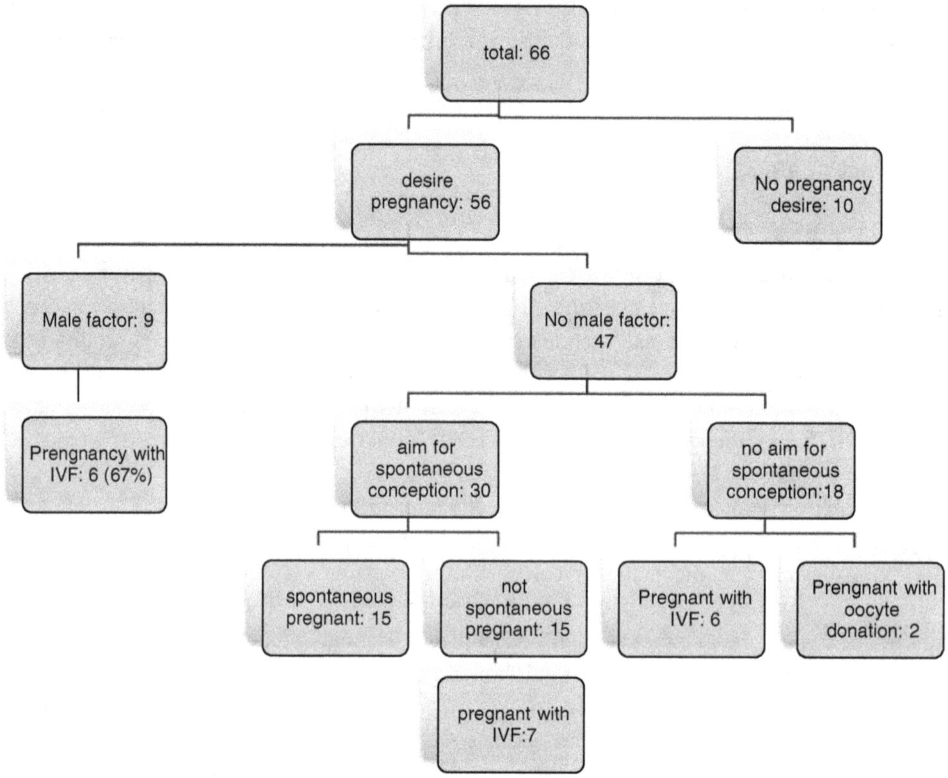

Fig. 1 Pregnancy outcome. Total = total of patients with follow-up of at least 1 year; male factor = abnormal sperm analysis; aim for spontaneous conception = no fertility treatment for at least 6 months; spontaneous pregnancy = pregnancy without fertility treatment

operation could be performed. Ten patients received GnRH-agonist treatment for 3 months postoperatively. Six of them were given because they were referred for immediate starting of in vitro fertilization (IVF) treatment and in four patients because on MRI, adenomyosis was suspected.

Only patients with a follow-up of at least 1 year were included for further analysis. Eight patients were lost of follow-up and excluded. Mean follow-up was 776 days (SD=465).

In six patients recurrence of symptoms was noted (8 %). The mean time of recurrence was 540 days. In four patients an endometriotic cyst was visualised on ultrasound. In three patients a second laparoscopy was performed. Two laparoscopies showed invasion in the bowel serosa. One laparoscopy showed only recurrence of an endometriotic cyst. In one patient with a cyst on ultrasound, an aspiration of the cyst was performed. One patient had only recurrence of symptoms without obvious pathology; thus, no laparoscopy was performed.

We also evaluated the pregnancy outcome after surgery (Fig. 1). Ten patients did not try to conceive. In the rest of the group, we noted an overall pregnancy rate of 63 %. In nine couples a male factor was present. Those patients were immediately referred for IVF. In this group a mean of 7.7 oocytes were retrieved with a fertilization rate of 65 %. They reached a pregnancy rate of 67 %. In the group with no male factor, some patients were advised not to opt for a spontaneous pregnancy. These were older patients or patients with previous infertility treatments. They were directed towards IVF (n=16) or oocyte donation (n=2). In the patients for IVF treatment, a mean of six oocytes were retrieved with a fertilization rate of 61 %. In this group a pregnancy rate of 37 % was reached. If no ovarian endometriosis was present, a mean of 7.5 oocytes were retrieved. In those patients where only one ovary had endometriosis, a mean of 7.4 oocytes could be retrieved. If both ovaries had ovarian endometriosis, a mean of eight oocytes were retrieved at oocyte pick-up. Two patients were poor responders in the IVF treatment and they started an oocyte donation treatment. The ages of these two patients were 34 and 38 years.

Thirty couples were advised to aim for a spontaneous pregnancy. The mean age of these patients was 29.7 years. The spontaneous pregnancy rate was 50 % in this study. In those patients with associated ovarian endometriosis, the spontaneous pregnancy rate was also 50 % (Table 2). The mean time to spontaneous conception was 7.4 months.

Table 2 Spontaneous pregnancy according to localisation of the lesion in patients with desire of pregnancy and no male pathology

Localisation of the lesion	Number[a]	Spontaneous pregnancy
Ovarian endometriosis	16	8
Rectosigmoid	24	11
Solitary vaginal	2	1

[a] Infertility without any symptoms of pain

Conclusions

Our study provides information regarding the outcome related to the shaving technique for patients with deep endometriosis. Over the last decade, it seems to have been widely accepted that complete excision of deep endometriosis is the treatment of choice. The idea is that the excision should be complete in order to achieve maximal pain relief and minimal recurrences. To our knowledge, however, there are no data to substantiate this. The decision to perform bowel resection seems to be based on attitude rather than on data. The argument used by some gynaecologists and surgeons to defend bowel resection is that this procedure is more 'radical'. But, even with bowel resection, the margins are not free of disease in more than 10 % of cases [15, 19]. Other studies have shown that residual lesions in the muscularis of the rectum do not evolve and remain constant for a long time [14]. The question remains as to whether complete long-term relief of pain systematically requires complete resection of the digestive foci, when taking into consideration the risk of postoperative complications and unpleasant functional symptoms. The 'price to pay' for segmental bowel resection is presented by possible complications. It should also be pointed out that colorectal segmental resection is a complex procedure, sometimes resulting in pelvic nerve damage and unpleasant urinary and digestive symptoms [15, 20]. A review [21] of 34 articles of bowel resections for deep endometriosis showed an overall complication rate of 22 %. Major complications occurred in 11 % of women, that is 6.4 % with severe bowel complications (leakage rate, 1.9 %; fistula rate, 1.8 %; and severe obstruction rate, 2.7 %), 2.5 % with haemorrhage and 1 % with infections. Minor complications occurred in 14.7 % of the women, with an incidence of temporary bowel dysfunction of 3.6 % and of bladder dysfunction of 8 %. Another review of Payá [9] concluded that when surgical treatment does not include intestinal resection, the rates of surgical complications are low, in the majority of papers not reaching 5 %, with bladder and intestinal dysfunction practically non-existent. They conclude that segmental bowel resection should be performed in selected cases. The indication for bowel resection might be represented by important bowel stenosis. Also in our study, low surgical complication rate of 1.4 % is reached. We cannot exclude that the fact that the patients were mainly infertility patients and not pelvic pain patients, which influenced these results. The study of Fanfani et al. compared postoperative complications to the patient satisfaction and recurrence rates between two laparoscopic techniques (discoid versus segmental resection) [18]. They conclude that the complication rate is lower in the discoid resection group, but patient satisfaction and recurrence rate are comparable in both groups.

In most cases, perirectal periviscеritis may be left in place. The residual lesion in the muscularis of the rectum does not seem to evolve and remains constant for a long time. Patients are usually free of symptoms, so we can consider that systematic bowel resection in case of perirectal visceritis and rectal muscularis involvement is unnecessary. Moreover, such surgery increases morbidity and is responsible for more adhesions resulting from extensive lateral dissection. In case of bowel occlusion and rectal bleeding with rectal mucosa involvement, resection of the rectosigmoid junction can be performed.

Little data are available on the fertility and pregnancy outcome after surgery for deep infiltrating endometriosis. Some studies have shown a higher pregnancy rate for minimally invasive procedures (shaving and discoid resection) compared with segmental resection [22]. As we are a fertility unit, most of our patients present with infertility. The results of this study demonstrate that even in this subfertile population, a good spontaneous pregnancy rate can be achieved after conservative surgery. The spontaneous pregnancy rate of 50 % in our study was similar as reported in other studies (Darai, Marpeau et al. 2005; Donnez and Squifflet 2010). Compared to our overall IVF population, the number of oocytes retrieved was slightly lower (7.3 versus 8.9). The fertilization rates were identical (63 versus 62.3 %). But the pregnancy rates are higher than the general IVF population (57 versus 39.6 %). Of course these groups are not comparable in a lot of aspects, but it is an indication of the pregnancy outcome with IVF treatment after conservative surgery for deep endometriosis. These results are comparable as the results found by other authors [23, 24].

Conservative surgery for deep endometriosis in young women means preservation of organs, nerves, vascular blood supply and fertility. There is therefore a need for further strong and energetic debate to weigh up the benefits of shaving versus radical surgery. Feasibility is not always synonymous with efficacy.

Conflict of interest The authors report no conflicts of interest. The authors alone are responsible for the content and writing of the paper.

References

1. Koninckx PR, Meuleman C, Demeyere S, Lesaffre E, Cornillie FJ (1991) Suggestive evidence that pelvic endometriosis is a progressive disease, whereas deeply infiltrating endometriosis is associated with pelvic pain. Fertil Steril 55(4):759–765
2. Fauconnier A, Chapron C, Dubuisson JB, Vieira M, Dousset B, Breart G (2002) Relation between pain symptoms and the anatomic location of deep infiltrating endometriosis. Fertil Steril 78 (4):719–726

3. Pouly JL, Drolet J, Canis M, Boughazine S, Mage G, Bruhat MA, Wattiez A (1996) Laparoscopic treatment of symptomatic endometriosis. Hum Reprod 11(Suppl 3):67–88
4. Macafee CH, Greer HL (1960) Intestinal endometriosis. A report of 29 cases and a survey of the literature. J Obstet Gynaecol Br Emp 67:539–555
5. Koninckx PR, Martin DC (1992) Deep endometriosis: a consequence of infiltration or retraction or possibly adenomyosis externa? Fertil Steril 58(5):924–928
6. Brouwer R, Woods RJ (2007) Rectal endometriosis: results of radical excision and review of published work. ANZ J Surg 77 (7):562–571. doi:10.1111/j.1445-2197.2007.04153.x
7. Chapron C, Chopin N, Borghese B, Foulot H, Dousset B, Vacher-Lavenu MC, Vieira M, Hasan W, Bricou A (2006) Deeply infiltrating endometriosis: pathogenetic implications of the anatomical distribution. Hum Reprod 21(7):1839–1845. doi:10.1093/humrep/del079
8. Abrao MS, Podgaec S, Dias JA Jr, Averbach M, Silva LF, Marino de Carvalho F (2008) Endometriosis lesions that compromise the rectum deeper than the inner muscularis layer have more than 40 % of the circumference of the rectum affected by the disease. J Minim Invasive Gynecol 15(3):280–285. doi:10.1016/j.jmig.2008.01.006
9. Payá V, Hidalgo-Mora JJ, Diaz-Garcia C, Pellicer A (2011) Surgical treatment of rectovaginal endometriosis with rectal involvement. Gynecol Surg 8(3):269–277. doi:10.1007/s10397-011-0663-y
10. Dousset B, Leconte M, Borghese B, Millischer AE, Roseau G, Arkwright S, Chapron C (2010) Complete surgery for low rectal endometriosis: long-term results of a 100-case prospective study. Ann Surg 251(5):887–895. doi:10.1097/SLA.0b013e3181d9722d
11. Possover M, Diebolder H, Plaul K, Schneider A (2000) Laparascopically assisted vaginal resection of rectovaginal endometriosis. Obstet Gynecol 96(2):304–307
12. Keckstein J, Wiesinger H (2005) Deep endometriosis, including intestinal involvement–the interdisciplinary approach. Minim Invasive Ther Allied Technol 14(3):160–166. doi:10.1080/14017430510035916
13. Minelli L, Fanfani F, Fagotti A, Ruffo G, Ceccaroni M, Mereu L, Landi S, Pomini P, Scambia G (2009) Laparoscopic colorectal resection for bowel endometriosis: feasibility, complications, and clinical outcome. Arch Surg 144(3):234–239. doi:10.1001/archsurg.2008.555, discussion 239
14. Donnez J, Squifflet J (2004) Laparoscopic excision of deep endometriosis. Obstet Gynecol Clin North Am 31(3):567–580. doi:10.1016/j.ogc.2004.06.006, ix
15. Roman H, Loisel C, Resch B, Tuech JJ, Hochain P, Leroi AM, Marpeau L (2010) Delayed functional outcomes associated with surgical management of deep rectovaginal endometriosis with rectal involvement: giving patients an informed choice. Hum Reprod 25(4):890–899. doi:10.1093/humrep/dep407
16. Kavallaris A, Köhler C, Kühne-Heid R, Schneider A (2003) Histopathological extent of rectal invasion by rectovaginal endometriosis. Hum Reprod 18(6):1323–1327
17. Remorgida V, Ragni N, Ferrero S, Anserini P, Torelli P, Fulcheri E (2005) The involvement of the interstitial Cajal cells and the enteric nervous system in bowel endometriosis. Hum Reprod 20 (1):264–271. doi:10.1093/humrep/deh568
18. Fanfani F, Fagotti A, Gagliardi ML, Ruffo G, Ceccaroni M, Scambia G, Minelli L (2010) Discoid or segmental rectosigmoid resection for deep infiltrating endometriosis: a case–control study. Fertil Steril 94 (2):444–449. doi:10.1016/j.fertnstert.2009.03.066
19. Anaf V, El Nakadi I, De Moor V, Coppens E, Zalcman M, Noel JC (2009) Anatomic significance of a positive barium enema in deep infiltrating endometriosis of the large bowel. World J Surg 33 (4):822–827. doi:10.1007/s00268-008-9903-3
20. Slack A, Child T, Lindsey I, Kennedy S, Cunningham C, Mortensen N, Koninckx P, McVeigh E (2007) Urological and colorectal complications following surgery for rectovaginal endometriosis. BJOG 114(10):1278–1282. doi:10.1111/j.1471-0528.2007.01477.x
21. De Cicco C, Corona R, Schonman R, Mailova K, Ussia A, Koninckx PR (2011) Bowel resection for deep endometriosis: a systematic review. BJOG 118(3):285–291. doi:10.1111/j.1471-0528.2010.02744.x
22. Mohr C, Nezhat FR, Nezhat CH, Seidman DS, Nezhat CR (2005) Fertility considerations in laparoscopic treatment of infiltrative bowel endometriosis. JSLS 9(1):16–24
23. Donnez J, Squifflet J (2010) Complications, pregnancy and recurrence in a prospective series of 500 patients operated on by the shaving technique for deep rectovaginal endometriotic nodules. Hum Reprod 25(8):1949–1958. doi:10.1093/humrep/deq135
24. Bianchi PH, Pereira RM, Zanatta A, Alegretti JR, Motta EL, Serafini PC (2009) Extensive excision of deep infiltrative endometriosis before in vitro fertilization significantly improves pregnancy rates. J Minim Invasive Gynecol 16(2):174–180. doi:10.1016/j.jmig.2008.12.009

21

Gynaecological robotic surgery in an Irish setting—cost analysis

O. E. O'Sullivan · M. O'Carroll · M. Hewitt · B. A. O'Reilly

Abstract Robotic surgery is associated with reduced hospital stay compared with open surgery. While the initial outlay is expensive, the increased number of patients amenable to this minimal access approach compared with conventional 'keyhole surgery' has the potential for financial savings. Our aim was to show the cost per surgery and the potential for savings with increased caseload and reduced hospital bed stay. A cost analysis was performed incorporating an audit of robotic surgery over the initial 3 years. This was performed using prospectively acquired data completed after each robotically assisted case. Depreciation and maintenance on the robot accounted for an outlay of €260,000/annum. Due to the learning curves and hospital constraints, in year 1, an average of 1.5 cases were performed per week at a cost of €5,980/case, this cost reduced to €4,250 over the next 2 years with an increase to 2.4 cases/week. We projected that if maximum usage of nine cases/week was achieved the cost would reduce to €2,523/case. In 2010, 36 % of all hysterectomies were performed robotically. The average length of stay for robot-assisted cases was two nights compared to six to eight nights for open hysterectomy. The robotic approach is associated with savings of approximately €201,933/year compared with a similar tertiary referral hospital in Ireland with no robot. Purchasing a robot is costly but associated with greater cost savings when reduced length of stay is accounted for. Furthermore, maximisation of robotic use further decreases the cost per case.

Keywords Robotic surgery · Gynaecology · Cost analysis

O. E. O'Sullivan (✉) · M. O'Carroll · M. Hewitt · B. A. O'Reilly
Department of Obstetrics and Gynaecology, Cork University Maternity Hospital, Cork, Ireland
e-mail: scatterjack@gmail.com

Background

Surgery is an evolving science, aiming to improve patient outcome and reduce complication rates. Within the last 50 years, machines have been made to mimic human actions in order to perform specific tasks rather than to entertain and amuse. Furthermore, within the last 20 years, robotic technology has been applied to the practice of surgery. The goal of this technology has not been to replace the surgeon, but rather to enhance his or her performance with highly advanced tools [1]. At present, Intuitive Surgical® market the da Vinci® Surgical System (Intuitive Surgical, Inc., Sunnyvale, CA, USA), the only commercially available robot system with Food and Drug Administration (FDA) approval for use in gynaecology. Since gaining FDA approval in 2005, the role of the robot has increased with many traditional procedures now being performed with robot assistance. Within the gynaecological surgery setting, the robot has been used successfully for simple and radical hysterectomy, pelvic lymphadenectomy, tubal surgery, myomectomy, sacrocolpopexy/hysteropexy and interval cervical cerclage [2]. As with all new techniques, there is a learning curve associated with robotic surgery, this is divided into three stages: (1) the initial phase, (2) the plateau phase and (3) the mastery phase [3]. Each phase has been shown to be associated with a number of procedures performed. However, the learning curve varies from surgeon to surgeon and is influenced by the complexity of the case. In the study by Bokari, the initial phase is associated with the first 15 cases performed and the subsequent 10 cases are the plateau phase where the surgeon becomes more proficient with the techniques required prior to progressing to the mastery phase. During the mastery phase, the technical difficulty of the cases performed increases and accounts for the final 23 cases [3]. With specific regard to gynaecological surgery, the learning curves reported range 50 cases for benign hysterectomies [4] to 10 cases for sacrocolpopexy [5]. This should be borne in mind when conducting cost analysis involving theatre times and caseloads per day.

New technology comes with an economic burden for the healthcare system. This increased initial outlay cost is often offset by the benefits to the patient in terms of reduced hospital stay, blood transfusion and a reduction in complications. For the surgeon, there is the benefit of shortened operating times, an ability to perform more complex surgery using a minimally invasive technique [5]. It is therefore important for the hospital and the health system within each country utilising the new robotic technology to have a clear understanding of the costs associated with the adoption and implementation of this new technology. With increasing financial austerity, even more emphasis is being placed on cost reduction within the health sector.

The Cork University Maternity Hospital (CUMH) is a tertiary referral centre, which treats both benign, urogynaecological and oncology patients. The da Vinci® Surgical System is located in the purpose-built laparoscopic theatre, which is dedicated solely to gynaecological surgery. The aim of this study was to assess the initial cost of purchase and set up for the programme, the running costs and the cost benefits for the first 3 years of the programme, which commenced in 2008. We also endeavoured to implement a strategy of cost reduction within our hospital setting.

Materials and methods

Over the 3 years (July 2008–May 2011) since instigating the robotic programme in our unit, a prospective record was kept of surgical times, including setup time, docking time, anaesthetic time, operating time and recovery time. For each case, the procedure, surgeon, complication/conversion rate and indication were all recorded. Demographic details of each patient were recorded. A total of 281 cases were performed predominantly by three surgeons, with a further two surgeons records included in the data, these surgeons were closely supervised by the more experienced surgeons. The procedures performed included: benign and radical hysterectomy, sacrocolpopexy/hysteropexy, adnexal surgery, myomectomy and interval cervical cerclage.

Data was recorded on the costs generated in theatre including staff pay, surgical instruments: disposable, reusable and robot specific. Furthermore, the cost of procedure-specific instruments was also recorded. A cost model was set up to analyse the cost per operation and allow financial adjustments to be made to assess the cost implications of increasing caseloads. The robot purchasing cost, maintenance and depreciation were derived from hospital specific figures. The depreciation was valued over 10 years based on the life span of the robot. Using the Health Service Executive (HSE) Ready Reckoner 2011, a specific cost per night hospital stay was recorded and a weighted average used per case based on the diagnosis-related group.

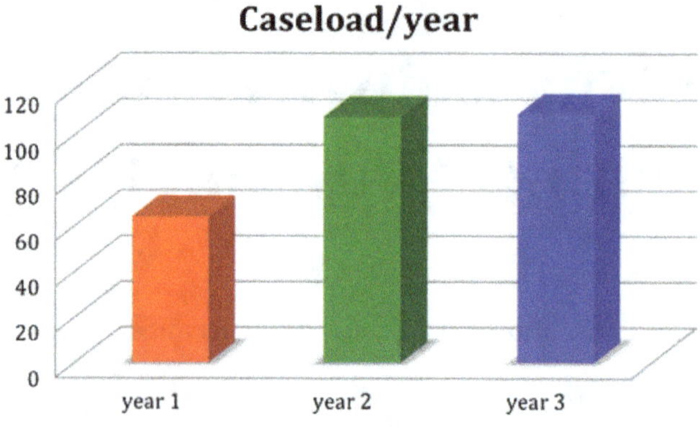

Fig. 1 Caseload per year

Findings

Two hundred and eighty one robotic procedures were performed by five surgeons from July 2008–May 2011 in our unit. The breakdown of cases was as follows: 76 % of cases were hysterectomy (simple and radical)±adnexal surgery, 18 % of cases were sacrocolpopexy/hysteropexy and the remaining 6 % were made up of interval cervical cerclage, myomectomy and endometriotic surgery (Fig. 1).

The cost of purchasing the da Vinci® Surgical System in 2008 was €1.35 million, with a current residual trade-in value of €800,000. The life expectancy is quoted as 7–10 years; however, many of the original systems in other units are still functioning 12 years since being commissioned. The maintenance contract is €125,000/year with an 'as new' policy. This incorporates all service and repair costs of the robot. Within the HSE, depreciation on machinery is

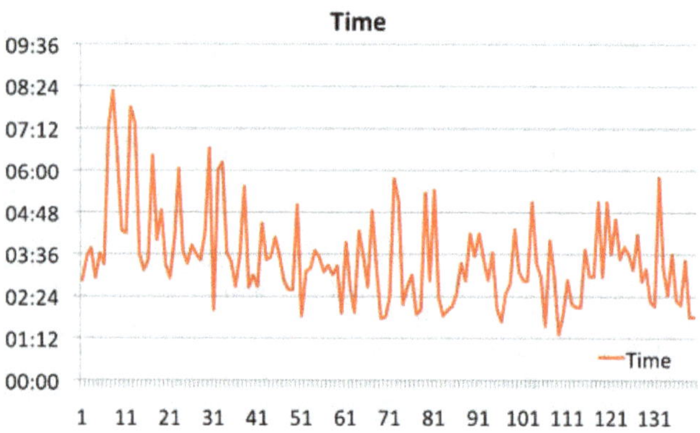

Fig. 2 Operative times over the course of the study for surgeon A

Table 1 The operative times per year of programme

	Operations/week	Mean in-theatre time per surgery type			Range of time
		Overall	Hysterectomy	Sacrocolpopexy	
Year1	1.4	4:25	4:26	4:01	2:40–9:30
Year2	2.3	3:11	3:24	3:01	1:50–5:45
Year3	2.4	3:04	3:10	2:56	1:18–5:39

10 % straight line giving an annual cost of €135,000 based on a 10-year life expectancy. The total cost for maintenance and depreciation per annum is €260,000. Furthermore, the operative sets, including trocars and light cables cost €6,418. Four sets were constructed to allow time for sterilisation. The initial expenditure includes the cost of disposable trocars for the camera and the assistant (€94.78 per operation). Instrument costs varied according to the operation performed, as different instruments were required to perform the operation. The instrument cost was then assessed by type of operation—the sacrocolpopexy/hysteropexy cost €1,612 while all other operations cost €1,979 (Appendix A).

The surgical learning curves were evaluated and a per-year breakdown of procedures performed analysed (Fig. 2). As expected, the number of operations performed per week increased per year and the operative time decreased (Table 1). The CUMH is a training centre and during this period, three specialists registrars were trained using the system to the level of performing simple hysterectomies 'unassisted'. Furthermore, a recognised gynaecological robotic fellowship was commenced and the first graduate completed their training in the 2010. The instrument cost per annum based on caseload was calculated (Table 2). Using these figures, we calculated an average cost per operation, which incorporated the depreciation and maintenance costs. This overall cost decreases with increased caseload per year.

Using our cost model to calculate, the cost per operation if the caseload increased to a maximum of nine cases per week. In so doing the cost reduced from €4,250 to 2,523.

We analysed the cost benefit with regard to length of stay comparing open midline, lower transverse, laparoscopic, vaginal and robotic cases in our centre where the length of stay was eight (5–18), six (3–14), 3 (1–5), three (1–5) and two (0–4) nights, respectively. We then compared our hysterectomy caseload for 2010 to that of another tertiary referral teaching hospital in Ireland with similar inpatient capacity but no facility for robotic surgery. As expected, there were similar rates for vaginal hysterectomy at 45 % in both units, the reference unit performed more laparoscopic hysterectomies (20 vs. 5 %), and our unit performed fewer hysterectomies via the abdominal approach (14 vs. 35 %). We performed 36 % of our hysterectomies using the robot. When we compared our hysterectomy figures for 2009 to 2010, we found the abdominal approach had reduced from 24 to 10 % (Fig. 3a and b). This reduction in open cases is associated with a reduction in cost for length of stay. Using the HSE Ready Reckoner 2011, it was calculated that the weighted average based on the case mix treated for one night of stay is €534.19. We predict if the rate of open procedure falls by a further 10 % as it did between 2009 and 2010, we would save €201,932 due to bed day reduction (Table 3a and b).

Comments

Health Technology Assessments assess the clinical benefits of the new technique in relation to the cost of its implementation. Two recent health technology assessments (HTA) concluded that robot-assisted surgery is an emerging technology that could be promising in ideal circumstances and given adequate training and experience of the surgical team performing the interventions [6] and may have a significant impact on many clinical outcomes in patients undergoing prostatectomy, partial nephrectomy or hysterectomy; however, benefits vary between indications [7]. Robotically performed surgery is costly compared with open and laparoscopic approaches. The investment made in acquiring this technology is significant, and institutions that choose to

Table 2 Cost per year for robotic instruments

	Hysterectomy Total number/year	Sacrocolpopexy Total number/year	Instrument cost Hysterectomy	Instrument cost Sacrocolpopexy	Total cost/year
Year1	57	7	112,845.75	11,287.50	124,133.25
Year2	89	19	176,197.75	30,637.50	206,835.25
Year3	83	26	164,319.25	41,925.00	206,244.25

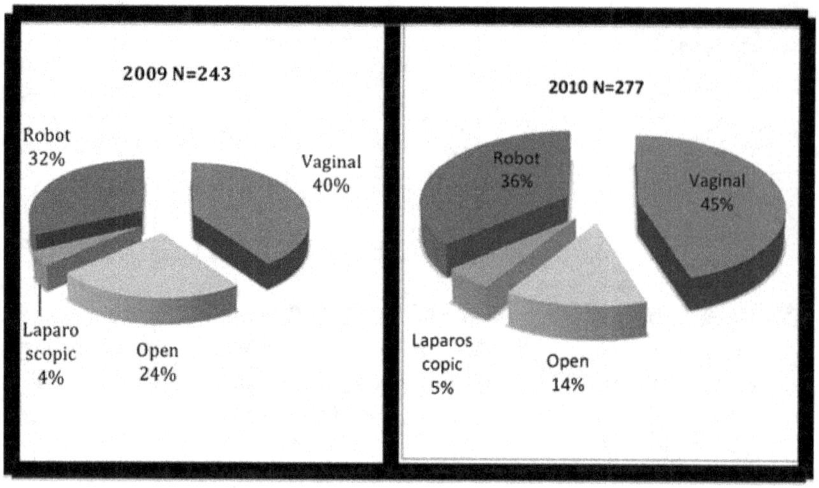

Fig. 3 Comparison of mode of hysterectomy in CUMH in 2009 and 2010

adopt it should make efforts to monitor its costs and outcomes in order to maximise cost-effective use within their own centre. To decrease costs, centres should maximise caseloads, consider keeping the robot operational for longer durations if possible, and use the technology for multiple indications, particularly those with greater potential impact on important patient outcomes and savings on institutional costs [7]. Furthermore, the increased bed usage and throughput of patients would decrease waiting lists and eliminate the need for national treatment purchasing fund to purchase treatment in private hospitals for these patients. The knock-on effect is to reduce the number of gynaecological emergency admissions by patients on long waiting lists. There would also be social savings such as reduced post-operative sick leave and earlier return to work.

In 2009, the American Congress of Obstetricians and Gynecologists released a statement recommending vaginal hysterectomy as the approach of choice for benign hysterectomies due to reduced operating times when compared to the laparoscopic approach [8]. However, they note that laparoscopic surgery is an alternative where vaginal hysterectomy is not feasible or indicated. Increasing the rate of vaginal surgery decreases the cost of surgery compared to the open approach due to reduced length of stay. Consideration must be given to the fact that not all surgeries are amenable to the vaginal approach. Our figures showed that during 2009–2010, our vaginal hysterectomy rate increased from 40 to 45 % in association with the decrease in open hysterectomies. Our rate of vaginal hysterectomy was equal to that of another tertiary referral unit in Ireland. However, as a tertiary referral centre providing oncology care, the robotic approach allows complicated and radical hysterectomies be performed using a minimal access approach. Our rates of open hysterectomy were almost three times lower (14 vs. 35 %) when compared to a similar sized tertiary referral centre in Ireland where robotic surgery is not available.

In conducting a cost analysis, there are direct, indirect and hidden costs, which need to be addressed. In this study, staffing costs were the same for all modes of surgery as irrespective of how and who performed the operation the same staff were employed to be present in theatre during normal working hours in the public sector. However, there is a cost saving potential in terms of staffing when using the da Vinci® Surgical System as a surgically trained assistants are not required, the scrub nurse can be trained to assist thus saving on salaries and leading to the redeploying of staff to

Table 3 Savings due to bed day reduction between 2009 and 2010

Types of hysterectomy	Number of cases/year	Average length of stay	Bed nights	Total cost per operation type	Accumulative cost
Predicted cost benefit for length of stay in CUMH (bed=534.19/night)					
Vaginal (45 %)	126	3	378	201,923.82	
Open (5 %)	14	6	84	44,871.96	
Laparoscopic (5 %)	14	3	42	22,435.98	
Robotic (45 %)	126	2	252	134,615.88	403,847.64
Predicted cost for length of stay in unit without robotic surgery (bed=534.19/night)					
Vaginal (45 %)	126	3	378	201,932.82	
Open (35 %)	98	6	588	314,103.72	
Laparoscopic (20 %)	56	3	168	89,743.92	605,780.46

another area. The central sterile supply department may require updating and new equipment and training required for staff dealing with the robot equipment, and finally the existing timetables for theatre may need to be adjusted to maximise robotic use. With regard to the indirect costs, many relate to the provision of the new programme including administrative staff, a programne co-coordinator/manager and data collection. The administration duties are conducted by current employees and data collection is performed by the theatre staff and the medical staff.

Historically, in Ireland, the length of stay has been higher than that of other European countries. While we are not aware of any studies that have examined factors which may influence the increased length of stay, possible influences include: reduced respite care, reduced provision for domiciliary visit by the public healthcare team and patients' expectations. To reduce the impact of patient and family expectation on length of stay, all patients are now counselled in the outpatients department as to their expected length of stay thereby reducing any misunderstanding by the patient and family regarding discharge days. Barnett et al. [9] used three different costing models and showed that laparoscopy was the least expensive surgical approach for the treatment of endometrial cancer. The robot is less costly than abdominal hysterectomy and is most economically attractive if disposable equipment costs can be minimised. When laparoscopic hysterectomy was compared with robot-assisted hysterectomy in terms of cost and clinical outcomes, there was no significant differences with regards to perioperative and postoperative events, but there was an increased per-case cost for the robot [10]

Conclusion

From the results of our study, we concur that the initial expenditure for the da Vinci® Surgical Systems is substantial, it is associated with the potential cost benefits of reduced length of stay, from 6 to 8 days for an open hysterectomy to 2 days for a robot-assisted hysterectomy. We are currently looking at outcome measures such as patient perception of recovery, with provisional results showing low post-operative pain scores and the majority of patients performed simple household chores within a week of surgery and 50 % were driving within 4 weeks of surgery. In this study, we have shown that maximising the caseload to nine cases per week reduces the overall cost of the operation, which would involve increasing our current caseload threefold. Based on these figures, a throughput of 450 robot-assisted operations would be required. In 2010, a total of 155 robot-assisted operations were performed, which would leave a shortfall of 300 cases. Clearly reducing the number of unwarranted open procedures would not increase the caseload to the required figure. Therefore, provision would need to be made to optimise the workload by opening the robot up to other specialties where the robot-assisted surgery has shown to be effective.

A recently published Irish HTA looked at the financial implications of robot-assisted surgery [11]. Using an economic model which was restricted to the HSE perspective and only incorporating direct costs, they showed the incremental cost of robot-assisted surgery (over the robot lifespan) if used for hysterectomy alone is €3,019 (95 % CI: €2,582–3,733), assuming a steady state volume of 300 cases per annum. However, when used for a combination of prostatectomy and hysterectomy procedures, it is €2,864 (95 % CI: €2,384–3,587). As expected, they found the increased cost of robot-assisted surgery was primarily due to the additional costs associated with the specific surgical equipment, purchase and maintenance and the cost of theatre staff due to longer operative times. They believe the costs are only partially offset by savings associated with shorter inpatient stays. Furthermore, based on the steady state volumes used in the model, use of one robot to assist surgery compared to standard surgical techniques will reduce the annual number of bed days by 565 days (95 % CI: 422–721) if used for hysterectomy alone and 558 days (95 % CI: 417–697) if used for a combination of prostatectomy and hysterectomy. Also, increasing the annual volume of cases per robot reduces the incremental cost of robot-assisted surgery, as does extending the lifespan of the robot. Interestingly the HTA concluded that the number of days to return to normal activity appears substantially shorter after robot-assisted surgery compared to open surgery and as such, robot-assisted surgery may offer a significant societal benefit.

Quality Adjusted Life Year (QALY) assessments are a standard to evaluate the outcomes of healthcare expenditure [12]. They offer a measure by which to ascertain which patient to treat and which treatment to use based on the quality of life benefit received by a certain form of intervention. It was not possible to assess the QALY for robotic surgery during our study and to date we are not aware of any studies which report this exercise. However, it would be beneficial to have a set of parameters by which to assess robotic outcomes further.

Acknowledgments We would like to thank Thomas O'Donovan from the purchasing department at Cork University Maternity Hospital for all his help in furnishing us with the costs for instruments used. We would also like to thank the hospital management for their foresight and cooperation in funding the purchase of the robot. Finally, we would like to thank the nurses in the theatre department without whom we could not have instigated a robotic surgical programme.

Declaration of interest Matthew Hewitt has received travel bursaries to attend educational meetings. He acts as a surgical proctor for Intuitive. All financial reimbursement from the company is placed in the department's research fund. Barry O'Reilly is a proctor for Intuitive. All financial reimbursement from the company are placed in the departments' research fund. The Cork University Maternity Hospital is an Intuitive recognised epicentre for robotic surgical training. All funds received from this are placed in the department's research fund.

Appendix A

Cost as per Cork University Maternity Hospital 2008

Table 4 Initial purchase cost and yearly cost

Product	Company	Model	Cost per unit	Life expectancy (years)	Maintenance	Residual value	Deprciation	Cost per year
Da Vinci Robot	Intuitive	Si Dual	2.1 m	7–10	165,000			
		Si Single	1.6 m	7–10	140,000			
		Cork model	1.35 m (2008)	7–10	125,000	800,000	10 % straight line	125,000+135,000=260,000

Table 5 Instrument cost per type of surgery

Product	Company	Quantity/ box	Cost per unit	Box quantity	Cost per box	Vat rate (%)	Total cost per unit	No of units per procedure	Hysterectomy	Sacrocolpopexy
All in One 1032P	3M	1	29.18	10	291.80	21	35	1	35	35
Robot Drapes	Intuitive	1	234.00	5	1,170.00	21	283	1	283	283
Endo Wrist Instrument	Intuitive	10 uses/ item								
Pro-grasp			220.00	1	2,200.00	21	2,662.00	1	266.20	266.20
Maryland Forceps			2,700.00	1	2,700.00	21	3,267.00	1		326.70
PK Dissector			2,900.00	1	2,900.00	21	3,509	1	350.90	
Monopolar Scissors			3,200	1	3,200	21	3,872	1	387.20	387.20
Fenestrated Bipolar Forceps			2,700	1	2,700	21	3,267	1	326.70	
Suture Cut Needle Holder			2,400	1	2,400	21	2,904	1	290.40	290.40
Cover for Scissors			20	10	200	21	24	1	24	24
Gyrius Cable		20 uses/ item	270	1	270	21	327	1	16.35	
Valleylab Black Mono polar Cable		Reusable	184.70	1	184.70	21	223	1	0	0
Valleylab Bipolar Disposable Cable		1	2.40	50	120.00	21	3	0		
SCD Sleeve	TYCO		22.00	5	110.00		22	0		
Total cost									€1,979.75	€1,612.50

Table 6 Cost for each operative set

Product	Company	Quantity/ box	Cost per unit	Box quantity	Cost per box	Vat rate (%)	Total cost per unit	No units per procedure	Total cost
Disposable Trocar		1	39.17	6	235.02	21	47.39	2	94.78
Metal Trocar		1	550	1	550		550	3	1,650
Obturator		1	550	1	550		550	2	1,100
Scope Target		1	500	1	500		500	1	500
Camera Adaptor		1	950	1	950		950	1	950
Camera Arm Adaptor		1	950	1	950		950	1	950
Light Cable		1	950	1	950		950	1	950
Monopolar Cord		1	184.70	1	184.70	21	223.49	1	223.49
									6,418.27

Table 7 Cost per operation depending on caseload

	Average cost/operation	Average operation/ per week	Maintainence/week	Maintainence/case	Depreciation cost	Ave cost/per operation
Year1	1,943.28	1.4	2,717.40	1,941.00	2,934.80/2,096.30	5,980.58
Year2	1,913.65	2.3	2,717.40	1,181.50	2,934.80/1,276.00	4,371.15
Year3	1,895.29	2.4	2,717.40	1,132.25	2,934.80/1,222.83	4,250.37
Projected figures						
	1,895.29	3	2,717.40	905.80	2,934.80/978.30	3,779.40
	1,895.29	6	2,717.40	452.90	2,934.80/489.20	2,834.40
	1,895.29	9	2,717.40	302.00	2,934.80/326.10	2,523.40

References

1. Ewing DR et al (2004) Robots in the operating room—the history. Semin Laparosc Surg 11(2):63–71
2. Advincula AP, Falcone T (2004) Laparoscopic robotic gynecologic surgery. Obstet Gynecol Clin North Am 31(3):599–609, IX-X
3. Bokhari MB et al (2011) Learning curve for robotic-assisted laparoscopic colorectal surgery. Surg Endosc 25(3):855–860
4. Lenihan JP Jr, Kovanda C, Seshadri-Kreaden U (2008) What is the learning curve for robotic assisted gynecologic surgery? J Minim Invasive Gynecol 15(5):589–594
5. Akl MN et al (2009) Robotic-assisted sacrocolpopexy: technique and learning curve. Surg Endosc 23(10):2390–2394
6. Camberlin C, S.A., Leys M, De Laet C (2009) Robot-assisted surgery: health technology assessment in Health Services Research (HSR). Brussels: Belgian Health Care Knowledge Centre
7. Ho, C.T., E. Tran, K. Cimon, et al (2011) Robot-assisted surgery compared with open surgery and laparoscopic surgery: clinical effectiveness and economic analyses. Ottawa: Agency for Drugs and Technologies in Health
8. ACOG Committee Opinion No. 444 (2009) Choosing the route of hysterectomy for benign disease. Obstet Gynecol 114(5):1156–1158
9. Barnett JC, JP JP, Wu JM et al (2010) Cost comparison among robotic, laparoscopic, and open hysterectomy for endometrial cancer. Obstet Gynecol 116(3):685–693
10. Pasic RP et al (2010) Comparing robot-assisted with conventional laparoscopic hysterectomy: impact on cost and clinical outcomes. J Minim Invasive Gynecol 17(6):730–738
11. HIQA (2012) Health technology assessment of robot-assisted surgery in selected surgical procedures. Dublin: H.I.a.Q. Authority
12. Singer P, McKie J, Kuhse H, Richardson J (1995) Double jeopardy and the use of QALYs in health care allocation. J Medical Ethics 21:144–150

22

Scar endometriosis after a caesarean section: a perhaps underestimated complication

B. M. E. Adriaanse · R. Natté · B. W. J. Hellebrekers

Abstract The exact incidence of scar endometriosis is unknown. The aim of this study is to determine the incidence of endometriosis in the abdominal wall following a caesarean section. Women who underwent surgery for scar endometriosis after a caesarean section and the total number of women with caesarean sections in The Haga Teaching Hospital, a gynaecologic centre in The Netherlands, were identified by the national obstetric registration and pathology archive in the period January 1995 to December 2008. Clinical data were collected from the existing hospital records. Twenty-nine women were diagnosed with scar endometriosis after a caesarean section, and 3,047 women underwent one or more caesarean sections, resulting in an incidence of scar endometriosis of 0.95 %. None of the women had a history of endometriosis. Symptoms were pain (94.0 %), cyclic with menstruation (50.0 %) and swelling of the scar (89.0 %). Mean time between caesarean delivery and symptoms was 4.1 years. No recurrence occurred. This study reveals a higher incidence of endometriosis in the scar of a caesarean section than described in current literature. To improve the detection rate, more attention to medical history and physical examination is mandatory. A higher incidence warrants research into the pathophysiology and prevention of endometriosis in the scar of a caesarean section.

Keywords Endometriosis · Scar · Caesarean section · Surgery · Incidence · Abdominal wall

B. M. E. Adriaanse (✉)
Department of Obstetrics and Gynaecology, VU University Medical Centre, PK 6Z 170, De Boelelaan 1117,
1081 HV Amsterdam, The Netherlands
e-mail: b.adriaanse@vumc.nl

R. Natté
Department of Pathology, Haga Teaching Hospital,
The Hague, The Netherlands

B. W. J. Hellebrekers
Department of Obstetrics and Gynaecology, Haga Teaching Hospital,
The Hague, The Netherlands

Introduction

Endometriosis is defined as functioning endometrium outside the cavum uteri and is found in 8–15 % of all menstruating women [1–3]. The most common site is the ovarium and less frequent sites include peritoneum, intestine, bladder, inguinal region, lungs, pleura, pancreas, central nervous system and vertebrae [1, 2, 4]. Furthermore, endometriosis can be seen in the abdominal wall after surgery, in particular, in women with a caesarean section in history. Currently, no exact incidence rate of scar endometriosis after a caesarean section has been described and rates range from 0.03–1.73 % [5–12] with an average rate of 0.50 % (see Table 1). There are, however, only five studies [6, 8–11] available that calculated the incidence rate in a study group of more than 3,000 women with caesarean sections each. When we combine the total number of cases with scar endometriosis from these studies, the average incidence rate is 0.15 %. It is generally believed that scar endometriosis is a rare complication of a caesarean section, but the question remains whether the actual incidence is as low as been stated in most of the current literature or that the complication is underestimated.

Symptoms of endometriosis are frequently not recognised which results in delay in the diagnosis and therapy of the scar endometriosis [13, 14]. A higher incidence justifies more attention to the diagnosis and requires research into pathophysiology and prevention. The aim of this study is to investigate the incidence of scar endometriosis after a caesarean section.

Methods

This retrospective observational cohort study was performed in the Haga Teaching Hospital, The Hague, The Netherlands. All women with the pathological diagnosis 'endometriosis in abdominal scar' were collected by searches in the nationwide pathology registry database Pathologic Anatomic National Automated Archive (PALGA). The following terms were used for the search: endometriosis, endometriosis cyst and external endometriosis. All women who were diagnosed in the period of 1995 until 2008 were selected. The number of women who delivered by caesarean section in the Haga Teaching Hospital in the same period was determined by data of the national obstetric registration. For detailed information, records of the selected women with scar endometriosis after caesarean section were examined. The following items were recorded: surgical history, number of caesarean deliveries in history, method of caesarean delivery (Pfannenstiel/median incision), age at time of caesarean delivery, body mass index (BMI) at time of caesarean delivery, endometriosis in history (yes/no), symptoms, time between the caesarean section and symptoms of scar endometriosis, specialist who diagnosed the scar endometriosis and operated the woman, size of endometrioma and recurrence of scar endometriosis (yes/no).

Results

In the Haga Teaching Hospital, 440 women underwent surgery for (external) endometriosis from 1995 until 2008. In this group, the endometriosis was located in the abdominal wall in 34 women (7.70 %). One woman with abdominal wall endometriosis had no surgical history, in one woman, the endometriosis was located in an abdominal scar with unknown cause, and in three women, the endometriosis was located in a scar of an operation other than caesarean section (appendectomy, umbilical hernia repair and episiotomy). Twenty-nine women were diagnosed with abdominal wall endometriosis after caesarean section and underwent surgery. In total, 3,047 women underwent one or more caesarean sections from 1995 until 2008, resulting in an incidence rate of scar endometriosis of 0.95 % (95 % CI, 0.61–1.29). Of these 29 women, 13 had their caesarean section in the Haga Teaching hospital and 16 in another hospital, leading to an incidence rate of 0.43 % (95 % CI, 0.20–0.66). The results of the women with scar endometriosis after a caesarean section are shown in Table 2. The mean number of caesarean deliveries in history was 1.3 (range, 1.0–4.0), and all caesarean deliveries were performed with a Pfannenstiel incision. The mean age of the women at time of the caesarean delivery was 26.7 years (range, 19.0–43.0), and the mean BMI was 28.4 kg/m^2 (range, 16.2–52.9).

Table 1 Overview of literature concerning incidence of scar endometriosis after caesarean section

Author	Year	Study population	Women with scar endometriosis	Reported incidence
Nominato et al. [10]	2010	18,083	46	0.25
Leite et al. [8]	2009	10,533	31	0.29
Minaglia et al. [9]	2007	46,250	37	0.08
Singh et al. [11]	1995	3,330	6	0.18
Bottino et al. [5]	1990	200	2	1.00
Wolf et al. [12]	1989	289	5	1.73
Chatterjee [6]	1980	3,736	1	0.03
Field et al. [7]	1962	425	2	0.47

None of the women had a history of previously diagnosed endometriosis. Symptoms were pain (94.0 %), 50.0 % cyclic with menstruation and swelling of the scar (89.0 %). Mean time between caesarean delivery and symptoms was 4.1 year (range, 0.0–7.0). The endometriosis was diagnosed in 18 women (62.1 %) by a gynaecologist and in 11 women (37.9 %) by a general surgeon. The resection of the endometriosis was performed 20 times (69.0 %) by a gynaecologist and 9 times (31.0 %) by a general surgeon. The mean size of the excised endometriomas was 2.7 cm (range, 1.0–5.0). No recurrences were diagnosed.

Discussion

Abdominal wall endometriosis is considered to be a rare complication of a caesarean section. This study describes a large series of women with scar endometriosis and reveals a higher incidence than published in current literature. Rates of

Table 2 Characteristics of women with abdominal wall endometriosis after caesarean section

	Mean	Range
Age (years)	26.7	19.0–43.0
BMI (kg/m^2)	28.4	16.2-52.9
Interval CS—symptoms (years)	4.1	0.0–7.0
Size endometrioma (cm)	2.7	1.0–5.0
CS in history (number)	1.3	1.0–4.0
	Pain	Swelling scar
Symptoms	94.0 %	89.0 %
	Gynaecologist	General surgeon
Diagnosed by	62.1 %	37.9 %
Operated by	69.0 %	31.0 %

Kg kilogramme, *m*^{2} metres square, *CS* caesarean section, *cm* centimetre scar endometriosis after a caesarean section range from 0.03–1.73 % [5–12] with an average rate of 0.50 % (see Table 2). There are, however, only five studies [6, 8–11] available that calculated the incidence rate in a study group of more than 3,000 women each. When we combine the total number of cases with scar endometriosis from these studies, the average incidence rate is 0.15 %. Many articles refer to studies from 1956–1995 [6, 7, 11, 15], see Table 1. They report an incidence rate of 0.03–0.47 % and refer to a study of Chatterjee [6] who described 17 cases in 1980 with an incidence of 0.03 % and Field et al. [7] who reported 0.47 % in 1962 based on only two women with scar endometriosis after a caesarean section. In the current study, we included 29 women with scar endometriosis after a caesarean section with an incidence rate

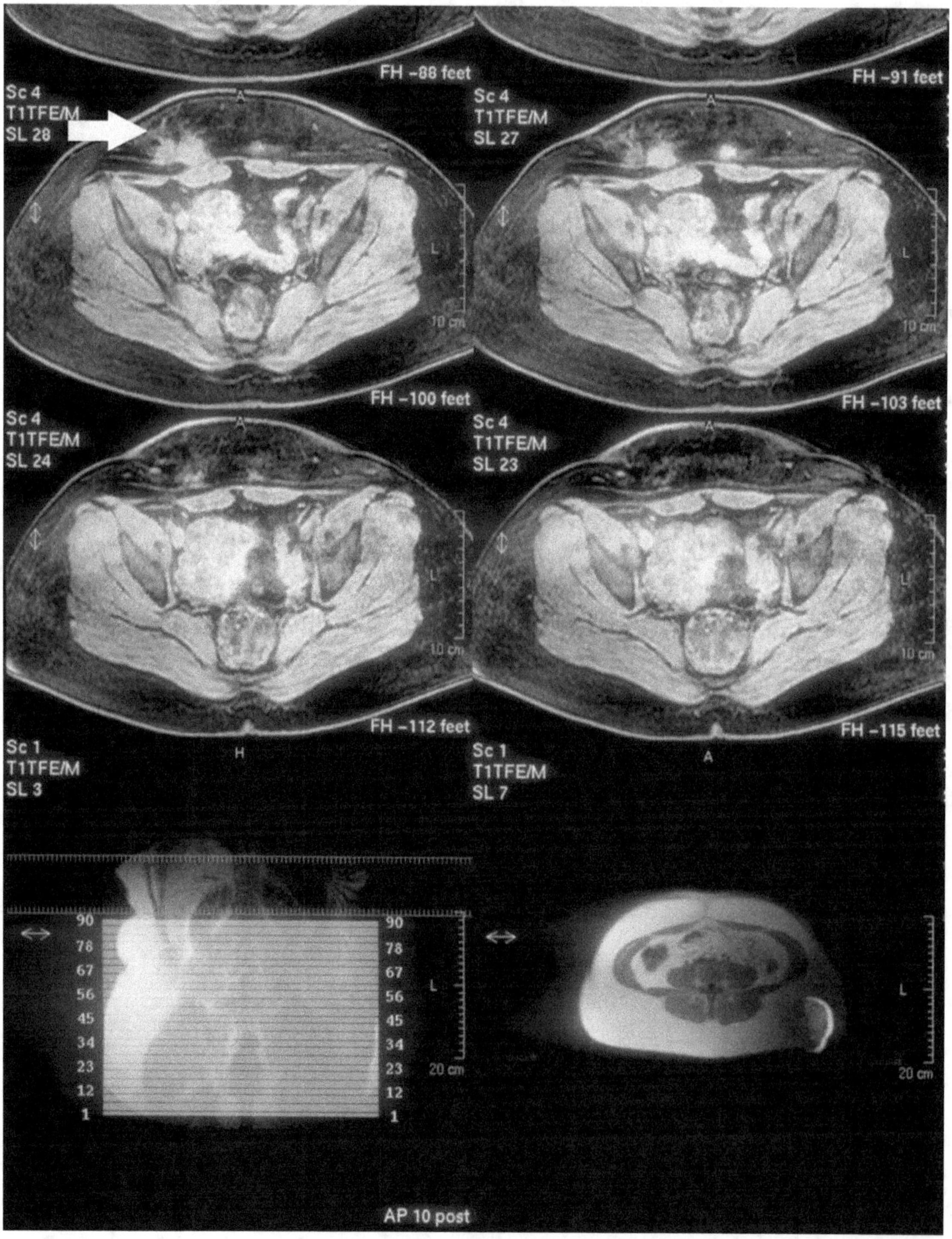

Fig. 1 MRI of a patient with scar endometriosis. Endometriosis depositions in the right part of the Pfannenstiel scar in the abdominal wall

of 0.95 % (95 % CI, 0.61–1.29). Importantly, our incidence rate is based on the pathological diagnosis. Women with endometriosis who did not undergo surgery are not included. This points to an even higher incidence rate of scar endometriosis after a caesarean delivery. A few other studies with more than 30 women with scar endometriosis after a caesarean section have been published. A large study of Minaglia et al. [9] reported an incidence of 0.08 % with 37 women with scar endometriosis from 1975 to 2005, and Leite et al. [8] calculated an incidence of 0.29 % with 31 women with scar endometriosis. Another large case series has been published by Bektas et al. [16] who studied retrospectively 36 cases of scar endometriosis after caesarean section. However, no incidence has been described in their study. Nominato et al. [10] described in a retrospective observational cohort study of 46 cases a lower incidence (0.25 %). Our study, however, covers a more recent study period (1995–2008) than the study of Nominato et al. (1978–2003) and Minaglia et al. (1975–2005). The higher incidence in our study might be explained by more awareness of scar endometriosis in the last decade and more accessible imaging possibilities. Also, the fact that 9 out of 29 women (31.0 %) were diagnosed and operated upon by a general surgeon might indicate that much of the burden of scar endometriosis happens not within the view of the gynaecologist. Although the incidence is still below 1.0 %, the incidence is higher than expected based on current literature, and, with this study, we want to emphasize that endometriosis should not be regarded as a rare complication of a caesarean section. Furthermore, a higher incidence requires more attention to this complication, in particular with increasing rates of caesarean sections [17–19].

Unfortunately, the pathophysiology is still not clear. Scar endometriosis after caesarean section is most likely caused by iatrogenic dissemination of decidual tissue. However, this will not explain the existence of endometriosis in the abdominal wall without any previous surgery. Different pathophysiological theories for abdominal wall endometriosis have been described. Sampson's theory postulated the implantation or retrograde menstruation hypothesis which states that endometrial tissue from the uterus is shed during menstruation and transported retrograde through the fallopian tubes, thereby gaining access to and implanting on pelvic structures [20–24]. Another theory suggests lymphatic or vascular dissemination, and a third explanation states that cells in the abdomen undergo metaplasia induced by hormonal manipulation [22]. Still, in our opinion, most of the cases can be explained by iatrogenic dissemination of decidual tissue.

The diagnosis of scar endometriosis can be difficult. In our study, women presented to the clinic with symptoms months to years after the caesarean section, as reported earlier in other studies [8, 10, 16]. Frequently, they presented with vague symptoms such as abdominal pain. The diagnosis of scar endometriosis should be based on symptoms of pain that coincides with the menstrual period or tumours in the scar after abdominal surgery [8]. This awareness applies to gynaecologists as well as to other specialists who are faced with these women, like general practitioners and surgeons. Other abnormalities should be excluded and differential diagnosis includes lipoma, haematoma, umbilical hernia, soft tissue sarcoma, abscess, carcinoma (primary), metastasis and corpus alienum. Diagnosis can be made by ultrasonography or MRI (not specific), see Fig. 1, and needle biopsy (specific) [25]. In particular, ultrasonography is a useful tool to detect scar endometriosis in an early stage [26, 27]. However, ultrasound accuracy is reduced in obese patients. Early diagnosis is of importance since delayed diagnosis creates repair problems during surgery, the possible need of meshes and can cause deformities. Histological diagnosis of endometriosis is based on the identification of characteristic endometrial glands and associated stromal cells outside the cavum uteri [28], as illustrated in Figs. 2 and 3. Therapy with oral anticonceptives, progestagens and androgens give reduction

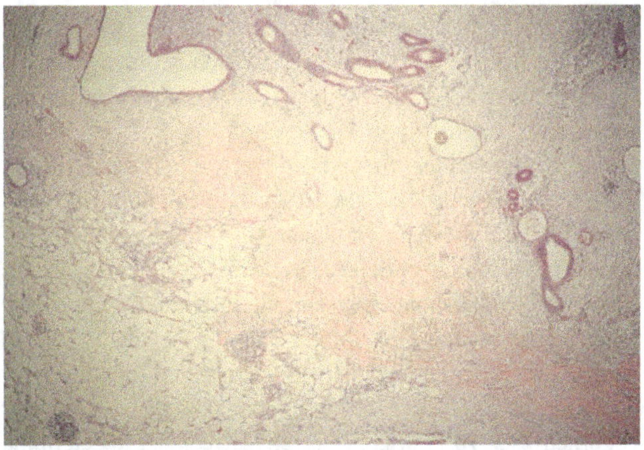

Fig. 2 Histology of scar endometriosis. Microscopy 40×. Disorderly arranged endometrial glands within densely collagenized stroma and fatty tissue. There is little endometrial stroma around the glands in the upper part of the figure

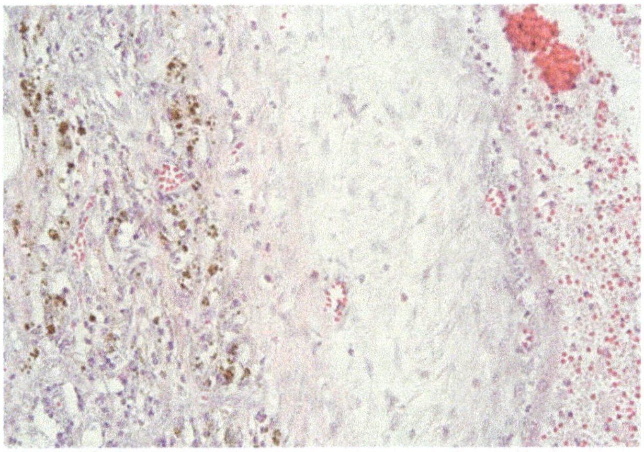

Fig. 3 Histology of scar endometriosis. Microscopy 400×. Characteristic iron deposition below endometrium epithelium as a sign of old haemorrhage

of the symptoms temporarily, with recurrence after discontinuation of the therapy. A wide surgical excision is usually curative [11, 16]. In none of the women in this study a recurrence occurred.

Removing decidual tissue from the wound before closing and cleansing with NaCl (normal saline solution) has been described as a preventive measure [29]. Intraoperative contamination of the surrounding tissue with the endometrial cells is a situation that should be taken into account during operations in the pelvis. Therefore, sweeping the uterus with a gauze during a caesarean delivery should be limited since it could be an important factor in the pathogenesis of scar endometriosis [16]. Further research is necessary to determine the exact role of this factor. In addition, preventive measures could have consequences for other types of surgery as oncologic surgery, where the mechanism of cancer recurrence in a scar, shows many similarities with scar endometriosis [30]. Given the magnitude of caesarean sections performed, studies on preventive measures could thus have importance for other fields of surgery.

A limitation of this study is the restriction of research to only one hospital in the Netherlands. Therefore, not all women with scar endometriosis had their caesarean section in the Haga Teaching Hospital. We assumed, however, that this number of women is comparable to the number of women who had their caesarean section in the Haga Teaching Hospital and surgery for scar endometriosis in another hospital. Moreover, this methodology was also used in the studies referred to in Table 2. This is the one of the first studies which described a higher incidence than has been established previously. Additional research by other groups is needed to confirm our data and conclusions. Furthermore, our study only describes the incidence of women who underwent surgery, not the women with scar endometriosis who did not undergo surgery. Therefore, the incidence is even higher than described in the present study.

In conclusion, this study reveals a higher incidence of endometriosis in the scar of a caesarean section than described in current literature. To improve the detection rate of scar endometriosis, more attention to medical history and physical examination is mandatory. The higher incidence warrants research into the pathophysiology and prevention of abdominal wall endometriosis after a caesarean section.

Conflict of interest No disclosure of interest.

References

1. Albrecht LE, Tron V, Rivers JK (1995) Cutaneous endometriosis. Int J Dermatol 34:261–262
2. Bergqvist A (1992) Extragenital endometriosis. A review. Eur J Surg 158:7–12
3. Patterson GK, Winburn GB (1999) Abdominal wall endometriomas: report of eight cases. Am Surg 65:36–39
4. DeSanto DA, McBirnie JE (1949) Endometriosis: a clinical and pathological study of 219 cases. Calif Med 71:274–279
5. Bottino G, Marinello M, Menna C, Torchio B, Vergano R (1990) Endometriosis of the lower abdominal wall. Report of two cases secondary to cesarean section. Minerva Ginecol 42:283–285
6. Chatterjee SK (1980) Scar endometriosis: a clinicopathologic study of 17 cases. Obstet Gynecol 56:81–84
7. Field CA, Banner EA, Symmonds RE (1962) Endometriosis of abdominal scar after cesarean section. Proc Staff Meet Mayo Clin 37:12–15
8. Leite GK, Carvalho LF, Korkes H, Guazzelli TF, Kenj G, Viana AT (2009) Scar endometrioma following obstetric surgical incisions: retrospective study on 33 cases and review of the literature. São Paulo Med J 127:270–277
9. Minaglia S, Mishell DR Jr, Ballard CA (2007) Incisional endometriomas after cesarean section: a case series. J Reprod Med 52:630–634
10. Nominato NS, Prates LF, Lauar I, Morais J, Maia L, Geber S (2010) Caesarean section greatly increases risk of scar endometriosis. Eur J Obstet Gynecol Reprod Biol 152:83–85
11. Singh KK, Lessells AM, Adam DJ, Jordan C, Miles WF, Macintyre IM, Greig JD (1995) Presentation of endometriosis to general surgeons: a 10-year experience. Br J Surg 82:1349–1351
12. Wolf GC, Singh KB (1989) Cesarean scar endometriosis: a review. Obstet Gynecol Surv 44:89–95
13. Nirula R, Greaney GC (2000) Incisional endometriosis: an underappreciated diagnosis in general surgery. J Am Coll Surg 190:404–407
14. Wolf Y, Haddad R, Werbin N, Skornick Y, Kaplan O (1996) Endometriosis in abdominal scars: a diagnostic pitfall. Am Surg 62:1042–1044
15. Nora E Sr, Meyer KA, Carbonera P (1956) Ectopic endometrium in abdominal scars following cesarean section. Am J Obstet Gynecol 71:876–884
16. Bektas H, Bilsel Y, Sari YS, Ersoz F, Koc O, Deniz M, Boran B, Huq GE (2010) Abdominal wall endometrioma: a 10-year experience and brief review of the literature. J Surg Res 164:e77–e81
17. Blanchette H (2011) The rising cesarean delivery rate in America: what are the consequences? Obstet Gynecol 118: 687–690
18. O'Dwyer V, Hogan JL, Farah N, Kennelly MM, Fitzpatrick C, Turner MJ (2012) Maternal mortality and the rising cesarean rate. Int J Gynaecol Obstet 116:162–164
19. Wax JR, Cartin A, Pinette MG, Blackstone J (2004) Patient choice cesarean: an evidence-based review. Obstet Gynecol Surv 59:601–616
20. Sampson J (1927) Peritoneal endometriosis due to menstrual dissemination of endometrial tissue into the peritoneal cavity. Am J Obstet Gynecol 14:422–469
21. De Ziegler D, Borghese B, Chapron C (2010) Endometriosis and infertility: pathophysiology and management. Lancet 376:730–738
22. Horton JD, Dezee KJ, Ahnfeldt EP, Wagner M (2008) Abdominal wall endometriosis: a surgeon's perspective and review of 445 cases. Am J Surg 196:207–212
23. Gabriel A, Shores JT, Poblete M, Victorio A, Gupta S (2007) Abdominal wall endometrioma: case report and review. Ann Plast Surg 58:691–693
24. Seli E, Berkkanoglu M, Arici A (2003) Pathogenesis of endometriosis. Obstet Gynecol Clin N Am 30:41–61
25. Medeiros FC, Cavalcante DI, Medeiros MA, Eleuterio J Jr (2011) Fine-needle aspiration cytology of scar endometriosis: study of seven cases and literature review. Diagn Cytopathol 39:18–21

26. Francica G (2012) Reliable clinical and sonographic findings in the diagnosis of abdominal wall endometriosis near cesarean section scar. World J Radiol 4:135–140
27. Hensen JH, Van Breda Vriesman AC, Puylaert JB (2006) Abdominal wall endometriosis: clinical presentation and imaging features with emphasis on sonography. AJR Am J Roentgenol 186:616–620
28. Pathan SK, Kapila K, Haji BE, Mallik MK, Al-Ansary TA, George SS, Das DK, Francis IM (2005) Cytomorphological spectrum in scar endometriosis: a study of eight cases. Cytopathology 16:94–99
29. Wasfie T, Gomez E, Seon S, Zado B (2002) Abdominal wall endometrioma after cesarean section: a preventable complication. Int Surg 87:175–177
30. Reilly WT, Nelson H, Schroeder G, Wieand HS, Bolton J, O'Connell MJ (1996) Wound recurrence following conventional treatment of colorectal cancer. A rare but perhaps underestimated problem. Dis Colon Rectum 39:200–207

23

Trends in first-generation endometrial ablation procedures performed in a district general hospital, 1995–2005

Vincent Boama · Tania Dexter

Abstract Heavy menstrual bleeding is a common presenting complaint and can significantly affect the quality of life of affected women. The 2007 National Institute for Clinical Excellence guideline on heavy menstrual bleeding states that in women with heavy menstrual bleeding alone, endometrial ablation should be considered preferable to hysterectomy. The choice of the type of endometrial ablation procedure would depend on several factors including the availability of first-, second- or even third-generation endometrial ablation equipment, clinician experience and preference as well as patient choice and if procedure is intended to be performed as an office procedure without the use of general anaesthetic where second- or third-generation endometrial ablation equipment would be used. The number of first-generation endometrial ablation procedures being performed is expected to decrease over time. This is as a result of clinicians' preference, due to reported higher operative complication rates in some studies, even though a meta-analysis of individual patient data has found it to be as effective as the second-generation techniques for heavy menstrual bleeding. We performed a retrospective clinical audit to investigate the trend from January 1995 to December 2005 in the use of first-generation endometrial ablation techniques performed at a district general hospital in the UK. We found that the general trend is of a rapidly decreasing number of first-generation endometrial ablation procedures being performed. We also found that the operative complication rates are low and similar to rates in the published literature. The long-term hysterectomy rate after first-generation endometrial ablation procedure in our audit population is also low and similar to the rates in the published literature. We conclude from our audit data that first-generation endometrial ablation techniques such as transcervical resection of the endometrium for heavy menstrual bleeding are effective and in experienced hands have fairly low operative complication rates and long-term hysterectomy rates. These are similar to rates in the published literature for second-generation endometrial ablation techniques. We recommend that until further larger scale randomised controlled trials comparing first generation and the newer second-generation endometrial ablation techniques are performed which would provide clinicians with better evidence, first-generation endometrial ablation equipment should not yet be condemned to gather dust in hospital storage facilities and become 'museum pieces'. Rather, a concerted effort must be made to increase training opportunities in the use of first-generation endometrial ablation techniques especially in institutions that have already made the financial investment and are in possession of perfectly functioning equipment. This would ensure that the valuable clinical skill in the use of available first-generation endometrial ablation technique is not lost over time.

Keywords Trends · First-generation endometrial ablation · Second-generation endometrial ablation · Heavy menstrual bleeding

T. Dexter
49, Kennedy Road, Horsham, West Sussex RH13 5DB, England, UK
e-mail: tania.dexter13@gmail.com

V. Boama (✉)
Department of Obstetrics and Gynaecology, Hampshire Hospitals NHS Foundation Trust, Aldermaston Road, Basingstoke, Hampshire RG 24 9FT, UK
e-mail: vincent.boama2015@gmail.com

Background

Heavy menstrual bleeding (HMB) is a significantly common health problem in women of reproductive age. The 2007 National Institute for Clinical Excellence (NICE) guideline on heavy menstrual bleeding states that in women with HMB alone, with a uterus no bigger than a 10-week pregnancy, endometrial ablation should be considered preferable to hysterectomy [1]. First-generation endometrial ablation methods considered the 'gold standard' include trans-cervical resection of endometrium (TCRE), roller ball and laser ablation [2]. The NICE guideline also states that women considering endometrial ablation for heavy menstrual bleeding should have access to second- generation ablation techniques such as microwave endometrial ablation (MEA), thermal balloon endometrial ablation and impedance-controlled bipolar radiofrequency ablation [1]. The choice of the type of endometrial ablation technique used would depend on many factors including availability of equipment, clinician experience and preference as well as patient choice. Avoidance of use of general anaesthetic and even local anaesthetic for office procedures using second- and third-generation endometrial ablation techniques is gaining popularity with clinicians and patients alike.

A survey in 2008 of 1,460 UK gynaecologists showed that second- generation endometrial ablation devices were preferred and used by most compared to first-generation devices [3]. The clinician's preferred choice of second-generation endometrial ablation techniques over first-generation techniques is likely influenced by published literature that indicate fewer operative complications, a shallow learning curve, quicker and technically easier as well as less need for general anaesthesia when second-generation endometrial ablation techniques are used compared to first-generation ablation techniques.

At the Royal Cornwall Hospital, Truro (RCHT), only one consultant at the time of this clinical audit performed first-generation endometrial ablation procedures. The expectation therefore is that the number of first-generation endometrial ablation procedures performed for heavy menstrual bleeding will decrease over time due to the availability and widespread use of second-generation and third-generation endometrial ablation techniques. The clinical skill in the use of first-generation endometrial ablation technique is at risk of becoming lost over time.

A randomised controlled trial (RCT) that compared second-generation endometrial ablation–MEA with a first-generation endometrial ablation–TCRE with a minimum 10-year follow-up showed that both techniques achieve significant and comparable improvements in menstrual symptoms, health-related quality of life and high rates of satisfaction. Bleeding and pain score reductions were significantly reduced and similar amenorrhea rates of up to 88 % were achieved in both groups. The only difference found in this randomised controlled trial was a significantly higher hysterectomy rate after 10 years of 28 % in the TCRE arm compared to 17 % in the MEA arm [4].

An individual patient data meta-analysis of existing randomised controlled trials and population-based retrospective cohort study based on record linkage found that more women were satisfied after hysterectomy than after endometrial ablation [5]. They concluded that, although the most cost-effective strategy, hysterectomy may not be considered an initial option owing to its invasive nature and higher risk of complications.

A further individual patient data meta-analysis supplemented with cost and outcome data from published sources taking a National Health Service (NHS) perspective showed that hysterectomy is the preferred strategy for the first intervention for heavy menstrual bleeding. They demonstrated that although hysterectomy is more expensive, it produces more quality adjusted life years relative to other remaining strategies like first- and second-generation endometrial ablation techniques and the Mirena intrauterine system and is therefore likely to be considered cost effective. The authors did argue that the incremental cost-effectiveness ratio for hysterectomy compared with second-generation ablation per additional quality adjusted life year was £970.00. Using a mathematical cost-effectiveness model based on costs associated with treatment for heavy menstrual bleeding in the UK at 2008 prices, this article did demonstrate marginally higher quality adjusted life years with second-generation- compared to first-generation endometrial ablation techniques [6].

The Cochrane Systematic review shows an overall favourable comparison in terms of the success rates and complication profiles of the second-generation techniques compared to first-generation techniques. Despite this however, the review also concludes that the rapid development and introduction of a number of new second-generation methods of endometrial ablation techniques make it difficult to systematically compare them to the 'gold standard' [7]. A meta-analysis of individual patient data found that second-generation endometrial ablation techniques were at least as effective as first-generation techniques [8]. A recent network meta-analysis of 19 randomised controlled trials involving 3,287 women who had different types of second-generation endometrial ablation techniques performed for heavy menstrual bleeding did show relatively low but variable rates of heavy bleeding across the studies such as 0–32 % for thermal balloon ablation and 8–18 % for bipolar radiofrequency ablation. This network meta-analysis did also look at trends in types of second-generation endometrial ablation procedures performed in England, 2004–2011, and indicates a sharper rise in number of bipolar radio frequency ablative technique compared to other second-generation techniques [9].

The current state of the global economy and financial state of the national health service in UK and the need for efficiency savings in health care make it essential to review the cost-effectiveness of every medical procedure.

Second-generation endometrial ablation techniques have marginally lower costs associated with treatment compared to first-generation techniques [10, 11]. However, the cost-effectiveness calculations in these studies are based on relatively lower purchase price and operational costs compared to the current significantly higher purchase price and operational costs for available second- and third-generation endometrial ablation equipment. The recent exponential increases in purchase price and operational costs for these newer second-generation endometrial ablation techniques are multifactorial and may include the effects of the global economic downturn and the falling value of the Pound Sterling. It may therefore be reasonably prudent for NHS Trusts not to abandon in a knee jerk attitude their available and fully functioning first-generation endometrial ablation equipment. There is clearly the need for large-scale, well-designed RCT's that would compare cost-effectiveness across the many new and emerging second- and third-generation endometrial ablation techniques with first-generation techniques.

The apparent decreasing number of first-generation endometrial ablation techniques being performed across the nation may lead to decreasing training opportunities and loss of this clinical skill in the near future.

This clinical audit was therefore undertaken to clearly determine the trend in first-generation endometrial ablation techniques performed at a district general hospital in England.

Aims of this study include the following:

1. Primarily to audit the trend at RCHT of first-generation endometrial ablation procedures for heavy menstrual bleeding from January 1995 to December 2005.
2. Secondarily to audit the intra-operative and post-operative complication rates as well as the long-term hysterectomy rate.
3. To ensure compliance with local guidelines and NICE guidelines in the management of women with heavy menstrual bleeding who opt for endometrial ablation procedure

Methods

This is a retrospective clinical audit. The clinical audit was registered with the Clinical Effectiveness, Quality and Safety Department at the RCHT and allocated a clinical audit number 1459.

A formal request was sent to the Information Services Department at RCHT using the Information Gateway Process for the clinical record numbers of all patients who had undergone TCRE as coded between January 1995 and December 2005. The following search words were used: endometrial resection, hysteroscopic resection of endometrium, TCRF, and TCRE. At the Royal Cornwall Hospital, the only first-generation endometrial ablation technique available since 1995 is TCRE. This is performed solely by one senior consultant gynaecologist between 1995 and 2005. Second-generation endometrial ablation techniques such as microwave endometrial ablation (recently withdrawn) and bipolar radiofrequency ablation (NOVASURE) are performed by most of the rest of the consultant body at RCHT on a regular basis.

A proforma was produced for data gathering of all patients who satisfied the inclusion criteria of trans-cervical resection of endometrium performed for heavy menstrual bleeding. A total of 710 patient notes were retrieved based on the search words by the Information Services department. All the 710 patient notes were reviewed by the two authors (TD and VB) with respect to the proforma. Following data collection, Microsoft Excel software was used for computing and analysis of data.

Findings

We reviewed 710 notes for eligibility based on the list of all clinical record numbers generated by RCHT Information Services Department. One hundred eighty-five satisfied the inclusion criteria and 525 were excluded. The mean age of patients was 45 years of age. Twenty-three (12 %) of these patients were lost to follow-up; however, the majority (162 patients, 88 %) were followed up for a minimum of 3 months after their procedure. One patient in the reviewed group fell pregnant a few years following the procedure. The indications for the procedure were (1) HMB only (87 patients, 47 %), (2) HMB and pain (51 patients, 27 %), (3) peri-menopausal bleeding (20 patients, 11 %) or other reasons including inter-menstrual bleeding, post-coital bleeding, irregular bleeding or combinations of these after full investigations (27 patients, 15 %).

The following graph (Fig. 1) demonstrates the number of first-generation endometrial ablation procedures performed at RCHT over the 10-year period (1995–2005).

The mean recorded pre-procedure bleeding in these patients was 8 days which reduced to 2 days post-procedure. Treatment options tried before ablation included the Mirena intrauterine system, non-steroidal anti-inflammatory drugs, the combined oral contraceptive pill, progestogens, gonadotropin releasing hormone analogues, fibroid embolisation,

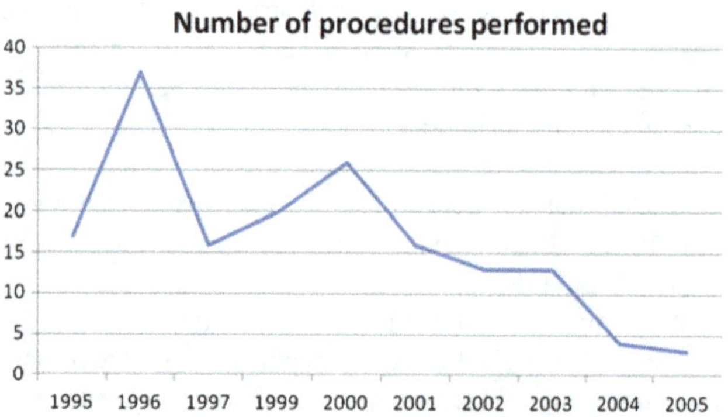

Fig. 1 Number of TCRE performed at RCHT between 1995 and 2005

myomectomy and other treatments such as herbal remedies and other self medications. Intra-operative and short-term complications were uncommon but included uterine perforation (three cases—1.6 %), excessive bleeding (seven cases—3.7 %), excessive (>800 ml deficit) fluid absorption (six cases—3.2 %), hysterectomy (two cases—1 %), uterine infection requiring antibiotics (four cases—2 %), failed attempt of procedure (one case—0.5 %) and ventricular ectopic beats during surgery (one case—0.5 %). Nine (4.9 %) patients required overnight admission for minor complaints such as nausea and vomiting or pain.

Eighty-one percent (44 %) of patients reported being satisfied with their procedure, 63 (34 %) were unsatisfied and satisfaction was not recorded for 18 (10 %) patients. Ten patients (5 %) required additional medical treatment in the long term after ablation and 60 (32 %) required an additional surgical treatment in the long term.

These additional surgical procedures were carried out in a time range of 2 weeks to 9 years following the initial ablation. The mean time between procedures was 3 years. They are summarised in Table 1:

Table 1 Additional surgical procedures performed after initial TCRE

Procedure	Number of patients
Hysterectomy (excluding the 2 performed intra-operatively)	38 (21 %)
First-generation ablation	19 (10 %)
Second-generation ablation	3 (2 %)
Uterine artery embolisation	1 (<1 %)

Conclusions

The general trend is that of a rapidly decreasing number of first-generation endometrial ablation procedures being performed at RCHT. Despite this, the minor and major operative complication rates for first-generation endometrial ablation technique at RCHT are low and similar to rates in the published literature. The long-term hysterectomy rate of 21 % after TCRE in our audit population is similar or lower than the published figures in the region of 28 %.

First-generation endometrial ablation procedures in well-trained hands are comparatively safe and have low patient dissatisfying rates in the long term compared to second-generation endometrial ablation methods. There is a great need for well-designed multi-centred large randomised controlled studies that would compare the many new and emerging second- and third-generation endometrial ablation techniques to the 'gold standard'. Until there is stronger evidence in favour of second- and third-generation endometrial ablation techniques over the first-generation ablation techniques, we recommend that Hospital Trusts take a moment's pause and not rush to condemn their existing perfectly functioning first-generation endometrial ablation equipment as a 'museum piece' to gather dust in a storage facility. Increasing the number of first-generation endometrial ablation techniques performed would also increase training opportunities and enhance the acquisition of this clinical skill by both trainees and consultants.

Acknowledgments We thank Mr D Byrne for his guidance and assistance with the clinical audit.

Declaration of interest We the authors, Vincent Boama (VB) and Tania Dexter (TD), report of no conflict of interest.

Informed consent Informed consent from patients was not required for this clinical audit. The audit was registered with and approved by the clinical effectiveness and audit department of the hospital.

References

1. NICE. (2007). Heavy menstrual bleeding. CG44. [Online] www.nice.org.uk/CG044fullguideline. Accessed 13 April 2013
2. Papadopoulos NP, Magos A (2007) First-generation endometrial ablation: roller-ball vs loop vs laser. Best Pract Res Clin Obstet Gynaecol 21(6):915–929
3. Deb S, Flora K, Atiomo W (2008) A survey of preferences and practices of endometrial ablation/resection for menorrhagia in the United Kingdom. Fertil Steril 90(5):1812–1817
4. Sambrook AM, Bain C, Parkin DE, Cooper KG (2009) A randomised comparison of microwave endometrial ablation with transcervical resection of the endometrium: follow up at a minimum of 10 years. BJOG 116(8):1033–1037
5. Bhattacharya S, Middleton LJ, Tsourapas A, Lee AJ, Champaneria R et al (2011) Hysterectomy, endometrial ablation and Mirena® for heavy menstrual bleeding: a systematic review of clinical effectiveness and cost-effectiveness analysis. Health Technol Assess 15(19):iii-xvi, 1-252.
6. Roberts TE, Tsourapas A, Middleton LJ, Champaneria R, Daniels JP, Cooper KG et al (2011) Hysterectomy, endometrial ablation, and levonorgestrel releasing intrauterine system (Mirena) for treatment of heavy menstrual bleeding: cost effectiveness analysis. BMJ 342:d2202
7. Lethaby A, Hickey M, Garry R, Penninx J (2009) Endometrial resection/ablation techniques for heavy menstrual bleeding. Cochrane Database Systematic Reviews. Vol. 4
8. Middleton LJ, Champaneria R, Daniels JP (2010) Hysterectomy, endometrial destruction and Levonorgestrel IUS for heavy menstrual bleeding. Systematic review and meta-analysis of data from individual patients. BMJ 341:C3929
9. Daniels JP, Middleton LJ, Champaneria R, Khan KS, Cooper K, Mol BWJ, Bhattacharya S (2012) Second generation endometrial ablation techniques for heavy menstrual bleeding: network meta-analysis. BMJ 344:e2564
10. Cameron IM, Mollison J, Pinion SB, Atherton Naji A, Buckingham K, Torgerson D (1996) A cost comparison of hysterectomy and hysteroscopic surgery for the treatment of menorrhagia. Eur J Obstet Gynecol Reprod Biol 70:87–92
11. Garside R, Stein K, Wyatt K, Round A, Price A (2004) The effectiveness and cost effectiveness of microwave and thermal balloon endometrial ablation for heavy menstrual bleeding: a systematic review and economic modelling. Health Technol Assess 8:iii, 1-155

24

The effectiveness of outpatient Thermachoice endometrial balloon ablation: a long-term 11-year outcome study

Vinod Kumar · Janesh Kumar Gupta

Abstract The aim of this study was to evaluate the long-term treatment outcomes of outpatient Thermachoice balloon endometrial ablation under a direct local anaesthetic cervical block (LA-Thermachoice). This paper is a prospective cohort study and a postal questionnaire survey in a UK teaching hospital with the participation of 253 women with heavy menstrual bleeding (HMB) undergoing LA-Thermachoice over an 11-year period between 2001 and 2011. Treatment success was measured by postoperative bleeding patterns, improvement in dysmenorrhoea, patient satisfaction and post-procedure hysterectomy rates. LA-Thermachoice was completed in 98 % of women. The survey response rate was 78 %. The median follow-up interval was 71 months (SD 42). Seventy-nine percent of the responders reported significant improvement in HMB with 40 % amenorrhoea rate and 86 % improvement in dysmenorrhoea. Eighty-one percent felt that the benefit of procedure was maintained over a long period of time. Eighty-six percent of women were satisfied with the outcome of their procedure. The case notes of non-responders were examined to check if any had undergone hysterectomy since the LA-Thermachoice procedure. In total, only 16 % of women had a hysterectomy. This study represents the largest published series of local anaesthetic thermal endometrial ablation, reporting clinical outcomes with 11 years (median 71 months) of post-treatment follow-up. It demonstrates that the patient satisfaction with LA-Thermachoice is high, and is maintained over a long period of time after the procedure.

V. Kumar
Community Sexual and Reproductive Healthcare, University Hospitals Birmingham NHS Foundation Trust, Birmingham, UK

J. K. Gupta (✉)
Clinical and Experimental Medicine, University of Birmingham, Birmingham Women's NHS Foundation Trust, Edgbaston, B15 2TG Birmingham, UK
e-mail: j.k.gupta@bham.ac.uk

Keywords Thermachoice endometrial ablation · Surgical management · Heavy menstrual bleeding · Questionnaire · Patient satisfaction

Background

Heavy menstrual bleeding (HMB) as a symptom is a very common gynaecological problem affecting 20 % of women of reproductive age [1, 2]. It can be managed medically with drugs such as tranexamic acid, mefenamic acid, oral contraceptive pills, or the levonorgestrel intrauterine system (LNG-IUS, Mirena™) [3] or surgically with procedures such as endometrial ablation or hysterectomy.

While hysterectomy still remains the definitive surgical treatment for HMB, endometrial ablation in contrast is less invasive and associated with shorter hospital stay and recovery, significant less pain, and fewer complications [4–7]. Currently, there is a variety of endometrial ablation techniques used worldwide, which are well-established alternatives to hysterectomy for the management of women with HMB [5, 8].

Thermachoice endometrial ablation (Gynecare; ethicon Inc., Somerville, NJ, USA) is a non-hysteroscopic ablation technique, involving a heated fluid-filled balloon to thermally ablate the endometrial tissue. This system has undergone significant improvement from the first generation Thermachoice (TBEA) to a third generation Thermachoice III (TBEA-III) in 2003, with the key differences including replacement of the latex balloon with a compliant silicone balloon and introduction of an impeller device for active fluid circulation to enable equal heat distribution to the entire endometrial surface area.

We previously compared the clinical outcome and effectiveness of TBEA and TBEA-III devices and reported 3-years post-treatment follow-up results [9]. The results of that study indicated that the treatment satisfaction was high in both cohorts (combined satisfaction rate 76 %). However, TBEA-III was associated with a higher amenorrhoea rate (35 %) compared to the TBEA device (23 %) [9]. The primary aim of this study was to determine if the treatment success, measured by improvement in bleeding patterns, relief of dysmenorrhoea and patient satisfaction, was maintained over a prolonged period of time i.e., up to 11-year period after the LA-Thermachoice. The secondary aim was to determine if any further medical or surgical procedures such as repeat LA-Thermachoice, treatment with the LNG-IUS or hysterectomy were required to control symptoms since LA-Thermachoice.

Methods

This prospective cohort study was carried out in a large teaching hospital. The study population comprised of premenopausal women with heavy menstrual bleeding, refractory to medical treatment and no desire to retain fertility, and who opted for local anaesthetic thermal balloon endometrial ablation (LA-Thermachoice) between February 2001 and December 2011. All patients had preoperative endometrial sampling demonstrating benign histology. These women did not undergo hormonal endometrial thinning in the preoperative preparation. Informed consent for the procedure was obtained by the operating surgeon on the gynaecological ward prior to the procedure.

Women with submucosal fibroids sized >3 cm, undiagnosed abnormal vaginal bleeding, current lower pelvic infection or uterine abnormalities, atypical endometrial hyperplasia or endometrial cancer, past allergic reactions to local anaesthetic agents, or distorted uterine cavity due to large fibroid, were excluded from the study.

LA-Thermachoice was performed according to our previously described protocol using Thermachoice (Gynecare, Menlo Park, Calif., USA) at study commencement (February 2001–July 2003) and upgraded to Thermachoice III (Gynecare, Ethicon Inc., Somerville, N.J., USA) from August 2003 onwards [10]. The procedure was performed by three consultants over the study period. We maintained a computer database that was populated with the relevant peri-operative information from all patients undergoing LA-Thermachoice since 2001. Data were collected immediately post-procedure and updated once the patient was discharged, with any post procedural complications and analgesia requirements by the operating clinician.

All women were sent a postal questionnaire, including two further postal reminders 3 months apart to non-responders, between February 2012 and August 2012 to evaluate post-treatment symptoms and to determine the long-term effectiveness of therapy (Fig. 1).

Minimum follow-up interval post LA-Thermachoice was 12 months. Symptomatic improvement was assessed by asking women to grade the heaviness of their menstrual blood loss as none (amenorrhea), lighter than before (included spotting and vaginal discharge only), same as before, or heavier than before treatment. They were also asked to quantify their post-procedure menstrual pain, grade their satisfaction with the treatment on a 4-point ordinal scale (very satisfied, satisfied, dissatisfied, or very dissatisfied), and comment on any further

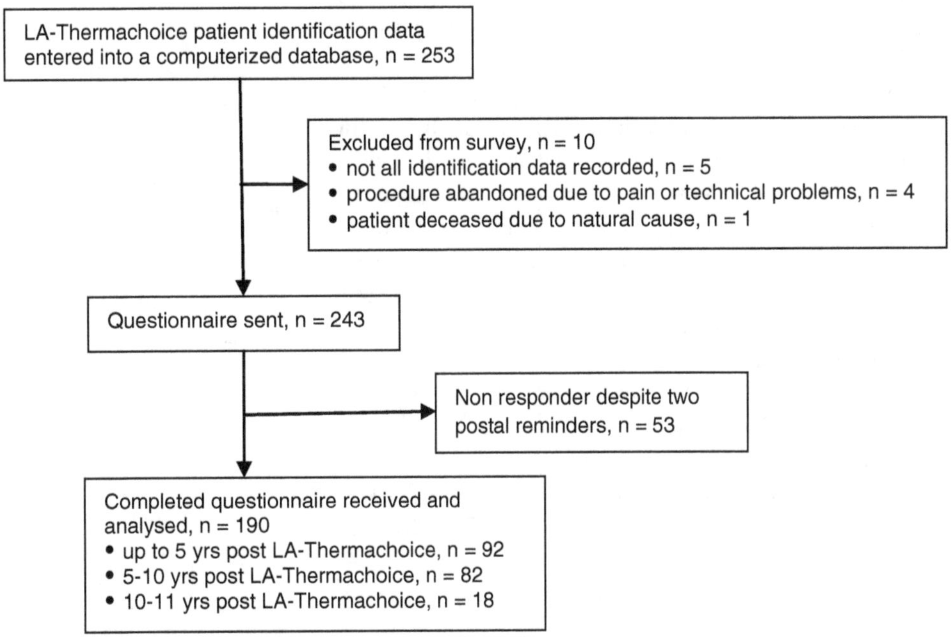

Fig. 1 Flowchart of the study population of patients treated with local anaesthetic thermal balloon endometrial ablation (LA-Thermachoice) between 2001 and 2011

medical or surgical procedures since LA-Thermachoice to control symptoms. All women were advised to quantify their period-related symptoms prior to hysterectomy procedures or menopause if they already had hysterectomy or achieved menopause since LA-Thermachoice. Case notes of non-responders were examined to check if any had undergone hysterectomy since the LA-Thermachoice procedure.

A formal ethics application was not required as the study was classified as a clinical service evaluation. Approval was obtained from the hospital research department to survey all patients who underwent the LA-Thermachoice procedure before the onset of data collection.

Categorical data were summarised as proportions and continuous data as means (±standard deviations (SD)) or medians (±range) where appropriate. Differences between proportions were analysed with the chi-square test with Fisher's exact test. A p value of <0.05 was considered as statistically significant. The collected data were analysed using Microsoft Office Excel 2007 and SPSS (version 16, IBM SPSS Statistics).

Findings

A total of 253 women (mean age 44 years, SD 4.7; BMI 30±7) underwent LA-Thermachoice between February 2001 and December 2011. The procedure was successfully completed in 249 (98 %) women. All baseline clinical characteristics and peri-procedure outcomes of the cohort studied are shown in Table 1.

Fully completed questionnaires were returned by 190 participants (78 %). One woman was deceased at the time of the first mailing. Median follow-up was 71 months (Range 8–134) (Table 2).

Seventy-nine percent of responders reported significant improvement in HMB and majority felt that the benefit of the procedure was maintained over a long period of time (Table 2). Ten (5 %) responders reported that they had undergone menopause since the LA-Thermachoice and of these, six (3 %) were using hormone replacement therapy (HRT). Twenty (11 %) responders reported that they had a hysterectomy. Both the above groups were excluded from the analysis for improvement in menstrual symptoms. Overall, 161 (86 %) reported that they were satisfied or very satisfied with the outcome and would recommend the procedure to a friend or a family member. The high satisfaction with endometrial ablation which was noticed in our previous study [9] was maintained for over an 11-years period of time (Table 2) since the procedure.

The satisfaction rates with the procedure in responders with up to 6 years follow-up ($n=96$) were similar to those in

Table 1 Demographics and intraoperative data of women undergoing local anaesthetic thermal balloon endometrial ablation (LA-Thermachoice) between 2001 and 2011, $n=253$

Variable	Number (%)
Age	
Mean	44
SD	4.7
BMI, $n=240$	
Mean	30
SD	6.8
Cycle phase, $n=247$	
Proliferative	93 (37 %)
Secretary	91 (37 %)
Menstruating	34 (14 %)
Mid cycle	15 (6 %)
Amenorrhoea due to drugs	14 (6 %)
Clinical findings (USS or hysteroscopic), $n=249$	
Normal	191 (77 %)
Intramural fibroid	39 (15 %)
Submucosal fibroid <3 cm	5 (2 %)
Polyp	7 (3 %)
Other	7 (3 %)
Uterine size, cm, $n=249$	
<10	184 (74 %)
≥10	43 (17 %)
Not recorded	22 (9 %)
Mean size	8.6
SD	1.2
Volume of fluid, ml	
Thermachoice, $n=51$	
Mean	24.1
SD	13.3
Thermachoice III, $n=185$	
Mean	19.1
SD	11.2
Intrauterine pressure, mm Hg	
Thermachoice, $n=51$	
Mean	157
SD	16
Thermachoice III, $n=188$	
Mean	179
SD	16
Mean visual analogue pain (VAS) immediately after procedure, $n=234$	
Mean	5.5
SD	2.7
Not severe (VAS ≤8)	200 (81 %)
Severe (VAS ≥9)	34 (14 %)

Data not reported in all cases; calculations were based on cases that were recorded

Table 2 Questionnaire survey depicting long-term outcomes in women undergoing local anaesthetic thermal balloon endometrial ablation (LA-Thermachoice) between 2001 and 2011

Variable	Varma et al. [9]	
	2001–2005 Up to 3-year f/up	2001–2011 Up to 11-year f/up
Response rate	n=88 (86 %)	n=190 (78 %)[a]
Mean follow-up time, months	30	62
Range	12–54	12–134
SD	13	42
Periods at review		
Amenorrhoea	27 (29 %)	106 (56 %)[b]
Lighter	51 (55 %)	75 (39 %)
No change or worse	15 (16 %)	9 (5 %)
Length of bleeding at review, n=188		
No bleeding		106 (56 %)
<3 days		26 (14 %)
3–5 days		27 (14 %)
6–7 days		16 (9 %)
8–10 days		6 (3 %)
>10 days		7 (4 %)
Dysmenorrhoea at review		
Less pain or no pain	64 (69 %)	167 (86 %)
No change	11 (12 %)	18 (9 %)
Worsening	18 (19 %)	10 (5 %)
Benefit maintained over time, n=185		
Yes		149 (81 %)
No		36 (19 %)
Further treatment (repeat ablation, drugs, LNG-IUS or hysterectomy), n=187		
No	83 (81 %)	166 (89 %)
Yes	19 (19 %)	21 (11 %)
Reason for further treatment, n=21		
Bleeding		6 (29 %)
Pain		8 (38 %)
Both		7 (33 %)
All types of further treatment		
No further treatment	74 (73 %)	156 (82 %)
LNG-IUS	3 (3 %)	4 (2 %)
Drugs (including HRT)	9 (9 %)	9 (5 %)
Repeat endometrial ablation	2 (2 %)	1 (0 %)
Hysterectomy[c]	14(14 %)	20 (11 %)
Satisfaction, n=186		
Very satisfied or satisfied	78 (76 %)	161 (86 %)
Dissatisfied	24 (24 %)	25 (14 %)

LNG-IUS=levonorgestrel releasing intrauterine system

[a] Data not recorded in all cases; calculations were based on cases that were reported

[b] Ten (5 %) responders reported that they had undergone menopause since the LA-TBEA

[c] Histology of the 16 hysterectomies reported adenomyosis, leiomyoma, both adenomyosis and leiomyoma, no histological pathology, and no data recorded in 6, 2, 3, 5, and 4 cases, respectively

responders between 6 and up to 11 years (n=90) follow-up (79 vs. 84 %, p>0.05).

Secondary treatment with the LNG-IUS (2 %), repeat TBEA (0.5 %), or hysterectomy (11 %) occurred in 34/190 (18 %) responders. Of the 20 (11 %) responders who indicated they had a hysterectomy following the LA-Thermachoice, 6 reported they were still satisfied with the initial procedure. These patients reported the main reason for the hysterectomy as dysmenorrhoea except for one responder who underwent a hysterectomy 10 years following the LA-Thermachoice due to a possible endometrial cancer.

In order to ensure a complete long-term follow-up, we examined the case notes of all non-responder patients for an entry of a hysterectomy operation over this period. In 15 patients, we cannot be sure if any additional surgery has been carried out elsewhere. Eighteen out of 53 (34 %) non-responders had a hysterectomy. Histology of these 18 hysterectomies reported adenomyosis (n=3), leiomyoma (n=2), adenomyosis with leiomyoma (n=4), and no histological abnormality (n=9). The remaining (n=20) patients have not had any surgical interventions since their LA-Thermachoice.

Therefore, in total, only 38 out of 243 (16 %) patients required hysterectomy post LA-Thermachoice to control their symptoms. The average time interval between LA-Thermachoice procedure and hysterectomy was 22 months (SD 17). Hysterectomy rate was higher in patients who underwent endometrial ablation with TBEA (n=15/51 i.e., 29 % users) compared to TBEA-III (n=23/192 i.e., 12 % users) device.

Discussion

This study represents the largest published series of local anaesthetic endometrial ablation. To the best of our knowledge, this is the first study to report clinical outcomes with 11 years (median 71 months) of post LA-Thermachoice follow-up. The study results show that the local anaesthetic outpatient thermal balloon endometrial ablation is an effective minimally invasive procedure for the management of women with symptoms of HMB. The results confirm that the patient satisfaction with LA-Thermachoice is high, and is maintained over a long period of time after the procedure. This study is important in that it provides further data on the long-term outcome and success of LA-Thermachoice.

Review of the literature data evaluating patient satisfaction and clinical outcomes with the LA-Thermachoice reveal a wide variation in results. Many of the studies are small and have a shorter follow-up time [11, 12]. It is important to follow the patients for longer periods, as some outcomes may change over time.

The main strength of this study lies in its long-term follow-up as we were able to cover a significant post-procedure follow-up time frame up to 134 months (median 71 months). The reported satisfaction rates with LA-Thermachoice in our study are in agreement with previously reported satisfaction rates (range 80–95 %) from women who underwent TBEA for HMB, proving the validity of the questionnaire survey [13–18].

There may be limitations in this study which lessens the reliability of its conclusions. The study population may be heterogeneous in relation to different heavy menstrual bleeding patterns. The study did not collect baseline quality-of-life data but we used established methods of assessing symptoms compared to pre-treatment. Also, it is possible that the 5 % of women who have subsequently undergone menopause would positively bias the results, but we were careful that we discounted these patients from the results which still showed significant improvement in patient outcomes. This could be particularly so as patients who underwent treatment from the TBEA device (older population of follow-up), which was shown to have a poorer outcome compared to TBEA-III device, have subsequently undergone the menopause [9]. All women were advised to quantify their period-related symptoms prior to menopause if they already had achieved menopause since LA-Thermachoice. To minimise this bias, we have reported our figures after excluding those women who had undergone the menopause. This therefore represents the most conservative but pragmatic situation regarding the long-term outcome following LA-Thermachoice. Another important issue for questionnaire research is responder and non-responder bias. To minimise this bias, we tried to increase our response rate by contacting eligible patients multiple times. We managed to receive a good response rate to our survey, with 78 % of women completing the survey, which was better than the mean response of other mail surveys [19]. The response rate may reflect women who are not willing to respond to postal questionnaires, those who may not recall their symptoms before LA-Thermachoice, natural loss of patients in long-term studies, and those where questionnaire was ultimately determined undeliverable due to incorrect address.

Conclusion

The study data confirms that patient satisfaction with LA-Thermachoice is high, and is maintained over a long period of time after the procedure. Furthermore, the data confirms that LA-Thermachoice is an effective treatment option for women with symptoms of HMB and a robust alternative to hysterectomy. This information is valuable when counselling patients regarding long-term satisfaction, success in reducing HMB and dysmenorrhoea with LA-Thermachoice, and potential need for further surgery after LA-Thermachoice.

References

1. Sculpher MJ, Bryan S, Dwyer N, Hutton J, Stirrat GM (1993) An economic evaluation of transcervical endometrial resection versus abdominal hysterectomy for the treatment of menorrhagia. Br J Obstet Gynaecol 100:244–252
2. Shapley M, Jordan K, Croft PR (2004) An epidemiological survey of symptoms of menstrual loss in the community. Br J Gen Pract 54:359–363
3. Gupta J, Kai J, Middleton L, Pattison H, Gray R, Daniels J (2013) Levonorgestrel intrauterine system versus medical therapy for menorrhagia. N Engl J Med 368:128–137
4. Cooper K, Lee A, Chien P, Raja E, Timmaraju V, Bhattacharya S (2011) Outcomes following hysterectomy or endometrial ablation for heavy menstrual bleeding: retrospective analysis of hospital episode statistics in Scotland. BJOG 118:1171–1179
5. Pados G, Athanatos D, Tsolakidis D, Stamatopoulos P, Tarlatzis B (2011) Treatment options for dysfunctional uterine bleeding: evaluation of clinical results. GynecolSurg 8:385–393
6. Middleton LJ, Champaneria R, Daniels JP et al (2010) Hysterectomy, endometrial destruction, and levonorgestrel releasing intrauterine system (Mirena) for heavy menstrual bleeding: systematic review and meta-analysis of data from individual patients. BMJ 341:c3929
7. Clark TJ, Samuels N, Malick S, Middleton L, Daniels J, Gupta J (2011) Bipolar radiofrequency compared with thermal balloon endometrial ablation in the office: a randomized controlled trial. Obstet Gynecol 117:1228
8. Matteson KA, Abed H, Wheeler TL, Sung VW, Rahn DD, Schaffer JI, Balk EM (2012) A systematic review comparing hysterectomy with less-invasive treatments for abnormal uterine bleeding. J Minim Invasive Gynecol 19:13–28
9. Varma R, Soneja H, Samuel N, Sangha E, Clark TJ, Gupta JK (2010) Outpatient Thermachoice endometrial balloon ablation: long-term, prognostic and quality-of-life measures. Gynecol Obstet Invest 70:145–148
10. Clark TJ, Gupta JK (2004) Outpatient thermal balloon ablation of the endometrium. Fertil Steril 82:1395–1401
11. Jarrell A, Olsen ME (2003) Patient satisfaction with thermal balloon endometrial ablation. A retrospective review. J Reprod Med 48:635–636
12. Vilos GA, Fortin CA, Sanders B, Pendley L, Stabinsky SA (1997) Clinical trial of the uterine thermal balloon for treatment of menorrhagia. J Am Assoc Gynecol Laparosc 4:559–565
13. Cash C Jr, Garza-Leal J, Donovan A et al (2012) Clinical evaluation of long-term safety and effectiveness of a third-generation thermal uterine balloon therapy system for heavy menstrual bleeding. J Minim Invasive Gynecol 19:469–476
14. Chapa HO, Antonetti AG, Venegas G, Sandate J, VanDuyne CP (2010) Menstrual and dysmenorrhea outcomes after ThermaChoice III: a 2-year prospective study. J Gynecol Surg 25:233–236
15. Cooley S, Yuddandi V, Walsh T, Geary M, McKenna P (2005) The medium- and long-term outcome of endometrial ablative techniques. Eur J Obstet Gynecol Reprod Biol 121(2):233–5
16. Hazard D, Harkins G (2009) Patient satisfaction with thermal balloon ablation for treatment of menorrhagia. Am J Obstet Gynecol 200:e21–e23
17. Andersson S, Mints M (2007) Thermal balloon ablation for the treatment of menorrhagia in an outpatient setting. Acta Obstet Gynecol Scand 86:480–483
18. Kleijn JH, Engels R, Bourdrez P, Mol BW, Bongers MY (2008) Five-year follow up of a randomised controlled trial comparing NovaSure and ThermaChoice endometrial ablation. BJOG 115:193–198
19. Asch DA, Jedrziewski MK, Christakis NA (1997) Response rates to mail surveys published in medical journals. J Clin Epidemiol 50:1129–1136

Oliguria after prophylactic ureteric stenting in gynaecological surgery

Anita J. Merritt · Ilze Zommere · Richard J. Slade · Brett Winter-Roach

Abstract Ureteric injury is one of the most serious complications of gynaecological surgery. Use of prophylactic preoperative bilateral ureteric stents to reduce ureteric injury is established in colorectal surgery and becoming commonplace in complex gynaecological surgery. The safety of the procedure has been questioned due to reports of stent-induced complications including a rare but serious phenomenon of stent-induced transient obstructive oligo-anuria termed reflex anuria, a response to manipulation and irritation of the ureters. A retrospective case-note review of patients who had bilateral ureteric stents placed prior to gynaecological surgery at Salford Royal Hospital, UK, from 2007 to 2011 was performed to identify cases of oligo-anuria post-stenting, which were not related to hypovolaemia, nephrotoxic drugs or a radiologically evident obstruction. All patients had their stents removed immediately at the end of surgery before leaving the operating theatre. Three out of 439 patients (0.7 %), who had preoperative bilateral ureteric stents, developed post-operative oligo-anuria despite relatively normal radiological assessment. In these three cases outlined below, one self-resolved, and two required urgent re-stenting to relieve obstruction. Use of ureteric stents for major gynaecological surgery can expedite intraoperative identification of the ureters to help reduce accidental ureteric injury but can directly cause complications. These three cases have contributed to knowledge of the complications of ureteric stents during major gynaecological surgery. Awareness of reflux anuria as a possible root cause of post-operative acute renal failure is important for guiding appropriate and timely management to preserve renal function.

A. J. Merritt (✉) · I. Zommere · R. J. Slade · B. Winter-Roach
Department of Gynaecology, Salford Royal Hospitals NHS Trust, Stott Lane, Salford M6 8HD, UK
e-mail: anita.merritt@doctors.org.uk

Keywords Ureteric stents · Catheterization · Reflex anuria · Renal failure

Background

Ureteric injury during gynaecological surgery can be associated with significant morbidity [1]. This injury rate is approximately 1 % but is particularly associated with abdominal hysterectomies and more complex surgery involving exenterative procedures [2]. Preoperative insertion of ureteral catheters/stents to aid identification of the ureters and avoid injury and/or enhance intraoperative recognition of injury and repair is becoming more common in gynaecology and other surgical disciplines.

Whether or not the use of stents actually helps prevent ureteric injury is controversial. Some studies have found that using stents reduced the injury rate [3], whereas others do not find any clear benefit [4, 5]. A large randomised controlled trial of 3,141 women who were randomised to prophylactic bilateral ureteral catheterization versus no catheters showed a similar low incidence of ureteral injury in both groups; however, severe injury was less common in women with ureteral catheterization [5].

The procedure of catheterization and stent insertion *per se* is associated with complications [6]. Urinary tract infection is common but can be reduced by perioperative antibiotics and early stent removal. Macrohaematuria, dysuria, urgency, pain and fever are particularly associated by stents left in for increased time. There are also rare reports of anuria and acute renal failure as a complication of ureteric catheterization.

During a 5-year period from 2007 to 2011, 439 patients had prophylactic ureteric stents prior to major gynaecological surgery at Salford Royal Hospital, UK. All stented patients had the stents removed immediately at the end of the surgery. Of these, three (0.7 %) developed anuria and acute renal failure not linked to hypovolaemia or acute tubular necrosis, but of a transient obstructive nature, but with relatively normal radiological assessment. These three cases are described.

Case 1

An 82-year-old lady with obesity, hypertension ischemic heart disease and diabetes presented with post-menopausal bleeding. Investigations confirmed an endometrial carcinoma, and she underwent total abdominal hysterectomy and bilateral salpingo-oophorectomy with preoperative bilateral ureteric stenting.

There were no intraoperative complications and no difficulties during stent insertion, but directly after the stents were removed at the end of surgery, gross haematuria was noted. On day 1, post-op haematuria persisted but urine output, vital observations and biochemistry investigations were within normal limits.

On day 2, the patient complained of bilateral groin pain and had persistent haematuria, and despite intravenous fluid challenges, urine output declined to 20 ml/h, (24 h fluid balance: 3,224 ml in/490 ml out). She then developed pulmonary oedema, and investigations revealed metabolic acidosis, urea 7.9 mmol/l, and creatinine 184 μmol/l. A renal tract ultrasound scan showed only mild bilateral hydronephrosis with no site of obstruction or ureteric dilation, and the cause of the oliguria was unclear (Fig. 1b).

Day 3 was a worsening clinical picture (24 h fluid balance: 1,450 ml in/49 ml out, creatinine 339 μmol/l, urea 15.55 mmol/l), and since post-renal obstruction was considered the most likely cause of the acute renal failure, cystoscopy with bilateral ureteric stenting was performed. The stents were inserted with ease and resulted in dramatic diuresis (7 l over 24 h) and much improved renal function tests. The ureteric stents were left in situ for 10 weeks, after which they were removed without further complications.

Case 2

A premenopausal woman with a high grade ovarian malignancy was admitted for total abdominal hysterectomy with right salpingo-oophorectomy with preoperative bilateral ureteric stenting. The stents were removed at the end of surgery. On day 1, post-op urine output was within normal limits (24 h fluid balance: 3,300 ml in/2,310 ml out), and there was no evidence of haematuria. On day 2, post-op urine output decreased (24 h fluid balance: 2,550 ml in/480 ml out), and the patient complained of severe abdominal and back pain, associated with nausea and vomiting, pyrexia, and rise in creatinine to 202 μmol/l and urea to 5 mmol/l. A CT scan of the abdomen and pelvis showed mild prominence of the pelvicalyceal collecting system and proximal ureters bilaterally tapering to normal calibre in the upper third with no evidence of obstruction or extrinsic compression (Fig. 1a).

In light of the clinical and biochemical findings, and experience from case 1 (above), an obstruction of the renal tract was still suspected, and she underwent cystoscopy and bilateral ureteric stents on day 3 post-op, after which the creatinine and urea rapidly decreased to 66 μmol/l and 3.6 mmol/l, respectively, and the normal urine output returned (24 h fluid balance: 3,200 ml in/1,726 ml out). The stents remained in situ for 3 weeks, after which her renal function remained normal.

Case 3

A lady in her 70s' with endometrial cancer was admitted for laparotomy, hysterectomy and bilateral oophorectomy with

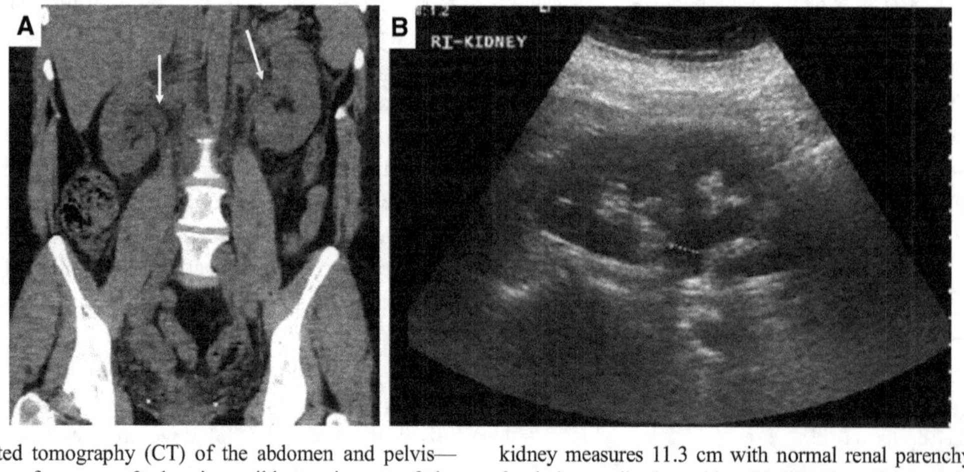

Fig. 1 **a** Computed tomography (CT) of the abdomen and pelvis—unenhanced image, from case 2 showing mild prominence of the pelvicalyceal collecting system and proximal ureters bilaterally (*arrows*), with no evidence of perinephric, peri-ureteric, intra-abdominal or pelvic collections. **b** Ultrasound scan of right kidney from case 1. The right kidney measures 11.3 cm with normal renal parenchyma and no large focal abnormality but with mild dilatation of the pelvicalyceal collecting system. The renal pelvis measures approximately 10.9 mm at the pelvo-ureteric junction (*dotted line*), consistent with mild hydronephrosis. Similar findings were observed for the left kidney (not shown)

preoperative cystoscopy and bilateral ureteric stenting. There were no intraoperative complications, and stents were inserted with ease and removed at the end of surgery. Post-operatively, she passed 1,800 ml of gross haematuria (24 h fluid balance: 2,000 ml in/1,800 ml out) but then became oliguric for 3 days (day 1 post-op 24 h fluid balance: 3,050 ml in/180 ml out, day 2: 2,200 ml in/10 ml out, day 3: 450 ml in/375 ml out), and biochemistry investigations revealed a creatinine of 537 μmol/l and a urea of 16.6 mmol/l. A renal ultrasound performed on day 3 post-op showed no evidence of obstruction and only mild hydronephrosis. Both ureters were not noted to be dilated. She passed 3,700 ml of urine on day 4 (day 4 post-op 24 h fluid balance: 1,300 ml in/3,700 ml out) and 400 ml on day 5 (day 5 post-op 24 h fluid balance: 1,450 ml in/400 ml out) but then again became oliguric for the next 2 days (day 6 post-op 24 h fluid balance: 1,400 ml in/100 ml out, day 7 post-op 24 h fluid balance: 2,500 ml in/0 ml out) (creatinine 602 μmol/l and urea 23.8 mmol/l). Fortunately, she passed 7 l of urine on day 8, and her renal failure was self-resolved without the need for dialysis or further intervention.

Discussion

We describe three case reports of patients who had bilateral ureteric stents placed prior to gynaecological cancer surgery and developed post-operative oligo-anuria with clinically obstructive renal failure despite relatively normal radiological assessment. One case was self-resolved, and two cases required urgent re-stenting to relieve obstruction and regain normal renal function.

Development of oligo-anuria has been occasionally documented as a complication of ureteral catheterization, thought to be caused by transient ureteric obstruction following stent removal [7], and has been estimated as a rate of 0–7.6 % for routine prophylactic ureteric catheterizations [8]. This transient obstructive phenomenon has been described as 'reflex anuria' defined as 'cessation of urine output from both kidneys in response to irritation or trauma to one kidney or ureter or severely painful stimuli to other organs' [9].

The mechanism for the oligo-anuria is not fully understood, but there is evidence that ureteric manipulation can result in reduced renal blood flow and glomerular filtration rate or a reflex spasm of renal arterioles [10]. Other studies suggest ureteric oedema as the cause of uretovesical junction obstruction and resulting anuria [6]. This theory would explain how re-stenting bypasses the oedema, relieves the obstruction and restores renal function. The majority of studies, however, involved colorectal surgery where ureteric stenting has a longer history and such complications are known to those surgeons. There are only two reports of reflex anuria involving ureteric stents in gynaecological surgery. Abu-Rustum et al. reported that 2 out of 38 hysterectomy cases had a transient rise in post-operative creatinine attributed to distal ureteric oedema and one needed re-stenting to resolve the anuria [3], whereas Wood et al. reported that 7 out of 92 patients had post-operative oligo-anuria [11]. In contrast, Kuno et al. reported 0 out of 469 patients with reflux anuria post-gynaecological surgery [12].

Our case series provides further evidence for transient obstructive renal failure as a complication of ureteric catheterization in gynaecological surgery at a rate of 0.7 %. Whilst we cannot be absolutely certain of the exact aetiology of the oligo-anuria, we consider these to be cases of reflex oligo-anuria as (1) radiologically there was either no abnormality or only mild hydronepthrosis without organic obstruction of the urinary tract, (2) it was rapidly resolved by re-stenting or self-resolving causing a large diuresis, and (3) it was not associated with hypovolaemia or nephrotoxic drugs and did not respond to fluid challenges. As routine prophylactic ureteric stenting prior to gynaecological surgery becomes more widespread, it is crucial that gynaecologists are aware of the more serious complications so as to take appropriate, timely action.

To aid in identification of cases of reflux anuria, post-operative measurement of serum urea and electrolytes may be useful to help evaluate ureteric patency; however, these parameters are commonly affected by factors other than obstruction, such as intraoperative blood loss, fluid replacement and nephrotoxic drugs. It is important to first try to exclude those causes of acute renal failure by fluid challenge and cessation of nephrotoxic drugs.

One way to reduce the possibility of reflux anuria is to use staged removal of stents over a 24-h period or longer [6]. Bothwell used staged removal of stents over 24 h (i.e. removal of the right stent immediately post-operatively and the left stent 24 h later) for 92 colorectal surgery patients and reported no cases of anuria [4], whereas Chou et al. removed bilateral ureteric catheters at the end of surgery for 1,583 patients and reported no complications directly related to the catheters [5]. The timing of stent removal is likely to be an important factor in the development of reflux anuria. Leaving the stents in for longer may indeed reduce complications but may require a longer post-operative stay or readmission for stent removal may incur increased cost and inconvenience for the patient. It may be that time of stent removal should be made on an individual case or individual institution basis taking into account all the above factors.

Whether or not ureteric stents should be used routinely prior to gynaecological surgery is still under debate. Nevertheless, for surgeons using stents either routinely or on a case-by-case basis, awareness of serious complications of stenting such as the oligo-anuria described here is essential to guide appropriate, timely action and preserve renal function.

Conflict of interest Anita Merritt, Brett Winter-Roach, Ilze Zommere and Richard Slade declare that they have no conflict of interest.

For studies with human subjects, please include the following statement:

Declaration of consent All procedures followed were in accordance with the ethical standards of the responsible committee on human experimentation (institutional and national) and with the Helsinki Declaration of 1975, as revised in 2000 (5). Informed consent was obtained from all patients for being included in the study. No identifying information about the patients is included in the article.

Co-author's contributions AJM, IZ and BWR are responsible for the concept and design and execution of the study, AJM wrote the manuscript, and IZ, RJS and BWR were responsible for manuscript editing.

References

1. Carley ME, McIntire D, Carley JM, Schaffer J (2002) Incidence, risk factors and morbidity of unintended bladder or ureter injury during hysterectomy. Int Urogynecol J Pelvic Floor Dysfunct 13(1):18–21
2. Jha S, Coomarasamy A, Chan K (2004) Ureteric injury in obstetric and gynaecological surgery. Obstet Gynaecol 6:203–208
3. Abu-Rustum N, Sonoda Y, Balck D, Chi D, Barakat R (2006) Cystoscopic temporary ureteral catheterization during radical vaginal and abdominal hysterectomy. Gynecol Oncol 103:729–731
4. Bothwell W, Bleicher R, Dent T (1994) Prophylactic ureteral catheterization in colon surgery. Dis Colon Rectum 37:330–334
5. Chou M, Wang C, Lien R (2009) Prophylactic ureteral catheterization in gynaecologic surgery: a 12-year randomized trial in a community hospital. Int Urogynecol J Pelvic Floor Dysfunct 20:689–693
6. Sheik F, Khubchandani I (1990) Prophylactic ureteral catheters in colon surgery – how safe are they? Dis Colon Rectum 33:508–510
7. Levine R, Pollack H, Banner M (1982) Transient ureteral obstruction after ureteral stenting. Am J Roentgenol 138:323–327
8. Bienek J, Meade P (2012) Reflux anuria after prophylactic ureteral catheter removal: a case description and review of the literature. J Endourol 26:294–296
9. Sirota J, Narins L (1957) Acute urinary suppression after ureteral catheterization: the pathogenesis of 'reflex anuria'. N Engl J Med 257:1111–1113
10. Maletz R, Berman D, Peele K, Bernard D (1993) Reflex anuria and uremia from unilateral ureteral obstruction. Am J Kidney Dis 22:870–873
11. Wood EC, Maher P, Pelosi MA (1996) Routine use of ureteric catheters at laproscopic hysterectomy may cause unnecessary complications. J Am Assoc Gynecol Laparosc 3:393–397
12. Kuno K, Menzin A, Kauder H (1998) Prophylactic ureteral catheterization in gynecologic surgery. Urology 52:1004–1008

The risk of uterine rupture after myomectomy

J. Claeys · I. Hellendoorn · T. Hamerlynck · J. Bosteels · S. Weyers

Abstract Fibroids may give rise to specific obstetrical complications such as pain due to degeneration, fetal malpresentation, or placenta previa. For all these reasons, surgical resection of the fibroid may be indicated before a pregnancy is pursued. The occurrence of a uterine rupture is a rare but severe complication of myomectomy. This study seeks to review the risk of uterine rupture during pregnancy and/or labor after laparoscopic myomectomy in comparison with laparotomic myomectomy. A systematic search of the literature through search strategies in MEDLINE (PubMed) and Embase (Embase.com) from January 1970 up to March 2013 was performed. We used the following MeSH terms and free text words: gynecologic surgical procedures, gynecologic surgery, leiomyoma, fibromyoma, fibroids, myoma, uterine tumors, and pregnancy complication. Our data show that the risk of uterine rupture during labor and delivery is low (0.75 %). Compared with traditional open myomectomy, the risk of uterine rupture during pregnancy is not significantly higher after a laparoscopic approach (P=0.119). More elective cesarean sections are performed after laparoscopic myomectomy compared with the conventional open technique (P= 0.001). Our conclusions are supported by statistical pooling of observational studies of generally low methodological quality. The risk of uterine rupture after myomectomy is low (0.75 %). The available evidence in the literature does no allow discouraging attempts for childbirth per viam naturalem after previous myomectomy, regardless of the technique used. Randomized studies are needed before definitive evidence-based recommendations can be given.

J. Claeys and I. Hellendoorn contributed equally to this manuscript.

J. Claeys · I. Hellendoorn · T. Hamerlynck · S. Weyers (✉)
Department of Obstetrics and Gynecology, Ghent University Hospital, Ghent, Belgium
e-mail: steven.weyers@ugent.be

J. Bosteels
Department of Obstetrics and Gynecology, Imelda Hospital, Bonheiden, Belgium

Keywords Myomectomy · Pregnancy · Uterine rupture

Introduction

During pregnancy, fibroids may cause pain due to degeneration, fetal malpresentation, or placenta previa. Therefore, surgical resection of the fibroid may be necessary before allowing women with fibroids to conceive. A laparotomic or laparoscopic approach will, in most cases, cause a scar in the myometrium, which may lead to weakening of the muscular wall and, by consequence, may increase the risk for the obstetric calamity of the sudden uterine rupture [1]. Nevertheless, it is at the present unclear whether an elective cesarean section may prevent all cases of uterine rupture during labor after previous scarring of the uterus [2].

For unselected pregnant women, the prevalence of uterine rupture is significantly lower in community-based studies (median 0.05, range 0.02–0.30 %) versus hospital-based studies (median 0.31, range 0.01–2.90 %) [3]. Since most women suffering from severe pain after a previous myomectomy will be admitted in the emergency department of a hospital, the hospital-based studies are likely to reflect the true incidence of the problem under study. In women with a history of cesarean section, the prevalence rate is about 1 % [3]. The frequency of uterine rupture is generally lower in developed countries versus undeveloped countries, as defined by the United Nations. The World Health Organization (WHO) recommends doing further clinical research to estimate the incidence of uterine rupture and to distinguish clearly between ruptures with or without previous surgery on the uterus.

This study aimed to measure the likelihood of uterine rupture after myomectomy. We want to investigate if there are differences in the risk for this serious adverse event during pregnancy versus during the active labor stage. Moreover, we aimed to study if there are significant differences in the incidence of uterine rupture in women treated by laparoscopy versus classic open surgery.

Materials and methods

A systematic research of MEDLINE (PubMed) and Embase (Embase.com) for publications from January 1970 to March 2013 on the occurrence of uterine rupture after surgical myomectomy during pregnancy or labor was performed by using a combination of MeSH terms and free text words: gynecologic surgical procedures, gynecologic surgery, leiomyoma, fibromyoma, fibroids, myoma, uterine tumors, and pregnancy complication (Appendix 1). The results of the search are described in the attached PRISMA flowchart and checklist (Appendixes 2 and 3).

After removal of duplicates, 227 potentially useful publications were retained. The selection of potential studies to be included was done by reviewing the titles and abstracts by two authors (J.C. and J.B.) simultaneously and independently. Non-English articles were only used if an English abstract was available. If there was doubt, arbitration by the third review author (SW) was sought until consensus was reached. Finally, we included 56 articles for this meta-analysis [1, 4–58]. There was no selection based on the study methodology so that various types of articles were included, such as randomized controlled trials, case studies, case series, systematic and narrative reviews, comments, and letters to the editor.

The data extraction was performed by means of a standardized data extraction form (Appendix 4).

The data collected included the method of myomectomy, technique of suturing, location and size of the removed fibroids, time to pregnancy, setting of the study, and, for the published ruptures, the outcome of mother and child. In the absence of important information related to the type of surgery and the outcome of the mother or child, the authors were contacted in order to obtain this information.

If a single article stated that "no major obstetric complications happened," we assumed that no rupture had occurred. A statistical analysis was carried out on the data using Fisher's exact test in the statistical program SPSS.

Results

In the 56 included articles, a total number of 3,685 pregnancies after myomectomy were described, the majority of which (2,017) following laparoscopic myomectomy, while 705 pregnancies occurred after laparotomic myomectomy and 484 pregnancies after other methods of myomectomy (hysteroscopic resection, myolysis, etc.). In 479 pregnancies, we failed to obtain any data on the method of myomectomy; these were excluded from further analysis.

Within these 3,685 pregnancies, 29 cases of uterine rupture were reported (0.79 %), one during labor and 28 prior to the onset of labor. There was a trend for an increased occurrence of uterine rupture following laparoscopic myomectomy (24 events/2,017 or 1.2 %) versus following laparotomic myomectomy (3 events/705 or 0.4 %); the differences were not statistically significant (P=0.119) (Fig. 1). There was one case of uterine rupture after hysteroscopic myomectomy, while in one case (the one rupture during labor), the mode of myomectomy was unknown [35]. The 28 ruptures during pregnancy occurred between 17 and 40 weeks of gestation, with 80 % of the ruptures occurring between 28 and 36 weeks.

The number of planned vaginal deliveries and primary cesarean sections in the laparoscopic group was 401 and 544, respectively, as compared to 124 and 101 cases, respectively, in the open surgery group. The likelihood of a primary cesarean section was significantly increased following a laparoscopic versus a classic open myomectomy (P=0.001).

Of the 401 women who attempted vaginal birth after laparoscopy, a large majority (373 women or 93 %) eventually experienced a successful vaginal delivery, while only 28 (7 %) women were delivered by secondary cesarean section. In the group of 124 women attempting vaginal delivery after myomectomy by an open approach, 109 (88 %) delivered vaginally compared to 15 (12 %) who needed to be delivered by secondary cesarean section. There were no significant differences for the risk of secondary cesarean section between women treated by laparoscopic versus classic open myomectomy (P=0.090).

Just over 50 % of the removed fibroids leading to a rupture of the uterine wall in a subsequent pregnancy were localized in the intramural part of the womb (13/24 or 54 %). The median size of the fibroid was 5 cm. We found no clear correlation between the risk for a uterine rupture and location of the fibroid and suturing technique or whether the operation was done in a university or a non-university hospital.

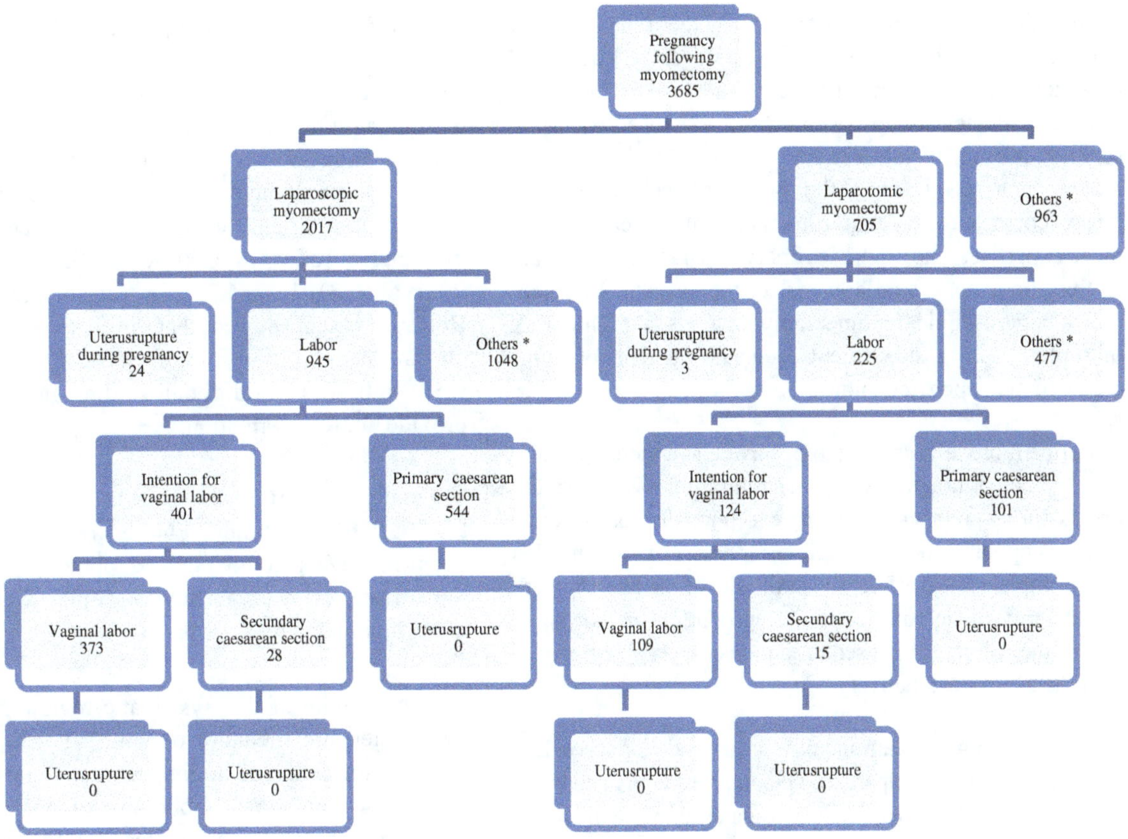

*Others: missing data, lost to follow-up, miscarriage, abortion, ectopic pregnancy

Fig. 1 Summary of pregnancies following myomectomy

When information on maternal and fetal outcome after rupture was unknown, we tried to contact the author. By doing this, we were able to obtain additional information in 75 % of the contacted cases (three out of four). No difference was found in outcome of mother and child in relation to the setting (university versus non-university hospital). There were eight (33 %) neonatal deaths following a uterine rupture (five in the laparoscopic and three in the open surgery group). Our search failed to retrieve any report on maternal deaths following uterine rupture. This finding illustrates the high risk of publication bias associated with adverse events in the medical literature.

Discussion

A uterine rupture is very exceptional in developed countries and more frequent in developing countries due to prolonged labor caused by fetomaternal disproportion or second-stage disorders [2]. In developed countries, uterine rupture is almost exclusively observed following a previous cesarean section or previous surgery on the uterus, including myomectomy [59].

Our present systematic review identified pregnancies following myomectomy reported in the medical literature of the past four decades. We aimed to measure the incidence of uterine rupture after myomectomy in women wishing to conceive.

The prevalence of uterine rupture following myomectomy—all types of surgery—(0.79 %) is comparable with that after cesarean section. Based on the available evidence, there is no significant difference between the incidences of a rupture during pregnancy following a laparoscopic (1.2 %) versus an open myomectomy (0.4 %).

We observed a higher primary cesarean section rate after laparoscopic than after open myomectomy (P= 0.001). This observation may be partially explained by confounding: between 1970 and 2013, there has been an overall increase in the cesarean section rates leading to a higher primary C-section rate in the last two decades (the "era of laparoscopy") compared to the era of open surgery. Indeed, in the last two decades, the laparoscopic approach has become the preferred technique, with laparoscopic suturing requiring more than average technical expertise. The higher primary cesarean section rate in this group may similarly reflect the surgeon's anxiety that a laparoscopic myomectomy beholds a higher risk of rupture during subsequent pregnancy and labor compared to the open technique.

Furthermore, it is striking to observe that a uterine rupture in a woman following a myomectomy almost exclusively occurs during pregnancy and very exceptionally during active labor, as opposed to following a prior cesarean section. This can be explained to differences in the site of the incision with the majority of myomectomies being done in the corporeal part of the womb as opposed to the lower uterine segment in the case of cesarean delivery.

There is no significant increase in the risk for secondary cesarean section after laparoscopic compared with open myomectomy (P=0.090). Attempts at vaginal birth seem equally highly successful following a laparoscopic or an open myomectomy (about 90 %). Moreover, none of the cases of secondary cesarean section was reportedly done for an impending uterine rupture. This finding should be interpreted with great caution, given that in the majority of published reports, no fully described reason for the secondary cesarean section was mentioned.

Furthermore, the occurrence of uterine rupture during labor was analyzed. There was one case of rupture during labor. Unfortunately, there were no data available whether this happened after laparotomic or open myomectomy. An attempt to obtain information from the primary study authors was not successful. It is important to note that this rupture during labor occurred under high-dose oxytocin administration, which, according to the author, could also have caused a rupture in an intact uterus [35].

It is clear that the location and size of the fibroids might affect the likelihood of uterine rupture following previous myomectomy. The limited number of events is too small to present definitive evidence on this subject. The same goes for the study of the relationship between the used suturing technique and the risk of uterine rupture. Also in the C-section literature, there is conflicting evidence about a possible increased risk of uterine rupture after closure of the wound in one layer, while a large multicenter case-control study demonstrated that a single-layer closure, as compared to a two-layer closure, might be associated with an increased risk of rupture [odds ratio (OR) 2.69, 95 % confidence interval (CI) 1.37–5.28]; a recent meta-analysis by Roberge et al. showed that only a locked single-layer closure leads to more ruptures (OR 4.96, 95 % CI 2.58, 9.52) [60, 61]. Additional studies in the future may provide more information.

Finally, most ruptures seem to occur in the mid-third trimester of pregnancy. Further research is needed to determine whether an adapted policy is needed in the third trimester of pregnancy in women who have undergone myomectomy.

The strength of this systematic review is that it is the first systematic literature review that was done to measure the incidence of uterine rupture following myomectomy based on the methodology of doing a systematic review of observational studies. Based on our findings, the risk of a uterine rupture following a myomectomy regardless of the technique used seems very rare (less than 1 % of the ongoing pregnancies). This estimation of the incidence might be used for counseling women wishing to conceive after a myomectomy, but it should be stressed that given the nature of our present research (systematic review (SR) and meta-analysis of observational studies) this should be done with utmost caution. It is clear that randomized studies are needed to study the effectiveness of laparoscopic myomectomy for the adverse outcome of uterine rupture before conclusive evidence can be used to present evidence-based recommendations for daily clinical practice.

Our research has several important limitations. First of all, we restricted our search to publications with an English abstract, which implies a high risk for selection bias. Secondly, the classically described systematic underreporting of iatrogenic complications is inevitably a potential source of publication bias. The observation that only 29 cases of uterine rupture during pregnancy after myomectomy were published and there were no maternal deaths is almost certainly a major underestimation of the true unknown incidence of this potentially life-threatening event. Thirdly, the risk of rupture after laparoscopic myomectomy during labor is possibly underestimated since obstetricians seem to be more apt to do a primary cesarean section for fear of medical litigation after laparoscopic myomectomy. This leads to a high risk of performance bias. In addition, many studies lacked detailed information on complications during pregnancy or labor. When "no major obstetric complications" were noted, it was assumed that no uterine rupture had occurred. This assumption might be a cause of reporting bias. Finally, the present research is based on observational studies only; this inevitably causes a high risk of bias. By consequence, our present calculation of the incidence of uterine rupture following myomectomy, although very clinically relevant and usable for counseling in daily practice, is, at the best, an estimation. The evidence presented in the present SR should therefore be graded as very low. The research question posed in this research is highly relevant for clinical practice. Randomized studies on this topic are eagerly awaited by the obstetrical community. These should not be considered as unethical, given the equipoise for the society, the pregnant women, and their treating physicians. It is clear that a large pragmatic multicenter randomized study could answer this present uncertainty.

Acknowledgments We would like to thank Jens De Groot, university librarian of the University of Leuven, for helping with the search strategy in this study and Prof. Georges Van Maele, professor in biostatistics of the University of Ghent, for his contribution to the statistical analysis.

Funding No external funding was sought for this study.

Conflict of interest J.C., I.H., T.H., J.B., and S.W. declare that they have no conflict of interest.

Appendix 1

Search strategy for MEDLINE

(("Gynecologic surgical procedures"[Mesh:NoExp] OR ((Gynecologic[tiab] OR Gynecological[tiab]) AND (Surgical[tiab] OR Surgery[tiab] OR Surgeries[tiab])))

AND

("Leiomyoma"[Mesh] OR Leiomyoma[tiab] OR Leiomyomas[tiab] OR Fibromyoma[tiab] OR Fibromyomas[tiab] OR Fibroid[tiab] OR Fibroids[tiab] OR ((Fibroid[tiab] OR Fibroids[tiab] OR fibromas[tiab] OR Myoma[tiab] OR Myomas[tiab]) AND (uterine[tiab] OR uterus[tiab] OR tumor[tiab] OR tumors[tiab])))

AND

("Pregnancy complications"[Mesh] OR ((Pregnancy[tiab] OR Pregnancies[tiab]) AND (Complications OR Complication)))

Search strategy for Embase

1. Leiomyoma/exp (12048)
2. Leiomyoma:ab,ti AND [embase]/lim (4821)
3. Leiomyomas:ab,ti AND [embase]/lim (2876)
4. Fibromyoma:ab,ti AND [embase]/lim (126)
5. Fibromyomas:ab,ti OR fibroid:ab,ti OR fibroids:ab,ti AND [embase]/lim (3310)
6. (Fibroid OR fibroids OR fibromas OR myoma OR myomas) NEAR/1 (uterine OR uterus OR tumor OR tumors) AND [embase]/lim (7611)
7. No. 1 OR no. 2 OR no. 3 OR no. 4 OR no. 5 OR no. 6 (20910)
8. "Gynecologic surgery"/de (8320)
9. (Gynecologic OR gynecological) NEAR/1 (surgical OR surgery OR surgeries) AND [embase]/lim (85423)
10. No. 8 OR no. 9 (86669)
11. "Pregnancy complication"/exp (91673)
12. ((Pregnancy OR pregnancies) NEAR/1 (complications OR complication)):ab,ti AND [embase]/lim (2256)
13. No. 11 OR no. 12
14. No. 7 AND no. 10 AND no. 13
15. Leiomyoma/exp OR (leiomyoma:ab,ti AND [embase]/lim) OR (leiomyomas:ab,ti AND [embase]/lim) OR (fibromyoma:ab,ti AND [embase]/lim) OR (fibromyomas:ab,ti OR fibroid:ab,ti OR fibroids:ab,ti AND [embase]/lim) OR ((fibroid OR fibroids OR fibromas OR myoma OR myomas) NEAR/1 (uterine OR uterus OR tumor OR tumors) AND [embase]/lim) AND (gynecologic surgery/de OR ((gynecologic OR gynecological) NEAR/1 (surgical OR surgery OR surgeries) AND [embase]/lim)) AND ((pregnancy OR pregnancies) NEAR/1 (complications OR complication)):ab,ti AND [embase]/lim

Appendix 2

PRISMA 2009 Flow Diagram

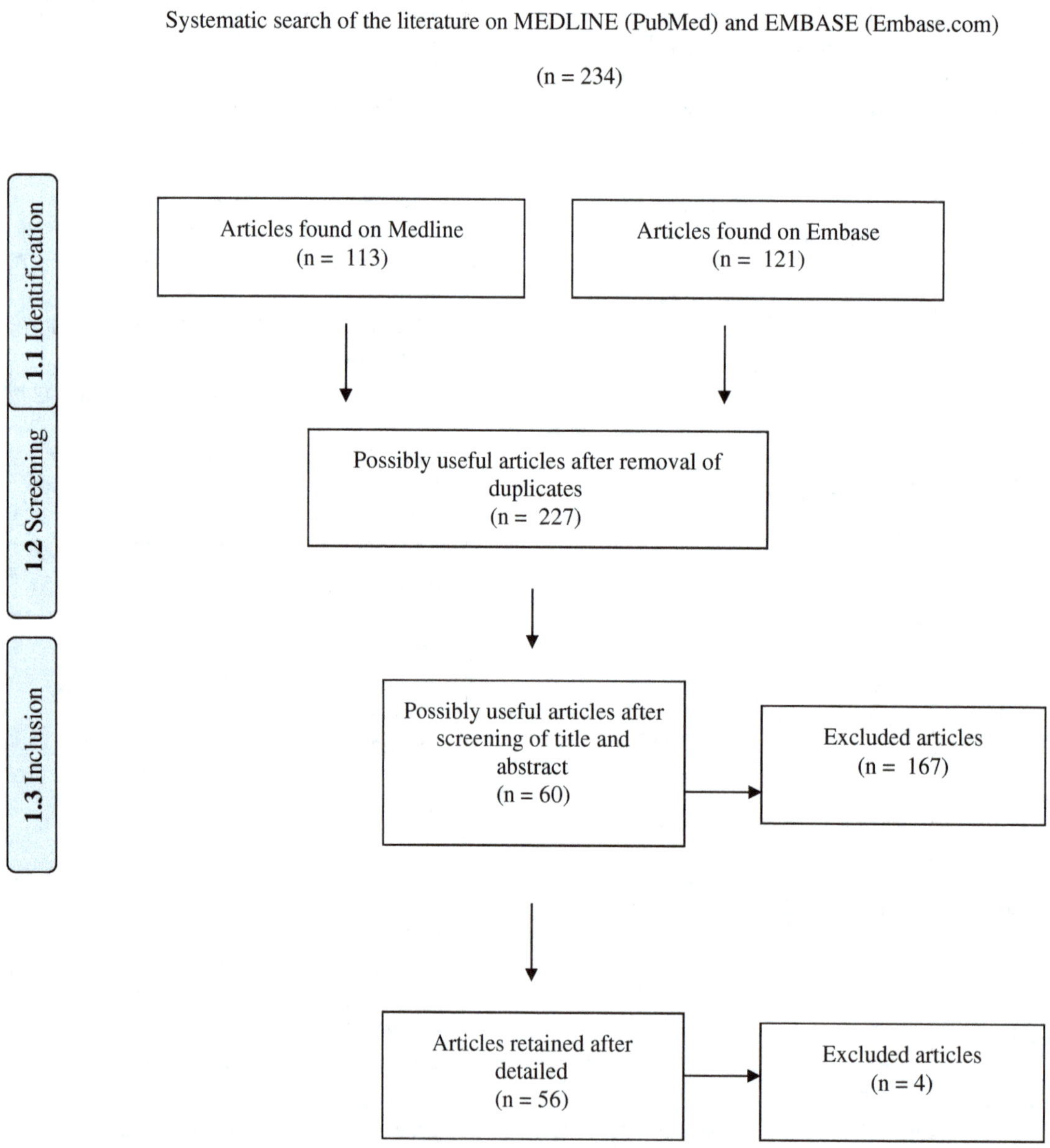

Appendix 3

PRISMA 2009 Checklist

Section/topic	#	Checklist item	Reported on page #
TITLE			
Title	1	Identify the report as a systematic review, meta-analysis, or both.	1
ABSTRACT			
Structured summary	2	Provide a structured summary including, as applicable: background; objectives; data sources; study eligibility criteria, participants, and interventions; study appraisal and synthesis methods; results; limitations; conclusions and implications of key findings; systematic review registration number.	2-3
INTRODUCTION			
Rationale	3	Describe the rationale for the review in the context of what is already known.	4
Objectives	4	Provide an explicit statement of questions being addressed with reference to participants, interventions, comparisons, outcomes, and study design (PICOS).	4
METHODS			
Protocol and registration	5	Indicate if a review protocol exists, if and where it can be accessed (e.g., Web address), and, if available, provide registration information including registration number.	4-5
Eligibility criteria	6	Specify study characteristics (e.g., PICOS, length of follow-up) and report characteristics (e.g., years considered, language,	4-5,27
		publication status) used as criteria for eligibility, giving rationale.	
Information sources	7	Describe all information sources (e.g., databases with dates of coverage, contact with study authors to identify additional studies) in the search and date last searched.	5
Search	8	Present full electronic search strategy for at least one database, including any limits used, such that it could be repeated.	5,20-21
Study selection	9	State the process for selecting studies (i.e., screening, eligibility, included in systematic review, and, if applicable, included in the meta-analysis).	5,27
Data collection process	10	Describe method of data extraction from reports (e.g., piloted forms, independently, in duplicate) and any processes for obtaining and confirming data from investigators.	5,27
Data items	11	List and define all variables for which data were sought (e.g., PICOS, funding sources) and any assumptions and simplifications made.	5,20-21
Risk of bias in individual studies	12	Describe methods used for assessing risk of bias of individual studies (including specification of whether this was done at the study or outcome level), and how this information is to be used in any data synthesis.	3,8-9
Summary measures	13	State the principal summary measures (e.g., risk ratio, difference in means).	5
Synthesis of results	14	Describe the methods of handling data and combining results of studies, if done, including measures of consistency (e.g., I^2) for each meta-analysis.	5-7
Section/topic	#	Checklist item	Reported on page #
Risk of bias across studies	15	Specify any assessment of risk of bias that may affect the cumulative evidence (e.g., publication bias, selective reporting within studies).	3,9

Additional analyses	16	Describe methods of additional analyses (e.g., sensitivity or subgroup analyses, meta-regression), if done, indicating which were pre-specified.	N/A
RESULTS			
Study selection	17	Give numbers of studies screened, assessed for eligibility, and included in the review, with reasons for exclusions at each stage, ideally with a flow diagram.	5,22
Study characteristics	18	For each study, present characteristics for which data were extracted (e.g., study size, PICOS, follow-up period) and provide the citations.	5-7,11-19
Risk of bias within studies	19	Present data on risk of bias of each study and, if available, any outcome level assessment (see item 12).	3,8-9
Results of individual studies	20	For all outcomes considered (benefits or harms), present, for each study: (a) simple summary data for each intervention group (b) effect estimates and confidence intervals, ideally with a forest plot.	5-7,17-19
Synthesis of results 21	21	Present the main results of the review. If meta-analyses are done, include for each, confidence intervals and measures of consistency.	5-7
Risk of bias across studies	22	Present results of any assessment of risk of bias across studies (see Item 15).	3,9
Additional analysis	23	Give results of additional analyses, if done (e.g., sensitivity or subgroup analyses, meta-regression [see Item 16]).	N/A
DISCUSSION			
Summary of evidence	24	Summarize the main findings including the strength of evidence for each main outcome; consider their relevance to key groups (e.g., healthcare providers, users, and policy makers).	7-9
Limitations	25	Discuss limitations at study and outcome level (e.g., risk of bias), and at review-level (e.g., incomplete retrieval of identified	8-9
		research, reporting bias).	
Conclusions	26	Provide a general interpretation of the results in the context of other evidence, and implications for future research.	2,9
FUNDING			
Funding	27	Describe sources of funding for the systematic review and other support (e.g., supply of data); role of funders for the systematic review.	2-3,10

Appendix 4

Data extraction form

1. Sources
   i. All sources available were used
2. Intervention
   i. Inclusion of laparoscopic myomectomy
   ii. Inclusion of laparotomic myomectomy
   iii. Inclusion of hysteroscopic myomectomy
   iv. Exclusion of electromyolysis
   v. Exclusion of a uterine embolization

   For each intervention

i. Suturing technique
ii. Number of pregnancies following the intervention
iii. Attempting vaginal birth of primary cesarean section
iv. When attempting vaginal birth: vaginal birth of secondary cesarean section
v. Reason for secondary cesarean section

3. Outcome
   i. Uterine rupture during pregnancy
   ii. Uterine rupture during labor

   For each rupture

i. When during pregnancy: week of pregnancy
   ii. Setting
   iii. Size of removed fibroids
   iv. Location of removed fibroids
   v. Outcome of child
   vi. Outcome of mother

References

1. Parker W, Einarsson J, Istre O, Duboisson J et al (2010) Risk factors for uterine rupture after laparoscopic myomectomy. J Minim Invasive Gynecol 17(5):551–554
2. Murphy D (2006) Uterine rupture. Obstet Gynecol 18:135–140

3. Hoffmeyr G, Say L, Gulmezoglu A et al (2005) WHO systematic review of maternal mortality and morbidity; the prevalence of uterine rupture. BJOG 112:1221–1228
4. Pritts EA (2001) Fibroids and infertility: a systematic review of the evidence. Obstet Gynecol Surv 56:483–491
5. Adesiyun A, Ojabo A, Durosinlorun-Mohmmed A et al (2008) Fertility and obstetric outcome after caesarean myomectomy. J Obstet Gynaecol 28(7):710–712
6. Bajekal N, Li T et al (2009) Fibroids, infertility and pregnancy wastage. Hum Reprod Update 6(6):614–620
7. Bernard G, Darai E, Poncelet C, Benifla J, Madelenat P et al (2000) Fertility after hysteroscopic myomectomy: effect of intramural myomas associated. Eur J Obstet Gynecol Reprod Biol 88:85–90
8. Bonito M, Gulemi L, Basili R, Roselli D et al (2007) Myomectomy during first and second trimester of pregnancy. Clin Exp Obstet Gynecol 34(3):149–150
9. Campo S, Campo V, Gambadauro P et al (2003) Reproductive outcome before and after laparoscopic or abdominal myomectomy for subserous or intramural myomas. Eur J Obstet Gynecol Reprod Biol 110:215–219
10. Celik C, Acar A, Cicek N, Gezginc K, Akyurek C et al (2002) Can myomectomy be performed during pregnancy? Gynecol Obstet Investig 53:79–83
11. Connolly G, Doyle M, Barrett T, Byrne P, De Mello M, Harrison R et al (2000) Fertility after abdominal myomectomy. J Obstet Gynaecol 20(4):418–420
12. Damiani A, Melgrati L, Marziali M, Sesti F et al (2003) Gasless laparoscopic myomectomy. J Reprod Med 48(10):792–798
13. Davies A, Hart R, Magos A et al (1999) The excision of uterine fibroids by vaginal myomectomy: a prospective study. Fertil Steril 71(5):961–964
14. Febo G, Tessarolo M, Leo L, Arduino S, Wierdis T, Lanza L et al (1997) Surgical management of leiomyomata in pregnancy. Clin Exp Obstet Gynecol 24(2):76–78
15. Gavai M, Hupuzi P, Papp Z et al (2006) Abdominal myomectomy as the alternative to hysterectomy: analysis of 504 cases. Orv Hetil 147(21):971–978
16. Gerli S, Baiocchi G, Favilli A, Di Renzo G et al (2011) New treatment option for early spontaneous rupture of a postmyomectomy gravid uterus. Fertil Steril 96(2):97–98
17. Goldberg J, Pereira L, Berghella V, Diamond J, Daraï E, Seinera P, Seracchioli R et al (2004) Pregnancy outcomes after treatment for fibromyomata: uterine artery embolization versus laparoscopic myomectomy. Am J Obstet Gynecol 191:18–21
18. Grande N, Catalano G, Ferrari S, Marana R et al (2005) Spontaneous uterine rupture at 27 weeks of pregnancy after laparoscopic myomectomy. J Minim Invasive Gynecol 12:131
19. Guillaume A, Benjamin F, Spitzer M et al (1998) Myomectomy performed concurrently with tuboplasty. J Reprod Med 43(6):483–486
20. Guillaume J, Benjamin F, Jean-Gilles M, Ajah M, Tabassi G, Kenel-Pierre C et al (2000) Myomectomy and tuboplasty performed at the same time in cases of distal tubal obstruction with associated fibroids. J Reprod Med 45(6):461–464
21. Hagnère P, Denoual I, Souissi A, Deswarte S et al (2011) Rupture uterine spontanée après myomectomie. À propos d'un cas et revue de la littérature. J Gynécol Obstét Biol Reprod 40:162–165
22. Jedrzejczak P, Pawelczyk L, Grewling K, Pelesz M, Serdynska M et al (2004) The assessment of the fertilization ability and the course of pregnancy in women after laparoscopic myomectomy. Przegl Lek 61(2):65–69
23. Kelly B, Bright P, MacKenzie I et al (2008) Does the surgical approach used for myomectomy influence the morbidity in subsequent pregnancy? J Obstet Gynaecol 28(1):77–81
24. Kucera E, Dvorska M, Krepelka P, Herman H et al (2006) Pregnancy after laparoscopic myomectomy—long-term follow-up. Ceska Gynekol 71(5):389–393
25. Kumakiri J, Takeuchi H, Kitade M, Kikuchi I, Shimanuki H, Itoh S, Kinoshita K et al (2005) Pregnancy and delivery after laparoscopic myomectomy. J Minim Invasive Gynecol 12(3):241–246
26. Kumakiri J, Takeuchi H, Itoh S, Kitade M, Kikuchi I, Shimanuki H, Kumakiri Y, Kuroda K, Takeda S et al (2008) J Minim Invasive Gynecol 15(4):420–424
27. Leidi L, Brusati M, Vespa M et al (2007) A treacherous scar. Am J Obstet Gynecol 197(5):553
28. Li T, Mortimer R, Cooke I et al (1999) Myomectomy: a retrospective study to examine reproductive performance before and after surgery. Hum Reprod 14(7):1735–1740
29. Lolis D, Kalantaridou S, Makrydimas G, Sotiriadis A, Navrozoglou I, Zikopoulos K, Paraskevaidis E et al (2003) Successful myomectomy during pregnancy. Hum Reprod 18(8):1699–1702
30. Malzoni M, Sizzi O, Rossetti A, Imperato F et al (2006) Laparoscopic myomectomy: a report of 982 procedures. Surg Technol Int 15:123–129
31. Malzoni M, Tinelli R, Cosentino F, Iuzzolino D, Surico D, Reich H et al (2010) Laparoscopy versus minilaparotomy in women with symptomatic uterine myomas: short-term and fertility results. Fertil Steril 93(7):2368–2373
32. Mara M, Maskova J, Fucikova Z, Kuzel D, Beslan T, Sosna O et al (2008) Midterm clinical and first reproductive results of a randomized controlled trial comparing uterine fibroid embolization and myomectomy. Cardiovasc Intervent Radiol 31(1):73–85
33. Marchionni M, Fambrini M, Zambelli V, Scarselli G, Susini T et al (2004) Reproductive performance before and after abdominal myomectomy: a retrospective analysis. Fertil Steril 82(1):154–159
34. Morita M, Asakawa Y et al (2006) Reproductive outcome after laparoscopic myomectomy for intramural myomas in infertile women with or without associated infertility factors. Reprod Med Biol 5: 31–35
35. Nezhat C, Nezhat F, Roemisch M, Seidman D, Tazuke S, Nezhat C et al (1999) Pregnancy following laparoscopic myomectomy: preliminary results. Hum Reprod 14(5):1219–1221
36. Obed J, Omigbodun A et al (1996) Rupture of the uterus in patients with previous myomectomy and primary caesarean section scars: a comparison. J Obstet Gynaecol 16(1):16–21
37. Okoro O, Onwere S et al (2007) Myomectomy during pregnancy. Pak J Med Sci 23(5):771–773
38. Pajszczyk-Kieszkiewicz T, Kazimierak W, Lech W, Lipecka-Kidawska E, Sieroszewski P, Kowalska-Koprek U et al (2002) Leiomyomas in pregnancy. Ginekol Pol 73(4):291–296
39. Park W, Jeon Y, Lee J, Shin S et al (2006) Subserosal pregnancy in a previous myomectomy site: a variant of intramural pregnancy. J Minim Invasive Gynecol 13(3):242–244
40. Persin J, Hanousek L et al (2006) Results of conservative surgery of uterine fibroids—5 years of follow-up. Ceska Gynekol 71(4):322–325
41. Ploszynski A, Gniadek R, Adamcio-Deptulska M, Mielnik J et al (1997) Myomectomy and long-term follow-up. Ginekol Pol 68(9): 423–426
42. Plotti G, Plotti F, Di Giovanni A, Battaglia F, Nagar G et al (2008) Feasibility and safety of vaginal myomectomy: a prospective pilot study. J Minim Invasive Gynecol 15(2):166–171
43. Ramarajan A, Achar S et al (2012) Successful pregnancy following extensive myomectomy in a case of uterine leiomyomatosis. Int J Gynecol Obstet 199:S459
44. Ribeiro S, Reich H, Rosenberg J, Guglielminetti E, Vidali A et al (1999) Laparoscopic myomectomy and pregnancy outcome in infertile patients. Fertil Steril 71(3):571–574
45. Rossetti A, Sizzi O, Chiarotti F, Florio G et al (2007) Developments in techniques for laparoscopic myomectomy. J Soc Laparoendosc Surg 11(1):34–40

46. Rovio P, Heinonen P et al (2006) Transvaginal myomectomy with screw traction by colpotomy. Arch Gynecol Obstet 273(4):211–215
47. Salfelder A, Lueken R, Gallinat A, Möller C, Busche D, Nugent W et al (1999) Laparoscopic myomectomy and pregnancy—results. Geburtshilfe Frauenheilkd 59(2):57–61
48. Sentilhes L, Sergent F, Berthier A, Catala L, Descamps P, Marpeau L et al (2006) Uterine rupture following operative hysteroscopy. Gynécol Obstét Fertil 34:1064–1070
49. Seracchioli R, Manuzzi L, Vianello F, Gualerzi B, Savelli L, Paradisi R, Venturoli S et al (2006) Obstetric and delivery outcome of pregnancies achieved after laparoscopic myomectomy. Fertil Steril 86(1): 159–165
50. Sinclair D, Gaither K, Mason T et al (2005) Fertility outcomes following myomectomy in an urban hospital setting. J Natl Med Assoc 97(10):1346–1348
51. Sizzi O, Rossetti A, Malzoni M, Minelli L, La Grotta F, Soranna L, Panunzi S, Spagnolo R, Imperato F, Landi S, Fiaccamento A, Stola E et al (2007) Italian multicenter study on complications of laparoscopic myomectomy. J Minim Invasive Surg 14(4):453–462
52. Skrablin S, Banovic V, Kuvacic I et al (2005) Letters to the editor—brief communication. Successful pregnancy after spontaneous rupture of scarred uterus following fundal myomectomy. Eur J Obstet Gynaecol Reprod Biol 121(2):251–253
53. Soriano D, Dessolle L, Poncelet C, Benifla J, Madelenat P, Daraï E et al (2003) Pregnancy outcome after laparoscopic and laparoconverted myomectomy. Eur J Obstet Gynecol Reprod Biol 108(2):194–198
54. Suwadinata F, Gruessner E, Owandho C, Tinneberg H et al (2008) Pregnancy-preserving myomectomy: preliminary report on a new surgical technique. Eur J Contracept Reprod Health Care 13(3):323–326
55. Tinelli A, Hurst B, Hudelist G, Tin D, Stark M, Mettler L, Guido M, Malvasi A et al (2011) Laparoscopic myomectomy focusing on the myoma pseudocapsule: technical and outcome reports. Hum Reprod 27(2):427–435
56. Walid S, Heaton R et al (2010) Laparoscopic myomectomy: an intent-to-treat study. Arch Gynecol Obstet 281(4):645–649
57. Wong K, Tan J, Ang C, Ngu A et al (2010) Myomectomy scar ectopic pregnancy. Aust N Z J Obstet Gynaecol 50(1):93–98
58. Zollner U, Classen V, Steck T, Dietl J et al (2001) Fertility and pregnancy outcome after myomectomy. Geburtshilfe Frauenheilkd 61(4):213–219
59. Zwart J, Richters J, Öry F, De Vries J, Bloemenkamp K, Van Roosmalen J et al (2009) Uterine rupture in the Netherlands: a nationwide population-based cohort study. Int J Obstet Gynaecol 116:1069–1080
60. Bujold E, Goyet M, Marcoux S et al (2010) The role of uterine closure in the risk of uterine rupture. Obstet Gynecol 116:43–50
61. Roberge S, Chaillet N, Boutin A et al (2011) Single- versus double-layer closure of the hysterotomy incision during cesarean delivery and the risk of uterine rupture. Int J Gynecol Obstet 115:5–10

27

Dilemmas in management of bilateral ectopic pregnancies

Arpita Ghosh · Daniel Borlase · Tosin Ajala · Anthony James Kelly · Zaky Ibrahim

Abstract Simultaneous bilateral ectopic pregnancies occurring spontaneously or following assisted conception techniques, although rare, present the clinician with diagnostic uncertainty and management dilemmas which may have an implication on the patient's future fertility. A review of available literature suggests that there is no universally accepted management strategy towards this condition, and care needs to be tailored to the needs of the patient, patient's preferences and the clinical picture. We report two such rare cases of simultaneous bilateral ectopic pregnancies with different management and outcomes highlighting the fact that these cases not only pose diagnostic and management challenges but also has complex ethical issues associated with it.

Keywords Bilateral ectopic · Salpingostomy · Salpingectomy

Introduction

Simultaneous bilateral ectopic pregnancies occurring spontaneously or following assisted conception techniques are rare, with an incidence reported to be between 1 in 725 to 1 in 1,580 of all extrauterine pregnancies Rondeau et al. [1]. Management of these rare cases presents the clinician with diagnostic and management dilemmas. This is primarily due to rarity of the condition posing diagnostic difficulties with ultrasonography and implication of its treatment on fertility of the women.

We report two such rare cases of simultaneous bilateral ectopic pregnancies with different management and outcome, highlighting the fact that these cases not only pose diagnostic and management challenges but also has complex ethical issues associated with it.

Case reports

Case 1

History

A 37-year-old lady self-referred to the Early Pregnancy Assessment Unit (EPAU) at our local hospital at approximately 6 weeks into a planned pregnancy (Fig. 1). She presented with vaginal spotting which self resolved 7 days before attending. She denied any abdominal pain. Her previous obstetric history was that of a forceps-assisted delivery in 2008 and an early miscarriage in 2012. There was no history of previous tubal problems, gynaecological surgery or pelvic inflammatory disease. Her Abdominal and pelvic examination was unremarkable.

A transvaginal ultrasound scan on the day she presented revealed an empty uterus with an endometrial thickness of 7 mm. The right ovary showed two small haemorrhagic cysts of about the same size (18 mm × 12 mm × 16 mm). Adjacent to the left ovary was a solid cystic lesion approximately 34 mm × 33 mm × 19 mm in size (Fig. 2). This lesion demonstrated no colour Doppler flow.

A. Ghosh (✉) · D. Borlase · T. Ajala · A. J. Kelly
Brighton and Sussex University Hospitals NHS Trust, Brighton, UK
e-mail: arpitagmc@yahoo.com

D. Borlase
e-mail: danielborlase@hotmail.com

T. Ajala
e-mail: Tosin.Ajala@bsuh.nhs.uk

A. J. Kelly
e-mail: Tony.kelly@bsuh.nhs.uk

Z. Ibrahim
Western Sussex Hospitals NHS Trust, West Sussex, UK
e-mail: Zaky.Ibrahim@wsht.nhs.uk

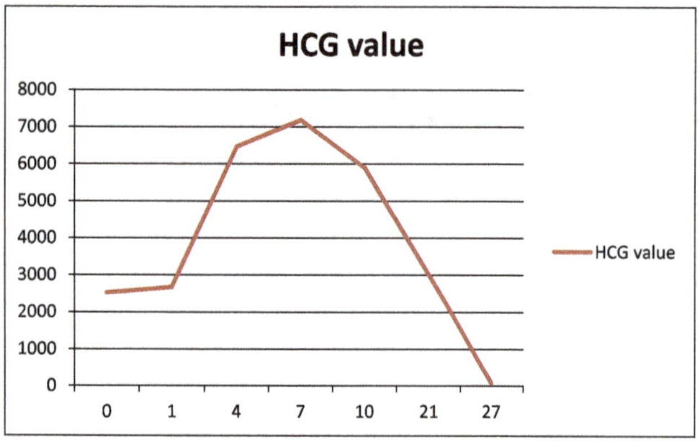

Fig. 1 Trend of HCG level in IU plotted against number of days

In view of her scan findings, particularly the empty uterus, blood was taken for serum levels of β-human Chorionic Gonadotrophin (β-hCG), progesterone and a full blood count. Her β-hCG was reported to be 2,512 IU with progesterone of 56.3 IU. Her Haemoglobin level was normal.

In view of her β-hCG level and scan findings, the decision was made to perform a diagnostic laparoscopy with a possibility of proceeding to salpingectomy as an emergency procedure. This was in line with the local guideline according to which laparoscopy is indicated in women with B-hCG more than 1,500 with no evidence of intrauterine gestation.

Laparoscopy revealed a 20-mm swelling in the mid-ampullary region covered with inflammatory material, suggestive of a chronic ectopic pregnancy. On further assessment, a smaller bean-shaped swelling of approximately 10 mm size in the mid-ampulla of the right tube was noticed (Fig. 3). This had the appearance of an acute tubal ectopic pregnancy. The options at this point were to do bilateral salpingectomy, salpingectomy and salpingostomy salpingectomy and methotrexate management or only methotrexate management. Due to the facts that the patient was asymptomatic, bilateral ectopic

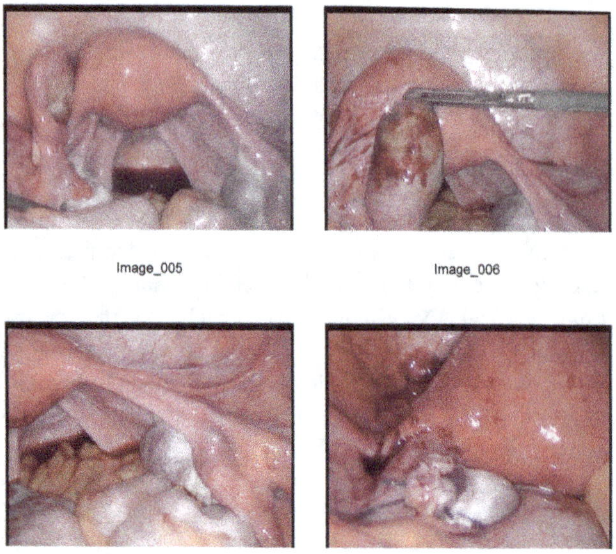

Fig. 2 Pictures showing left chronic tubal ectopic pregnancy case 1

pregnancy was an incidental finding, patient was not consented for further surgery, right tubal pregnancy was less than 3 cm in size and serum HCG was less than 3,000; the decision was made to perform salpingectomy only on the left side. Further management of right acute unruptured tubal pregnancy was deferred pending discussion with the patient pertaining to implications on her future fertility.

Postoperatively, the findings were explained to the patient, and the options were discussed which included conservative management, medical management with methotrexate and further laparoscopic surgery with a view to do salpingostomy. After a detail discussion, it was decided to manage this patient with methotrexate, which was given the day after her initial surgery. In line with the local protocol, plan was made to monitor her β-hCG levels on days 1, 4, 7 and 10 following methotrexate treatment.

Patient was clinical assessed after it was noted that β-hCG levels were rising on day 4 (see Fig. 1) after treatment with methotrexate. She was pain free and well. She was then treated with oral mifepristone 200 mg stat and was allowed home pending her further β-hCG level on day 7.

On day 7, her β-hCG levels were still rising, but she remained asymptomatic. At this point, the option of surgical management was re-discussed, and it was decided to continue to manage her conservatively. By day 10, 18 % decline in her HCG levels was noted. The mifepristone was repeated, and she was reviewed again 7 days later. Her β-hCG was still declining but not at a satisfactory rate. As the patient was still not complaining of any symptoms, it was decided to repeat the methotrexate regime. A steady decline in HCG levels was noted after the second cycle of Methotrexate treatment. The levels dropped down to 72 on day 10 following second cycle of methotrexate.

She was followed up in gynaecology outpatient clinic, and arrangements were made for her to under a go a laparoscopy and dye to test for tubal patency. At laparoscopy, the right tube had an appearance of chronic ectopic but her serum HCG at this point was less than 1. Hydrotubation revealed a free spillage of dye from the right tube confirming its patency.

Case 2

A 34-year-old woman with a BMI of 26 was referred to the infertility clinic with a 2-year history of primary infertility. No identifiable risk factors for sub-fertility were present in her and her partner. Her hormone profile did not reveal any abnormality. Hysterosalpingogram revealed bilaterally patent tubes with normal uterus.

Following the cycle of IUI, she presented at 5 weeks of gestation to the early pregnancy clinic with light per-vaginum bleeding and mild left iliac fossa pain. Pelvic ultrasound did not show any intrauterine gestation sac and reported the endometrial thickness of 10 mm with two small cystic areas

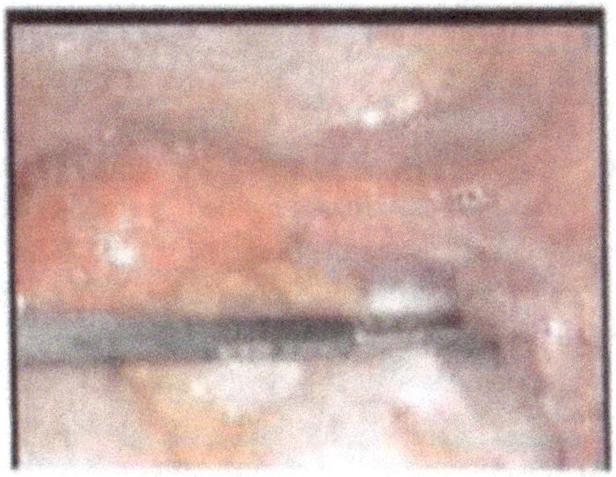

Image_002

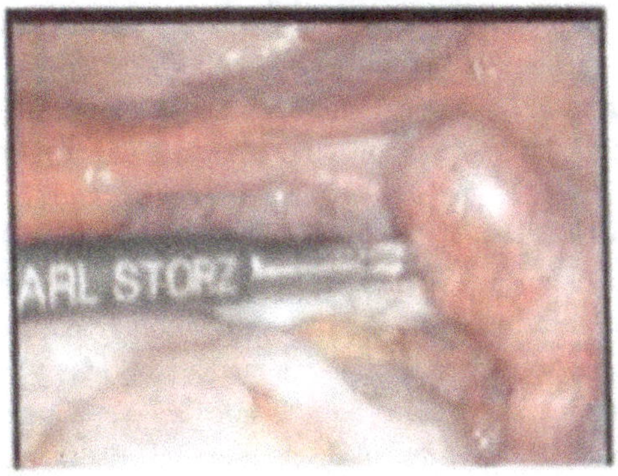

Image_003

Fig. 3 Pictures showing right acute tubal ectopic pregnancy case 1

near both ovaries suggestive of either a corpus luteal cyst or ectopic pregnancies. Her serum HCG level was 9,691 IU and she was haemodynamically stable. She was admitted to the hospital with a provisional diagnosis of 'pregnancy of unknown location', and the possibility of ectopic pregnancy was explained to her. A diagnostic laparoscopy was planned the following day, and the patient was counselled and consented for a possible salpingectomy.

Laparoscopy revealed bilateral haemorrhagic masses with a small amount of blood in the pouch of Douglas. As the patient was already seeking fertility treatment for unexplained infertility and the option of IVF was available to the couple if IUI treatment failed, the decision was made to perform bilateral salpingectomies and thereafter plan further IVF treatment. Histology confirmed the diagnosis of bilateral ectopic pregnancies. She and her partner were then offered IVF to help attain pregnancy. A year later, she had a successful intrauterine pregnancy following IVF treatment.

Discussion

Ectopic pregnancy is an important cause of maternal mortality and morbidity. Every 11 in 1,000 pregnancies are reported to be an ectopic (CEMACH report 2003–2005). The latest CEMACH report from 2003-2005 emphasise the importance of early recognition and diagnosis of such pregnancies to save mothers' lives. There has been a persistent failure to recognise ectopic pregnancy and hence one of the 'top ten' key recommendations from the latest CEMACH report is that there should be national guidelines for the management of pain and bleeding in early pregnancy. Comprehensive clinical guidelines for the treatment of ectopic pregnancy have been published by the Royal College of Obstetricians and Gynaecologists. Because of its rarity, bilateral ectopic pregnancy is not referred to in the guidelines, but the same principles of management can still be applied.

The main purpose of reporting these two cases of bilateral ectopic pregnancy is to highlight the two different management approaches for the same condition and to discuss the challenges and dilemmas faced by the clinicians while diagnosing and managing such rare cases. In both the above cases, the noninvasive diagnostic methods with transvaginal ultrasonography and serial serum HCG monitoring failed to establish conclusively the presence of bilateral ectopic pregnancy. Given the rarity of the condition, difficulties in interpretation of serum HCG and the limitations of ultrasonography, timely diagnosis can be difficult. However, its early diagnosis is imperative in preservation of future fertility of the woman.

A review of available literature reveals that in most cases, preoperative investigations with serum HCG and ultrasonography fail to diagnose the presence of bilateral ectopic pregnancy [2]. It is commonly diagnosed intraoperatively at the time of laparoscopy. In the majority of the cases, ultrasonography will diagnose the presence of ectopic pregnancy in one tube, with the subsequent unexpected finding of bilateral ectopics during laparoscopy. This emphasises the importance of maintaining a high index of suspicion and the importance of examining the contralateral tube carefully during the laparoscopy. It can be specially challenging for the clinicians making these complex decisions during an emergency procedure with limited time to discuss and think about the implications of different management options with regards to the women's future chances of conception and the desire for preservation of fertility.

A diagnosis of bilateral tubal ectopic pregnancy at laparoscopy presents the clinician with the dilemma that the curative approach, which is to perform a bilateral salpingectomy, will render the women infertile. Thereafter, the only option of conceiving is through assisted conception technique. This is an important consideration especially as in majority of the cases the condition is found incidentally at laparoscopy giving no time for a detailed discussion with the women regarding its implications. Most of the clinicians choose to attempt conserving at least one tube if not both. In the cases where both tubal ectopic pregnancies are found to be ruptured and patient is haemodynamically compromised, it may be reasonable to perform a bilateral salpingectomy as a lifesaving measure. Also, in cases where a woman is already considering an IVF treatment and performing a conservative tubal surgery would increase her risk of further ectopic pregnancy, bilateral salpingectomy can be considered as a treatment of choice provided that this has been discussed with the women. Loo et al. [3] reported the rare occurrence of spontaneous synchronous bilateral ectopic pregnancy in a haemodynamically unstable patient needing bilateral salpingectomy. Martinez J et al. reported one such case where bilateral salpingectomy was performed, and Marasinghe JP et al. reported a case where the patient needed emergency laparotomy in view of ruptured ectopic pregnancy.

However, in majority of the cases, it is either both ectopic pregnancies are unruptured or there is a unilateral ruptured ectopic pregnancy. Stamatellos I.et al. described a case of unrecognised bilateral ampullary ectopic pregnancy, and bilateral salpingostomy was performed for this. Eze JN et al. reported a case of spontaneous bilateral ectopic pregnancy with one ruptured and one unruptured ectopic pregnancy needing both salpingectomy and salpingostomy.

Conservative management poses further dilemma between performing a salpingostomy and opting for a medical management with methotrexate postoperatively. In haemodynamically stable patients with unruptured tubal pregnancy, systemic methotrexate and laparoscopic salpingostomy are both successful in treating the majority of cases, and there is no significant difference between the treatments in the homolateral patency rate. (Dr PJ Hajenius et al.).

Salpingostomy is a conservative tubal surgery, but it carries the risks of incomplete evacuation and persistence of gestational tissue post procedure. Moreover, salpingostomy is performed less frequently and consequently in the present system of training most of the clinicians are not trained enough to perform this competently, especially so in an emergency situation. This also re-emphasises the importance of pre-empting this rare condition so that the surgery could be as planned as possible with appropriate expertise available. Rammah A.M. reported a case of bilateral unruptured ectopic pregnancy following assisted conception technique, and the women had bilateral salpingostomy performed.

There was one report (Marcovici I.et al.) where methotrexate management was opted for bilateral ectopic pregnancy, but it failed and authors questioned the optimal dose of methotrexate to treat bilateral ectopic pregnancy. Methotrexate management postoperatively needs further monitoring of the patient with serial HCG and the risk of needing further surgery persists. However, it gives the clinician an opportunity to discuss treatment options with the women and have an informed consent to proceed with management decisions. While managing such rare but fatal cases, the clinician should carefully consider and weigh the risks and benefits of each of the treatment option in the light of individual patient's condition.

The incidence of simultaneous bilateral ectopic pregnancies is between 1 in 725 and 1 in 1,580 of all extrauterine pregnancies (Rondeau JA et al.) Although spontaneous bilateral ectopic pregnancies have also been reported, these are rare. The majority of such cases happen as a consequence of assisted conception techniques primarily with IVF. Reddy et al. [2] and Shetty JP et al. report cases of spontaneous bilateral ectopic pregnancy highlighting the diagnostic pitfalls and treatment options. Wali AS et al. also describe a similar case with diagnostic challenges and state that occurrence of bilateral ectopic pregnancies is on increase.

With the advent of artificial reproductive techniques, the risk of ectopic pregnancies has increased in the last few years. The risk of developing unilateral ectopic pregnancy following intrauterine insemination with ovarian stimulation is well recognised and is quoted to be between 4 and 8 % in literature (Azantee et al. [4] and Chang et al. [5]). However, simultaneous bilateral ectopic pregnancies following IUI is rare, and to our knowledge, there are only very few cases reported. Plotti et al. in [6] reported bilateral ovarian pregnancy after IUI. Shiau et al. in [7] reported a case of severe ovarian hyperstimulation syndrome with simultaneous bilateral tubal pregnancy following intrauterine insemination. Burgos San Cristobal D.J et al. and Woo I et al. each reports similar cases after IUI treatment. Khong et al. [8] and Mathew et al. [9] reported such cases after clomiphene ovulation induction.

Majority of bilateral ectopic pregnancies are reported after ART treatments like IVF and ICSI (intra cytoplasmic sperm injection). Bustos Lopez HH et al. reported two such cases and stated that attempts should be made to diagnose these rare conditions preoperatively using available noninvasive methods. Campo s et al. report a case of bilateral ectopic pregnancies after IVF treatment. These were the only two cases where a preoperative diagnosis of bilateral ectopic pregnancy was made based on transvaginal scan report. Sergent F et al., through their case report, have attempted to explain the reasons for an increase in rate of bilateral ectopic pregnancies in recent years and highlights the importance of thorough pelvic examination at the time of laparoscopy to avoid missing such rare condition. Klipstein S et al. and Reyad R.M. et al. report similar cases after IVF and ICSI treatment, respectively.

In summary, once bilateral ectopic pregnancies have been diagnosed, the management options include the following:

(a) Bilateral salpingectomy
(b) Salpingostomy and salpingectomy
(c) Salpingectomy and methotrexate management
(d) Bilateral salpingostomy
(e) Methotrexate management only

Therefore, the management option has chosen needs to be tailored to the needs of the patient, patient's preferences and the clinical picture, preferably after a detailed discussion with the patient.

Conclusion

Bilateral ectopic pregnancies occurring spontaneously or following assisted conception techniques, although rare, present the clinician with diagnostic uncertainty and management dilemmas. Available literature review suggests that most clinicians opt for a more conservative approach with salpingostomy if the ectopic pregnancy is unruptured, whereas the decision to perform bilateral salpingectomy is noted more in cases where patient is haemodynamically compromised with unilateral or bilateral ruptured ectopic pregnancies. Maintaining a high index of suspicion and examination of the contralateral tube carefully during the laparoscopy is imperative, as it can significantly influence management decisions that can have a long-term influence on the patient's fertility.

Conflict of interest Arpita Ghosh, Daniel Borlase, Tosin Ajala, Anthony James Kelly and Zaky Ibrahim declare that they have no conflict of interest.

Informed consent taken from both patients discussed above This article does not contain any studies with human or animal subjects performed by the any of the authors.

References

1. Rondeau JA, Hibbert ML, Nelson KM (1997). Combined tubal and cornual pregnancy in a patient without risk factors. A case report. J Reprod Med 42(10):675–677
2. Reddy AP, Chowdhary S, Saxena RK, Venkatesh S, Pandey P (2012) Spontaneous bilateral ectopic pregnancy. BJOG: Int J Obstet Gynaecol 119(151):1470–0328
3. Loo CY, Ng S, Rouse AM (2012) Spontaneous synchronous bilateral tubal ectopic pregnancy: a tale of caution. BJOG: Int J Obstet Gynaecol 119:217–218, 1470-0328
4. Azantee YW, Murad ZA, Roszaman R, Hayati MY, Norsina MA (2011) Associated factors affecting the successful pregnancy rate of intrauterine insemination at International Islamic University Malaysia (IIUM) Fertility Centre. Med J Malaysia 66(3):195–198
5. Chang MY, Huang HY, Lee CL, Lai YM, Chang SY, Soong YK (1993) Treatment of infertility using controlled ovarian hyperstimulation with intrauterine insemination: the experience of 343 cases. J Formos Med Assoc 92(4):341–348
6. Plotti F, Di Giovanni A, Oliva C, Battaglia F, Plotti G (2008) Bilateral ovarian pregnancy after intrauterine insemination and controlled ovarian stimulation. Fertil Steril 90(5):2015.e3–5
7. Shiau CS, Chang MY, Chiang CH, Hsieh CC, Hsieh TT (2004) Severe ovarian hyperstimulation syndrome coexisting with a bilateral ectopic pregnancy. Chang Gung Med J 27(2):143–147
8. Khong SY, Dimitry ED (2005) Bilateral tubal ectopic pregnancy after clomiphene induction. J Obstet Gynaecol 25(6):611–612
9. Mathew M, Saquib S, Krolikowski A (2004) Simultaneous bilateral tubal pregnancy after ovulation induction with clomiphene citrate. Saudi Med J 25(12):2058–2059

Further Reading

10. Aziz S, Al Wafi B, Al Swadi H (2011) Frequency of ectopic pregnancy in a medical centre, Kingdom of Saudi Arabia. J Pak Med Assoc 61(3):221–224
11. Martínez-Varea A, Hidalgo-Mora JJ, Payá V, Morcillo I, Martín E, Pellicer A (2011) Retroperitoneal ectopic pregnancy after intrauterine insemination. Fertil Steril 95(7):2433.e1–3
12. Bugatto F, Quintero-Prado R, Kirk-Grohar J, Melero-Jiménez V, Hervías-Vivancos B, Bartha JL (2010) Heterotopic triplets: tubal ectopic and twin intrauterine pregnancy. A review of obstetric outcomes with a case report. Arch Gynecol Obstet 282(6):601–606
13. Svirsky R, Maymon R, Vaknin Z, Mendlovic S, Weissman A, Halperin R, Herman A, Pansky M (2010) Twin tubal pregnancy: a rising complication? Fertil Steril 94(5):1910.e13–6
14. Ibrahim AG, Badawi F, Tahlak M (2009) Heterotopic pregnancy: a growing diagnostic challenge. BMJ Case Rep
15. Zadehmodarres S, Oladi B, Saeedi S, Jahed F, Ashraf H (2009) Intrauterine insemination with husband semen: an evaluation of pregnancy rate and factors affecting outcome. J Assist Reprod Genet 26(1):7–11
16. Childs AJ, Royek AB, Leigh TB, Gallup PG (2005) Triplet heterotopic pregnancy after gonadotropin stimulation and intrauterine insemination diagnosed at laparoscopy: a case report. South Med J 98(8):833–835
17. Chueh HY, Cheng PJ, Wang CW, Soong YK (2002) Inadvertent superovulation and intrauterine insemination during pregnancy: a lesson from an ectopic gestation. J Assist Reprod Genet 19(2):87–89
18. Berliner I, Mesbah M, Zalud I, Maulik D (1998) Report of a case with successful twin intrauterine gestation. J Reprod Med 43(3):237–239
19. Bontis J, Grimbizis G, Tarlatzis BC, Miliaras D, Bili H (1997) Intrafollicular ovarian pregnancy after ovulation induction/ intrauterine insemination: pathophysiological aspects and diagnostic problems. Hum Reprod 12(2):376–378
20. Kably Ambe A, Garza Rios P, Serviere Zaragoza C, Delgado Urdapilleta J (1992) [Heterotopic pregnancy in intrauterine insemination. Presentation of a case]. [Article in Spanish]. Ginecol Obstet Mex 60:110–111
21. Marcovici I, Scoccia B (1997) Spontaneous bilateral tubal ectopic pregnancy and failed methotrexate therapy: a case report. Am J Obstet Gynecol 177/6(1545-1546):0002–9378
22. Bustos Lopez HH, Rojas-Poceros G, Barron Vallejo J, Cintora Zamudio S, Kably Ambe A, Valle RF (1998) Conservative laparoscopic treatment of bilateral ectopic pregnancy. 2 case reports and review of the literature. [Spanish] Tratamiento laparoscopico conservador del embarazo ectopico bilateral. Informe de dos casos y revision de la literatura. Ginecol Obstet Mex 66(13-7):0300–9041, 0300-9041
23. Klipstein S, Oskowitz SP (2000) Bilateral ectopic pregnancy after transfer of two embryos. Fertil Steril 74/5(887-8):0015–0282, 0015-0282
24. Reyad RM, Aboulghar MA, Serour GI, Mansour RT, Amin YM, Momtaz M, Youssry I (1998) Bilateral ectopic pregnancy with an intact intrauterine pregnancy following an ICSI procedure. Middle East Fertil Soc J 3/1:1110–5690
25. Sergent F, Verspyck E, Marpeau L (2003) Management of ectopic pregnancies complicating in vitro fertilization: a remarkable case of bilateral ectopic pregnancy with independent courses of the pregnancies. [French] Prise en charge des grossesses extra-uterines apres fecondation in vitro: a propos d'un cas remarquable d'une grossesse extra-uterine bilaterale dont chacune des grossesses a evolue independamment. J Gynecol Obstet Biol Reprod 32/3 Pt 1(256-60):0368–2315, 0150-9918
26. Stamatellos I, Anagnostou E, Stamatopoulos P, Bontis I (2006) Unrecognized spontaneous bilateral ampullary pregnancy treated by laparoscopy. Gynecol Surg 3/3(218-219):1613–2076, 1613-2084

27. Burgos San Cristobal DJ, Agirregoikoa JA, Albisu M, Mieza J, Corcostegui B, Prieto B, Ramon O, Matorras R (2004) Simultaneous bilateral ectopic pregnancy after IUI [Spanish] Embarazo ectopico bilateral simultaneo tras IAC. Rev Iberoam Fertilidad Reproduccion Humana 21/5(349-353):1132–0249
28. Altinkaya SO, Ozat M, Pektas MK, Gungor T, Mollamahmutoglu L (2008) Simultaneous bilateral tubal pregnancy after in vitro fertilization and embryo transfer. Taiwan J Obstet Gynecol 47/3(338-40): 1028–4559, 1875-6263
29. Issat T, Grzybowski W, Jakimiuk AJ (2009) Bilateral ectopic tubal pregnancy, following in vitro fertilisation (IVF). Folia Histochem Cytobiol 47/5(S147-8):0239–8508, 1897-5631
30. Marasinghe JP, Condous G, Amarasinghe WI (2009) Spontaneous bilateral tubal ectopic pregnancy. Ceylon Med J 54/1(21-2):0009–0875, 0009-0875
31. Martinez J, Cabistany AC, Gonzalez M, Gil O, Farrer M, Romero JA (2009) Bilateral simultaneous ectopic pregnancy. South Med J 102/10(1055-7):0038–4348, 1541-8243
32. Shetty JP, Shetty B, Makkanavar JH, Chandrika (2011) A rare case of bilateral tubal pregnancy. J Indian Med Assoc 109/7(506-7):0019–5847, 0019-5847
33. Wali AS, Khan RS, Jcpsp NO (2012) Spontaneous bilateral tubal pregnancy. J Coll Physicians Surg Pak 22/2(118-9):1022–386X, 1681-7168
34. Woo I, Christianson M, Swelstad B, Yates M, Garcia J (2012) Bilateral ovarian ectopic pregnancies following intrauterine insemination after unsuccessful oocyte retrieval. Fertil Steril 97/3 SUPPL. 1(S31), 0015-0282
35. Rammah AM, Al Hijji JY, Amen AM, Chibber R, Ali SA (2012) Bilateral tubal ectopic pregnancy case presentation and review of literature. Int J Gynecol Obstet 119(S707-S708):0020–7292
36. Eze JN, Obuna JA, Ejikeme BN (2012) Bilateral tubal ectopic pregnancies: a report of two cases. Ann Afr Med 11/2(112-5): 0975–5764, 0975-5764
37. Hajenius PJ, Engelsbel S, Mol BWJ, van der Veen F, Ankum WM, Bossuyt PMM, Hemrika DJ, Lammes FB (1997) Randomised trial of systemic methotrexate versus laparoscopic salpingostomy in tubal pregnancy. Lancet 350(9080):774–779. doi:10.1016/S0140-6736(97)05487-1
38. Gazvani MR, Baruah DN, Alfirevic Z, Emery SJ (1998) Mifepristone in combination with methotrexate for the medical treatment of tubal pregnancy: a randomized, controlled trial. Hum Reprod 13(7):1987–1990. doi:10.1093/humrep/13.7.1987

28

NovaSure endometrial ablation

Patrick Campbell · Caitriona Monaghan · Michael Parker

Abstract The objective of this study is to review outcomes and factors predictive of patient satisfaction following NovaSure endometrial ablation in the treatment of menorrhagia. NovaSure endometrial ablation has been established as a safe and effective treatment for menorrhagia. The setting of a hospital that is the biggest user of NovaSure in Ireland, coupled with a stable population, provided a unique opportunity to obtain accurate long-term follow-up data on the largest sample size reported to date. This is a retrospective observational study of 400 women who attended for NovaSure endometrial ablation between December 2006 and December 2009. Information was collected from patient charts and followed up with postal and telephone questionnaires. Statistical analysis was performed using SPSS version 18. The mean age and parity of patients were 44 years and 2.84, respectively. Three hundred and sixty-eight patients underwent the procedure, with an average treatment time of 88 seconds. Eighty-seven percent of patients were satisfied with the procedure, with 59% achieving amenorrhoea. Subsequent hysterectomy was performed in 7.6%. The complication rate was 14% (32 abandoned procedures and 23 in-patient admissions following the procedure).

There were no uterine perforations. Women with longer uterine cavities were less likely to be satisfied with the procedure (p=0.045). Satisfaction rate at 1-year follow-up was 95%. NovaSure endometrial ablation is a highly effective treatment for menorrhagia. We recommend outpatient follow-up of women with longer cavities as further treatment may be necessary.

P. Campbell (✉) · C. Monaghan · M. Parker
Obstetrics & Gynaecology, Altnagelvin Area Hospital,
Londonderry, Northern Ireland, UK
e-mail: patrickcampbell@doctors.org.uk

Keywords NovaSure · Endometrial ablation

Introduction

One in 20 women aged 30–49 years in the UK consults her GP with menorrhagia each year [1]. NovaSure impedance control system has been established as a safe and effective second-generation technique for the treatment of this condition. [2–4] Five-year follow-up studies have reported amenorrhoea rates of 48–75% [3, 4]. The most commonly reported outcome measures in the current literature are amenorrhoea and hysterectomy rates, with a prospective follow-up of 200 cases representing the largest sample size [5]. Our study of 400 patients represents the largest sample size reported.

Most studies reporting outcomes following NovaSure have had strict inclusion criteria resulting in a selected group of women with normal-sized uterine cavities [2, 6, 7]. We hypothesised that NovaSure may be less effective when treating women with larger uterine cavities. We decided to assess this by examining whether patient satisfaction could be predicted on the basis of uterine cavity length.

NovaSure is primarily performed as a day-case procedure. It is therefore important to be aware of the rate of post-operative in-patient admission. We aimed to assess the number of post-operative admissions, and their indications, in our hospital.

Methods

A retrospective observational study was performed on women who underwent NovaSure endometrial ablation between December 2006 and December 2009 at a district general hospital in Northern Ireland. Inclusion criteria were simply any woman who was admitted for the procedure during the specified time period. No pre-treatment was given, and there were no exclusion criteria. The standard NovaSure technique was performed under general anaesthesia, as previously reported in the literature [5, 8, 9].

Four hundred patients were identified from theatre logbooks and their charts reviewed. A proforma was used to collect demographic data and procedural data (cavity measurements, time taken and power of the procedure). Cavity length was measured with a uterine sound; cornual width and power were calculated by the NovaSure device. Minor operative complications were classified as failure to complete the procedure or post-operative admission. Major complication was defined as uterine perforation. Outcome measures were amenorrhoea rate and patient satisfaction with the treatment ('yes' or 'no'). The rate of subsequent hysterectomy was determined for patients not satisfied. The post-operative histological data for these patients were examined. Follow-up information was obtained from gynaecology outpatient clinic letters. Those patients not reviewed at clinic were followed up by postal and telephone surveys.

Statistical analysis was performed with SPSS version 18. An independent-samples *t* test was conducted to compare uterine length with patient satisfaction ('yes' or 'no'), and Levene's test confirmed equal variances. Following this statistical test, we subsequently assessed satisfaction rates in women with uterine cavities measuring less than 5 cm, 5 to 6 cm and greater than 6 cm.

Results

Four hundred women were included in the study. Thirty-two procedures (8%) were not completed. Data were analysed on the remaining 368 patients. There were no missing data.

The mean age and parity were 44 years (range, 29–58 years) and 2.84 (range, 0–7), respectively. Cavity length ranged from 3.5 to 9.5 cm (mean 5.6 cm), and cornual width ranged from 2.5 to 5.2 cm (mean 4.1 cm). The mean time to complete the procedure was 88 s (range, 37 to 120 s).

The majority of the abandoned cases (28/32) were due to patient factors such as a uterine cavity that was too large or too small. Other rare causes included a sub-septate uterus, cervical stenosis and a lax cervix. The remaining four abandoned cases were due to mechanical failure of the NovaSure device. Hysteroscopy was performed in 16/32 cases with no confirmed uterine perforations. During the same operative session, thermal balloon ablation was performed in 11 cases and one patient had a Mirena coil inserted. Subsequent hysterectomy was performed in 13 patients. Of the remaining patients, five had no further treatment and two patients underwent successful repeat NovaSure endometrial ablation at a later date.

Three hundred and twenty-one women (87%) were satisfied with the procedure, and the overall amenorrhoea rate was 59% (217/368 cases). Of the 47 women not satisfied with the procedure, subsequent hysterectomy was performed in 28 cases—22 for menorrhagia and 6 for dysmenorrhoea—giving a total hysterectomy rate of 7.6%. Post-operative histological data were available on 21 of the 28 patients revealing ten cases of benign leiomyomas, two cases of adenomyosis, two benign endometrial polyps and one case of FIGO stage 1A endometrial carcinoma. The remaining six women had normal uteri (Fig. 1).

Twenty-three patients (6%) required post-operative in-patient admission from the day-case unit following the procedure. The most common indications for admission were pain (11 cases) and nausea (6 cases). Other indications were hypotension, dizziness and vasovagal episodes. Of the 368 women in whom the procedure was completed, there were no major intra-operative or post-operative complications. The overall complication rate, including failure to complete the procedure and requirement for post-operative admission, was 14% (55/400 cases).

Follow-up information was obtained from 172 patients reviewed at the gynaecology outpatient clinic. A postal questionnaire was delivered to the remaining 196 patients of whom 100 responded (59% response rate). The remaining patients were contacted by telephone. Follow-up data, which ranged from 4 months to 3 years, were available in 100% of cases. Long-term follow-up data (>1 year) were available mainly from those women who responded to the postal and telephone surveys. In this group, the satisfaction rate was 95% (135/142 women) at 1 year following the procedure and 91% (59/65 women) at 2 years (Fig. 2).

There was a statistically significant difference when uterine length was compared with patient satisfaction ($p = 0.045$) indicating that women with longer uterine cavities were more likely to be unsatisfied with the procedure. Further analysis revealed women with cavities less than 5 cm (147 patients) were satisfied in 91% of cases. Women with cavities measuring 5–6 cm (114 patients) had a satisfaction rate of 86%, and those with cavities greater than 6 cm (107 patients) were satisfied in 83% of cases.

Discussion

Many studies have published convincing evidence to confirm the safety and efficacy of NovaSure endometrial

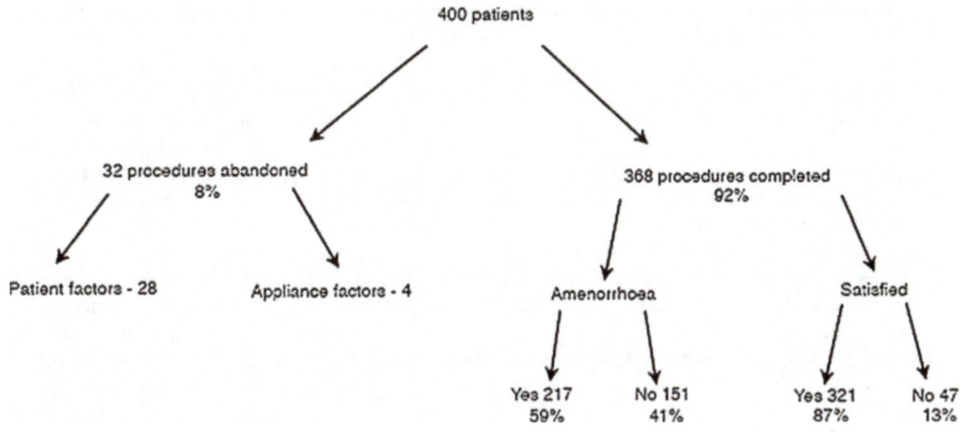

Fig. 1 Flow diagram summarising patient outcomes following NovaSure endometrial ablation

ablation in the treatment of menorrhagia. A recent survey reported that less than 10% of gynaecologists in the UK use the NovaSure device as their first choice endometrial ablative technique [10]. We were fortunate to be based in a Hospital where all seven consultants use NovaSure as their first choice endometrial ablative technique. In fact, our Hospital is the largest user of NovaSure in Ireland. This permitted a review of a large sample size over a relatively short time period. Follow-up data were achievable on all patients (100%), given that the local population is stable with minimal migration. Long-term follow-up greater than 1 year following the procedure was available in 56% of cases. Our results represent the largest sample size reported to date. Our findings of 59% amenorrhoea, 87% satisfaction and 7.6% hysterectomy rate are comparable with previous studies [4, 5, 8], suggesting that our sample is likely to be representative.

The overall complication rate of 14% was due to failure to complete the procedure (32 cases) or post-operative admission for symptom control (23 cases). There were no major complications such as uterine perforation. These findings are similar to those published by Cooper et al. [11] who reported a 13% complication rate with no perforations. Bongers et al. [6] reported no complications. It is possible that such a low complication rate in this study was the result of excluding abandoned procedures as complications and the use of strict inclusion criteria to ensure normal cavities. Given the retrospective nature of our study, we cannot confirm that patients underwent ultrasound assessment prior to treatment with NovaSure.

Statistical analysis revealed an inverse relationship between cavity length and overall patient satisfaction ($p = 0.045$). Further analysis revealed women with cavities less than 5 cm were satisfied in 91% of cases and those women with cavities measuring 5–6 cm and greater than 6 cm had satisfaction rates of 86% and 83%, respectively. These findings are supported by a recent study that reported an association between amenorrhoea and a total uterine length of less than 9 cm [12]. We propose that assessment of cavity length at the time of the procedure could be used as a measure of identifying those patients who are less likely to be satisfied. We recommend that patients with longer cavities may benefit from a post-operative review, as further treatment may be necessary.

We found that 6% of our patients required post-operative in-patient admission following the procedure. We considered that the administration of general anaesthesia might have accounted for many of the indications for admission, such as nausea, hypotension and vasovagal episodes. The recent advances in performing NovaSure under local anaesthesia [13], however, have comparable rates of post-operative in-patient admission (7%) [14].

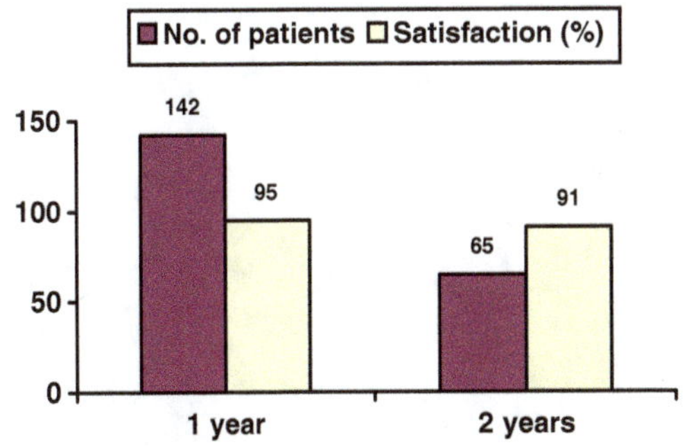

Fig. 2 Long-term follow-up of satisfaction rates following NovaSure endometrial ablation

Conclusion

This study highlights the effectiveness of NovaSure in the 'real life' setting of a district general hospital rather than a highly selected study population group. The results of our study reaffirm the place of NovaSure as a safe and effective treatment modality for women with menorrhagia.

Declaration of interest The authors report no conflicts of interest. The authors alone are responsible for the content and writing of the paper.

References

1. National Evidence Based Clinical Guidelines (2007) Heavy menstrual bleeding. Issue no. 4. Available at http://guidance.nice.org.uk/CG44. Accessed 1 Sept 2010
2. Gallinat A, Nugent W (2002) NovaSure impedence-controlled system for endometrial ablation. J Am Assoc Gynaecol Laparosc 9:283–289
3. Gallinat A (2007) An impedance-controlled system for endometrial ablation: Five year follow up of 107 patients. J Reprod Med 52:467–472
4. Kleijn J, Engels R, Bourdrez P, Mol B, Bongers M (2008) Five-year follow up of a randomised controlled trial comparing NovaSure and ThermaChoice endometrial ablation. BJOG 115 (2):193–198
5. Baskett T, Clough H, Scott T (2005) NovaSure bipolar radio-frequency endometrial ablation: report of 200 cases. J Obstet Gynaecol Can 27(5):473–476
6. Bongers M, Bourdrez P, Mol B, Heintz P, Brolmann H (2004) Randomised controlled trial of bipolar radio-frequency endometrial ablation and balloon endometrial ablation. BJOG 111:1095–1102
7. Fulop T, Rakoczi I, Barna I (2007) NovaSure impedance controlled endometrial ablation: long-term follow-up results. J Minim Invasive Gynaecol 14:85–90
8. Bongers M (2007) Second-generation endometrial ablation treatment: NovaSure. Best Pract Res Cl Ob 21(6):989–994
9. Gallinat A (2004) NovaSure impedance controlled system for endometrial ablation: Three-year follow-up on 107 patients. Am J Obstet Gynaecol 191:1585–1589
10. Deb S, Flora K, Atiomo W (2008) A survey of preferences and practices of endometrial ablation/resection for menorrhagia in the United Kingdom. Fertil Steril 90(5):1812–1817
11. Cooper J, Gimpelson R, Phillip L, Galen D (2002) A randomised multi-centre trial of safety and efficacy of the NovaSure system in the treatment of menorrhagia. J Am Assoc Gynaecol Laparosc 9:418–429
12. El-Nashar S, Hopkins M, Creedon D et al (2009) Prediction of treatment outcomes after global endometrial ablation. Obstet Gynecol 113:97–106
13. Penninx J, Mol B, Bongers M (2009) Endometrial ablation with paracervical block. J Reprod Med 54(10):617–620
14. Kalkat R, Cartmill R (2011) NovaSure endometrial ablation under local anaesthesia in an outpatient setting: an observational study. J Obstet Gynaecol 31(2):152–155

29

Surgical treatment of rectovaginal endometriosis with rectal involvement

**Vicente Payá · Juan José Hidalgo-Mora ·
Cesar Diaz-Garcia · Antonio Pellicer**

Abstract Rectovaginal endometriosis (RVE) is one of the most serious and incapacitating forms of presentation of this disease. Traditionally, medical treatment has not been considered effective for the majority of patients, being surgery the only reasonable and therapeutic choice in these cases. This exposes patients to a potentially serious morbidity, thus a careful evaluation should be done by a surgical board considering the impact of the disease as well as the quality of life of the patients. The main surgical techniques used are the shaving of the rectal wall affected by the endometriosic implants, the discoid excision of the front rectal wall, and the segmental intestinal resection, and there is no consensus concerning which is the most effective and suitable between them.

The bibliography published in the last 10 years relating to the surgical treatment of RVE is being reviewed with the intention of updating the knowledge base about the topic and looking for common ground between different studies, allowing us to come closer to reaching a consensus about treatment for this pathology.

Keywords Deep endometriosis · Deeply infiltrating endometriosis · Laparoscopy · Rectovaginal endometriosis · Surgery · Surgical management

V. Payá · J. J. Hidalgo-Mora (✉) · C. Diaz-Garcia · A. Pellicer
Department of Gynecology and Human Reproduction,
La Fe University Hospital,
Bulevar Sur,
46026 Valencia, Spain
e-mail: hidalmo@yahoo.es

Introduction

Endometriosis is a chronic illness defined by the presence of functional endometrial tissue outside of the uterus. It affects 6–10% of women of reproductive age, 50–60% of women and adolescents with pelvic pain, and up to 50% of infertile women [1, 2]. It is one of the pathologies that cause a large effect on the quality of life of young women, entailing a large social and economic impact on them and on the health care system [3].

Deep endometriosis is an aggressive form of endometriosis infiltrating more than 5 mm under the peritoneum. This term usually includes infiltrative forms involving structures such as bowel, ureters, bladder, and rectovaginal wall. Intestinal involvement occurs up to 12% of women with endometriosis, being its most common sites the rectosigmoid (65%), the ileocecal (20%) junctions, and the rectum (15%) [4, 5]. Rectovaginal endometriosis (RVE) is characterized by its effect on the vagina, rectum, rectovaginal septum, Douglas pouch, and sometimes even the ureters [6–8]. The rectum is affected on its anterior wall and rarely the whole thickness of the intestinal wall [9].

Clinically, although it involves a benign process, RVE can alter the quality of life for patients due to dysmenorrhea, dyspareunia, limitation of sexual activity, and the severe dyschezia that are provoked [10]. Pharmacological treatment is not very effective for the majority of patients. Surgery is the best therapeutic option for symptomatic RVE, even though it implies a greater morbidity. Laparoscopy is the chosen approach [11–16].

The preoperative diagnosis for RVE is crucial in order to establish the precise distribution of the deeply infiltrating endometriotic lesions, which is the most relevant tool to help the surgeon decide how to treat these patients.

Distinguishing retrocervical and rectovaginal involvement and the depth of lesions are important in the surgical management of patients. Clinical history, vaginal and rectal pelvic examination, transvaginal and transrectal ultrasounds, magnetic resonance imaging (MRI) and double-contrast barium enemas have been used for this purpose. Nevertheless, physical examination does not allow prediction of the extension of RVE, and the value of transvaginal sonography for assessment deep pelvic endometriosis is uncertain. Rectal endoscopic sonography has been recommended for detection of endometriosis in rectal, rectovaginal, uterosacral, or rectosigmoid locations, and MRI has demonstrated high sensitivity, specificity, positive and negative predictive values, and accuracy in prediction of the locations and in evaluation of the extension of lesions. The gold standard examination for classification of endometriosis is laparoscopy, and the diagnosis is confirmed by the histology obtained by laparoscopy or laparotomy or by the biopsy of visible endometriosic lesions in the posterior fornix [17–21]. The preoperative study should be done with an ultrasound of the urinary and kidney tracts, an intravenous pyelography to rule out an asymptomatic ureteral stenosis, and a rectosigmoidscopy to confirm the involvement of the rectal mucosa.

Several techniques have been proposed for the treatment of RVE with rectal involvement, with no consensus existing on which could be the best when the muscular rectal layer is affected [22]. In these cases, different surgical procedures have been described in terms of parameters, such as the size of the nodule and the affected bowel circumference, the depth of lesions on the rectal wall, the presence of other endometriosic foci, and the experience of the surgeon in the execution of each procedure [23, 24]. The most common surgical procedures used in the treatment of RVE are superficial thickness excision (shaving), the resection of the nodule with excision of the anterior side of the rectum (full thickness discoid resection) and the colorectal segmental resection.

At present, some gynecological surgeons prefer colorectal resection for symptomatic patients, as they are convinced that resection of all intestinal endometriosic foci is the choice of treatment to improve pain and to avoid relapses [5, 13, 25–27]. On the other hand, other groups prefer the excision of the endometriosic nodule to colorectal resection, since the rate of morbidity is lower and the recurrence of pain is similar [3, 28–30].

Until now, there has not been a randomized study that compares the different techniques, and few review articles have been published in relation to surgical treatment of RVE. If we add to this the great variety of results from observational studies and the lack of clinical trials, a review of the medical literature published on this topic over the last 10 years is valuable. The main objective of our paper is to assess, standardize, and analyze the data and results obtained in different studies regarding the surgical techniques employed in the treatment of RVE with rectal involvement.

Methods

The review of medical literature was done through an electronic search for articles in the databases of the US National Library of Medicine (PubMed database) and the Cochrane Library (Cochrane database). Its objective was to identify all of the observational studies, clinical trials, systematic and nonsystematic reviews, and meta-analysis published in English between January of 2000 and June of 2010 regarding the surgical treatment of endometriosis of the rectovaginal septum. The medical terms combined in the search included RVE, deep endometriosis, deeply infiltrating endometriosis, surgical management, surgical treatment, surgery, and laparoscopy. The complete text was obtained for all the selected articles and the list of bibliographic references for each one was reviewed with the aim of identifying other studies that could also be included in our review. Summaries of congress communications and scientific meetings were not included in the selected literature.

Articles in press whose text and complete results were available at the time of our search were included. To be selected, the studies needed to have a series of characteristics that were considered inclusion criteria: Patients must be diagnosed with RVE by means of physical examination, vaginal or transrectal ultrasound, MRI, and biopsy with histological confirmation; analysis of the results of one or more surgical techniques performed as treatment for RVE must be performed. The initial selection of the papers was done independently by two authors (VP and JJH) in terms of the title and abstract. In cases of discrepancy between the two authors, the decision to include or exclude the article was made by a third author (AP).

The year of publication, the type and design of the study, the number of patients, the surgical technique analyzed, and the primary and secondary results were taken from the selected papers. The studies were classified by their methodological design in observational studies, clinical trials, systematic and nonsystematic reviews, and meta-analysis. The two reviewers independently evaluated all the articles and produced a summary of each one according to a previously established format. The summaries were compiled into a single summary for each selected paper, reaching agreement by consensus in case of discrepancies.

This paper was not conceived as a systematic revision of the literature following QUOROM norms [31] since the different procedures described in the studies make it difficult to draw a direct comparison of the results. Moreover, the different papers do not provide results of the complications in detail or favorable effects of the surgery in terms of each technique. Therefore, we did not perform a qualitative analysis of the selected studies or a grouped analysis of the data obtained from them.

Forty one potentially relevant studies were identified. Of them, 36 corresponded to observational studies and five to nonsystematic revisions. No systematic revisions, clinical trials, or meta-analyses were identified.

Findings

The great heterogeneity of the studies in relation to the surgical treatment of RVE proves the difficulty of standardizing data collected and establishing general conclusions regarding the results. All of the analyzed studies are non-comparative observational studies with a limited number of patients. There were also five nonsystematic revisions published [3, 28, 32–34]. In some of the studies, a radical treatment was assessed [5, 13, 15, 25–27, 40–56], while others assessed a conservative one [57–63]. There were six nonrandomized papers in which groups of patients with different therapeutic options were compared [30, 35–39]. The follow-up time was not uniform within studies, neither were the criteria used to establish the diagnosis, the extent of the RVE, or the result variables.

In relation to the type of surgical approach, two main groups can be observed: those who propose a more aggressive approach and tend to defend the systematic intestinal resection under the premise that a more radical approach would be more effective (segmental resection of the rectum and/or sigmoid colon) and those that argue for a more conservative approach basing their argument on the lack of scientific evidence of better results with more radical techniques and the association of these techniques with higher long-term morbidity and a lower quality of life for patients (shaving of the rectal wall, disc excision of the anterior rectal wall).

In this review, the studies are grouped according to the surgical approach evaluated: a radical approach, a conservative approach, or a comparative approach between different treatment methods.

Radical surgery with intestinal resection

Surgery for endometriosis of the rectovaginal septum was described for the first time in 1991 by Reich et al. [64]. Initially, the majority of papers defended a conservative surgical approach directed toward the extirpation or ablation of the endometriosic lesions with minimal excisional surgery of the rectum [6, 12, 65–68]. However, in the last decade, multiple authors have proposed more aggressive techniques including intestinal resection, especially in those cases with an affected muscularis propia of the rectum but also in those having an intact mucosa [5, 13, 15, 25–27, 40–56]. The argument used for the practice of this radical surgery is that of achieving the greatest resection possible of the endometriosic lesions, diminishing the postoperative symptomatology and avoiding any early relapse of the disease [41, 42].

Most of the studies summarized in our review consider complications, symptomatic improvement (dysmenorrhea, dyspareunia, chronic pelvic pain, and dyschezia), rate of recurrence, and postoperative indices of gestation as main outcomes. The results of these studies are shown in Table 1.

The largest casuistry of colorectal resections by laparoscopy with 436 cases was published this year by the group in Verona [56]. In this long series, the rate of complications in the immediate postoperative period was 10.7%, with 3.2% being rectovaginal fistulas. In the later postoperative period, 9.5% of patients showed urinary retention and 4.2% constipation. The same authors published a previous report in 2009. In this publication, 357 cases were followed up for 20 months showing a recurrence rate of symptomatology of 6.3% and a recurrence rate of endometriosic nodules in 3.5% of the patients [27]. When they compared these results to those obtained after laparotomic colorectal resection, they found a similar rate of complications [51]. Keckstein and Weisinger [25] found a 7.4% complications rate and Daraï et al. [26] reported a 10% complications rate, with 6% being rectovaginal fistulas. When the laparotomic approach is used, Dousset et al. [5] reported a 16% complications rate, with 4% being rectovaginal fistulas. After 60 months follow-up, there were no relapses, but bladder and intestinal dysfunction reached 16% and 85%, respectively.

In 2006, Landi et al. [20] studied 45 women and compared the results of segmental intestinal resection by laparoscopy in two groups of patients according to whether (n=20) or not (n=25) neural preservation was done. While the surgical complications were not statistically significant between the groups, a difference was noted in favor of the group doing neural preservation in terms of recuperation time for urinary function (3 days compared to 12.5 days) as well as the level of subjective satisfaction among the patients during the follow-up period.

In 2008, Zanetti-Dällenbach et al. [53] compared a new combined technique, vaginal–laparoscopic–abdominal, done on 30 patients compared to the 18 intestinal resections performed using traditional techniques. The authors describe fewer complications in the group using the combined technique (10% vs. 39%) as well as lesser time of hospitalization (13.7 days compared to 15.8 days).

In 2009, Pereira et al. [54] analyzed the postoperative results of 168 women with RVE in which the intervention was conducted by gynecologists, without the initial

Table 1 Results from the main studies with radical surgical techniques on rectovaginal endometriosis

	Number (*n*)	Follow-up (months)	Technique	Complications	Improvement	Fertility	Relapse
Possover et al. [13]	34	16	Laparoscopic colorectal resection	CA: 6.6%		PR: 53% (8/15)	No
Redwine and Wright [40]	84	55	Laparoscopic colorectal resection	ID: 20%	Dysmenorrhoea: 68%, Dyspareunia: 66%, Pelvic pain: 78%	PR: 43% (12/28), SP: 25%, ART: 18%	
Darai et al. [44, 45]	40	24	Laparoscopic colorectal resection	RVF: 7.5%, PA: 2.5%, BD: 17.5%, ID: 37.5%	Dysmenorrhoea: 97%, Dyspareunia: 82%, Pelvic pain: 100%	PR: 45.5% (10/22), SP: 32%, ART: 13%	
Thomassin et al. [43]	27	15	Laparoscopic colorectal resection	BD: 7.5%, ID: 15%	Dysmenorrhoea: 96%, Dyspareunia: 75%, Pelvic pain: 100%, Dyschezia: 95%	SP: 15% (4/27)	
Fleisch et al. [46]	23	45	Laparoscopic/laparotomic colorectal resection	CA: 4%	Global: 91.3%	PR: 23.5% (4/17), SP: 17.5%, ART: 6%	Symptoms: 34.8%
Keckstein and Weisinger [25]	142		Laparoscopic rectal segmentary resection	CA: 6%	Dyspareunia: 87%, Pelvic pain: 96%, Dyschezia: 88%	PR: 50% (47/95)	
Seracchioli et al. [51]	22	42	Laparoscopic colorectal resection	CA: 4.5%, BD: 14%	Dysmenorrhoea: 86%, Dyspareunia: 78%, Pelvic pain: 50%, Dyschezia: 100%		No
Ford et al. [42]	60	12	Laparoscopic (n=48) or laparotomic (n=12) colorectal resection	CA: 3.3%	Global: 86%		Nodules: 13%
Dubernard et al. [47]	58	22	Laparoscopic colorectal resection	RVF: 10.3%, PA: 2%	Dysmenorrhoea: 92%, Dyspareunia: 88%, Pelvic pain: 80%, Dyschezia: 78%		
Minelli et al. [27]	357	20	Laparoscopic colorectal resection	RVF: 3.9%, CA: 3.1%, BD: 9.5%	Global: 93.7%	PR: 41.6% (47/113), SP: 9%, ART: 32.6%	Symptoms: 6.3%, Nodules: 3.5%
Dousset et al. [5]	100	60	Laparotomic subtotal (n=84) or total (n=16) rectal excision	RVF: 4%, CA: 2%, BD: 16%, ID: 85%	Global: 94%		No

RVF Rectovaginal fistula, *CA* complications of the anastomosis, *PA* pelvic abscess, *BD* bladder dysfunction, *ID* intestinal dysfunction, *PR* pregnancy rate, *SP* spontaneous pregnancy, *ART* assisted reproductive techniques participation of colorectal surgeons. In these patients, the interventions included shaving resection, discoid resection, and segmental resection. The results were comparable to the studies in which the intervention of the intestine was done by a colorectal surgeon, with a percentage of global complications of 7.3% and a significant improvement in all the assessed clinical parameters. The authors conclude that, after adequate training, endometriosis with intestinal involvement could be treated safely and efficiently by gynecologists who specialized in pelvic surgery.

The most frequent complication of the radical colorectal surgery is bladder and intestinal dysfunction. The first is defined in the majority of the studies as persistent urinary retention 30 days after the intervention, in the context of the denervation of the inferior hypogastric plexus. In some studies, the proportion of patients affected by this side effect of the surgery reaches 16–17% [5, 45]. Intestinal dysfunction in these patients is defined by the existence of constipation or diarrhea during several weeks after the surgery, due to a mechanical effect by rectal reduction as well as a neural disorder because of the denervation of the rectal plexus. This is the most frequent complication, being 15–20%, although it can reach 85% in some [5, 40, 45, 49, 56].

The second most frequent and very important complication due to its severity is the rectovaginal fistula, which reaches rates of 10% [45, 47]. Other complications that are normally described in these papers are related to alterations of rectal anastomosis and pelvic infectious processes (Table 1).

The indices of symptomatic improvement for patients treated with radical rectovaginal surgery in the majority of the analyzed studies stand around 90% as much in their global form as for each one of the assessed symptoms. This improvement is greater during the first year after the intervention, although it can stay above 70% of the patients after 3 and 5 years, especially for those specific intestinal symptoms such as dyschezia [46, 51].

In some reports, a subjective improvement is shown in the patients' global quality of life with respect to the time prior to the surgery [42, 45, 47, 48, 50]. Dubernard et al. [47] evaluated the quality of life in 58 women after laparoscopic colorectal resection using the validated questionnaire Medical Outcomes Study SF-36 and observed that all its items improved after surgery. Similar results were obtained by Ford et al. [42] in 60 patients following radical resection of RVE and by Lyons et al. [48] in seven patients undergoing laparoscopic colorectal surgery, both using the EQ-5D questionnaire.

Symptomatic recurrence was also analyzed by Fedele et al. [41] after following up 83 patients with RVE during 36 months. Thirty of them underwent laparotomic intestinal resection because of an involvement in the rectal wall. The rate of pain recurrence was 28%, and the necessity for new intervention and/or medical treatment was 27%. The factors which the authors correlated with a lessened probability of recurrence were pregnancy and intestinal resection. On the other hand, the youngest patients and those that had previously been treated for endometriosis showed a greater probability of recurrence. In the rest of the evaluated studies, the rate of relapse for the disease varies, ranging from some showing no reappearance of the disease to those that show 35% 4 years after the intervention [5, 46].

In the studies in which reproductive results were analyzed, a general improvement was noted in their gestation rate after radical surgery [13, 40, 44]. This rate varied between the studies depending on the antecedents of sterility or the wish to gestate, standing around 50% in the majority of the patients. In some studies, no difference has been noted upon comparing the expectant attitude with the surgical technique [36]. Moreover, it is not specified in each series if the gestations were achieved spontaneously or after reproductive assistance treatment, making the interpretation of the results difficult. What does appear uniform between the papers is the conclusion that improvement of reproductive function after surgery for RVE is greater the younger the patient and the earlier the intervention is made [44, 45, 55].

Conservative surgery without intestinal resection

The authors who propose conservative treatment of RVE point out as fundamental that it achieves lower indices of complications and similar rates of symptomatic improvement and preservation of fertility when compared with intestinal resection [68].

The most frequent conservative surgical techniques in the treatment of RVE are those aiming for simple lesional resection after separating the endometriosic nodule from the rectal wall [57], layer-to-layer excision shaving of the lesion without resecting the entire thickness of the intestinal wall [63], and discoidal resection with complete excision of the affected area of the intestinal wall by the endometriosic nodule [35]. In addition, in some papers, the technique proposed was in-block excision of the posterior vaginal fornix in an attempt as much to eliminate the greatest possible part of the disease as to avoid its progression [58, 60, 61]. This same proposal was done by Matsuzaki et al. [62] by studying histological samples from 61 patients after in-block resection for RVE. Every single sample was infiltrated by endometriosic tissue.

The main results of the papers, which assessed the conservative surgery for ERV, are shown in Table 2.

The largest casuistry using a conservative approach (the shaving technique) is that recently published by Donnez and Squifflet [63] with 500 cases. In this study, the rate of serious complications was 3.2%, the rate of relapse was

Table 2 Results from studies done with conservative surgical techniques for rectovaginal endometriosis

	Number (*n*)	Follow-up (months)	Technique	Complications	Improvement	Fertility	Recurrence
Chapron et al. [57]	29	12	Laparoscopic nodular resection	RVF: 3.5%	Dysmenorrhea: 91.7%, Dyspareunia: 100%, Pelvic pain: 93%		
Hollett-Caines et al. [58]	81	96	Laparoscopic shaving and posterior vaginal fornix resection	Fallopian tube abscess: 1.2%	Symptoms: 88%	PR: 57% (26/46), SP: 31%, ART: 26%	
Angioni et al. [60]	31	60	Laparoscopic nodular resection and posterior vaginal fornix resection		Dysmenorrhea: 60%, Dyspareunia: 70%, Pelvic pain: 60%		No relapse after 5 years follow-up
Kristensen and Kjer [61]	48	18	Laparoscopic rectovaginal septum and posterior vaginal fornix resection	Peritonitis: 2%, Bladder perforation: 2%, Vaginal rupture: 2%	Symptoms: 92%, Quality of life improvement: 73%		Nodules: 10%, Symptoms: 9%
Donnez and Squifflet [63]	500	36	Laparoscopic shaving	Rectal Perforation: 1.4%, Ureteral damage: 0.8%, BD: 0.8%		PR: 84% (328/388), SP: 57%, ART: 27%	Symptoms: 7.8%

RVF Rectovaginal fistula, *CA* complications of the anastomosis; *PA* pelvic abscess, *BD* bladder dysfunction, *ID*: intestinal dysfunction, *PR* pregnancy rate, *SP* spontaneous pregnancy, *ART* assisted reproductive techniques

8%, and 84% of women gestated after the intervention, 57% spontaneously. With this technique, there were no functional alterations of the bladder or intestine 1 month after the intervention.

The effectiveness of the discoidal resection technique was put in doubt by Remorgida et al. [59]. A segmental intestinal resection was done systematically after discoidal resection. The histological study of the enlarged piece, a priori free from disease, revealed that. in 7 of the 16 cases (43.8%), endometriosic tissue could still be found infiltrating up to the muscular intestinal layer, with a maximum distance of 2.6 cm from the edge of the nodulectomy, although other studies demonstrate that intestinal resection does not guarantee the complete elimination of endometriosic foci either [69, 70].

The in-block excision techniques of the posterior vaginal fornix are accompanied by resection of the endometriosic nodule and, as what happens with these techniques, there are low rates of complications and high rates of pain improvement [58, 60, 61]. In terms of fertility, the indices of gestation were 57% [58].

Comparative studies

Few studies have been published up until now comparing groups of patients with RVE treated with different therapeutic attitudes. All of them are observational studies in which the treatment option was not decided randomly; rather, it was made in terms of clinical criteria or in consensus with the patients [30, 35–39].

In four of these studies [30, 35, 37, 39], they compared the postoperative results between different techniques used for RVE. Although some of the outcomes and the way they were assessed are not directly comparable between papers, one can see a tendency that points to a similar symptomatic improvement among the different techniques and a greater rate of surgical complications among the most radical approaches.

The results for discoidal resection analyzed in comparative studies (Table 3) show that the rate of severe complications remains low, the symptomatic improvement stands around 90%, and the rate of relapse between 5% and 14% [30, 35, 37, 39]. Gestation rates, though low as they are, are still higher than those obtained with radical treatments [37, 39].

Fanfani et al. [39] compared two groups of symptomatic patients, with nodules smaller than 3 cm and stenosis of the intestinal lumen less than 60%, and observed that the group of 48 patients treated conservatively by laparoscopic discoidal resection showed less postoperative morbidity and similar rates of relapse when compared with the group of 88 patients treated via laparoscopic segmental intestinal resection. In another study, Roman et al. [30] achieved a

Table 3 Results of comparative studies between different surgical techniques for rectovaginal endometriosis

		Mohr et al. [35] (24 months)	Brouwer and Woods [37] (68 months)	Fanfani et al. [39] (32 months)	Roman et al. [30] (26 months)
Shaving	Number (*n*)	100	18		
	Complications	Total: 6%	Total: 17%, PA: 5.6%		
	Improvement	80%			
	Relapse		22.2%		
	Fertility	17%			
Discoidal excision	Number (*n*)	39	58	48	16
	Complications	Total: 23%, RVF: 3%, PA: 5%	Total: 2%, CA: 2%	Total: 31.4%, RVF: 2.1%, PA: 2.1%, ID: 2.1%	ID: 19%
	Improvement	92%		88.8%	86%
	Relapse		5.17%	13.8%	
	Fertility	11%			13%
Segmental intetinal resection	Number (*n*)	48	137	88	25
	Complications	Total: 38%, BD: 2%, CA: 6%	Total: 8%, PA: 1.4%, CA: 2.2%, BD: 1.4%, ID: 9%	Total: 59.7%, RVF: 3.4%, PA: 2.2%, BD: 14.7%, CA: 1.1%, ID: 4.5%	BD: 8%, ID: 64%
	Improvement	92%		93%	83%
	Relapse		2.19%	11.5%	
	Fertility	3%			12%

RVF Rectovaginal fistula, *CA* complications of the anastomosis, *PA* pelvic abscess, *BD* bladder dysfunction, *ID* intestinal dysfunction

lesser rate of urinary and intestinal disorders after discoidal resection even when they did not set up any nodule size limit.

Vercellini et al. [36] compared the effect of conservative nodulectomy through laparotomy and the expectant attitude in 44 and 61 infertile patients with RVE respectively, affirming that this type of surgery does not modify the reproductive outcome compared to the expectant attitude.

Conclusions

Endometriosis generally affects otherwise healthy young women with high expectations of well-being and quality of life. In this population, complications and side effects of surgery are tolerated with difficulty, and the recurrence of symptoms can be especially frustrating. In addition, the case of RVE is a complex pathology with difficult treatment, so that a careful and individualized evaluation in consensus with the patient must be taken into account at the time of choosing any surgical technique so that there is a balance between the expected benefit and the morbidity related to each technique. Surgical treatment of this form of endometriosis is necessary when the disease causes a reduction in the patients' quality of life, given that, in general, patients without symptoms will benefit from an expectant therapeutic attitude.

Laparoscopic treatment of RVE with rectal affectation through discoidal or segmental resection is safe and feasible, achieving similar or better results than laparotomic surgery [16, 27]. When surgical treatment does not include intestinal resection, the rates of surgical complications are low, in the majority of papers not reaching 5%, with bladder and intestinal dysfunction practically nonexistent. This lower morbidity is not accompanied by a greater rate of relapse [39]; therefore, colorectal resections should be reserved for those cases where the nodule is so large that it makes the suture of the intestine technically impossible or when the patient would like to gestate immediately, ruling out prolonged hormonal treatments [30].

Unanimity exists in that the preoperative symptoms as well as the quality of the patients' lives improve significantly in the years after RVE surgery. This improvement stands above 90% of patients, fundamentally with relation to pain symptoms (dysmenorrhoea, dyspareunia, dyschezia, and chronic pelvic pain), with no significant difference between resection surgery and conservative surgery.

Although the studies published to this point to assess the effect of different surgical techniques on the treatment of RVE show a great heterogeneity in their characteristics and methodology, we can say that, whenever technically possible, the more conservative techniques, shaving and discoidal intestinal resection, would be recommended since they present a lower rate of complications with similar recurrence and greater rates of gestation. Nevertheless, it would be worthwhile to develop randomized trials with a greater number of patients with longer-term follow-up to compare the results of intestinal resection and conservative treatment of rectovaginal endometriosis.

Conflicts of interest None.

References

1. Kennedy S, Bergquist A, Chapron C, D'Hooghe T, Dunselman G, Greb R et al (2005) ESHRE guideline for the diagnosis and treatment of endometriosis. Hum Reprod 20:2698–2704
2. Giudice LC (2010) Endometriosis. N Engl J Med 362:2389–2398
3. Vercellini P, Crosignani PG, Abbiati A, Somigliana E, Vigano P, Fedele L (2009) The effect of surgery for symptomatic endometriosis: the other side of the story. Hum Reprod Update 15:177–188
4. Bergqvist A (1993) Different types of extragenital endometriosis: a review. Gynecol Endocrinol 7:207–221
5. Dousset B, Leconte M, MD BB, Millischer AE, Roseau G, Arkwright S, Chapron C (2010) Complete surgery for low rectal endometriosis. Long-term results of a 100-case prospective study. Ann Surg 251:887–895
6. Koninckx PR, Timmermans B, Meuleman C, Penninckx F (1996) Complications of CO2-laser endoscopic excision of deep endometriosis. Hum Reprod 11:2263–2268
7. Martin DC, Batt RE (2001) Retrocervical, rectovaginal pouch, and rectovaginal septum endometriosis. J Am Assoc Gynecol Laparosc 8:12–17
8. Donnez J, Nisolle M, Squifflet J (2002) Ureteral endometriosis: a complication of rectovaginal endometriotic (adenomyotic) nodules. Fertil Steril 77:32–37
9. Chapron C, Fauconnier A, Dubuisson JB, Barakat H, Vieira M, Bréart G (2003) Deep infiltrating endometriosis: relation between severity of dysmenorrhoea and extent of disease. Hum Reprod 18:760–766
10. Vercellini P, Crosignani PG, Somigliana E, Berlanda N, Barbara G, Fedele L (2009) Medical treatment for rectovaginal endometriosis: what is the evidence? Hum Reprod 24:2504–2514
11. Redwine DB, Sharpe DR (1991) Laparoscopic segmental resection of the sigmoid colon for endometriosis. J Laparoendosc Surg 1:217–220
12. Nezhat C, Nezhat F, Pennington E (1992) Laparoscopic treatment of infiltrative rectosigmoid colon and rectovaginal septum endometriosis by the technique of videolaparoscopy and the CO2 laser. Br J Obstet Gynaecol 99:664–667
13. Possover M, Diebolder H, Paul K, Schneider A (2000) Laparoscopically assisted vaginal resection of rectovaginal endometriosis. Obstet Gynecol 96:304–307
14. Duepree HJ, Senagore AJ, Delaney CP, Marcello PW, Brady KM, Falcone T (2002) Laparoscopic resection of deep pelvic endometriosis with rectosigmoid involvement. J Am Coll Surg 195:754–758
15. Landi S, Ceccaroni M, Perutelli A, Allodi C, Barbieri F, Fiaccavento A, Ruffo G, McVeigh E, Zanolla L, Minelli L (2006) Laparoscopic nerve-sparing complete excision of deep endometriosis: is it feasible? Hum Reprod 21:774–781
16. Daraï E, Dubernard G, Coutant C, Frey C, Rouzier R, Ballester M (2010) Randomized trial of laparoscopically assisted versus open colorectal resection for endometriosis: morbidity, symptoms, quality of life, and fertility. Ann Surg 251:1018–1023
17. Fedele L, Bianchi S, Portuese A, Borruto F, Dorta M (1998) Transrectal ultrasonography in the assessment of rectovaginal endometriosis. Obstet Gynecol 91:444–448
18. Goncalves MO, Podgaec S, Dias JA Jr, Gonzalez M, Abrao MS (2010) Transvaginal ultrasonography with bowel preparation is able to predict the number of lesions and rectosigmoid layers affected in cases of deep endometriosis, defining surgical strategy. Hum Reprod 25:665–671
19. Kinkel K, Chapron C, Balleyguier C, Fritel X, Dubuisson JB, Moreau JF (1999) Magnetic resonante imaging characteristics of deep endometriosis. Hum Reprod 14:1080–1086
20. Landi S, Barbieri F, Fiaccavento A, Mainardi P, Ruffo G, Selvaggi L, Syed R, Minelli L (2004) Preoperative double-contrast barium enema in patients with suspected intestinal endometriosis. J Am Assoc Gynecol Laparosc 11:223–228
21. Del Frate C, Girometti R, Pittino M, Del Frate G, Bazzocchi M, Zuiani C (2006) Deep retroperitoneal pelvic endometriosis: MR imaging appearance with laparoscopic correlation. Radiographics 26:1705–1718
22. CNGOF Guidelines for the Management of Endometriosis Collège National des Gynécologues et Obstétriciens Français, 2006. http://www.cngof.asso.fr/D TELE/RPC endometriose en BM.pdf
23. Chapron C, Chopin N, Borghese B, Foulot H, Dousset B, Vacher-Lavenu MC et al (2006) Deeply infiltrating endometriosis: pathogenetic implications of the anatomical distribution. Hum Reprod 21:1839–1845
24. Abrao MS, Podgaec S, Dias JA, Averbach M, Silva LF, Marino de Carvalho F (2008) Endometriosis lesions that compromise the rectum deeper than the inner muscularis layer have more than 40% of the circumference of the rectum affected by the disease. J Minim Invasive Gynecol 15:280–285
25. Keckstein J, Wiesinger H (2005) Deep endometriosis, including intestinal involvement – the interdisciplinary approach. Minim Invasive Ther Allied Technol 14:160–166
26. Daraï E, Bazot M, Rouzier R, Houry S, Dubernard G (2007) Outcome of laparoscopic colorectal resection for endometriosis. Curr Opin Obstet Gynecol 19:308–313
27. Minelli L, Fanfani F, Fagotti A, Ruffo G, Ceccaroni M, Mereu L, Landi S, Pomini P, Scambia G (2009) Laparoscopic colorectal resection for bowel endometriosis: feasibility, complications, and clinical outcome. Arch Surg 144:234–239
28. Donnez J, Squifflet J (2004) Laparoscopic excision of deep endometriosis. Obstet Gynecol Clin N Am 31:567–580
29. Ret Davalos ML, De Cicco C, D'Hoore A, De Decker B, Koninckx PR (2007) Outcome after rectum or sigmoid resection: a review for gynecologists. J Minim Invasive Gynecol 14:33–38
30. Roman H, Loisel C, Resch B, Tuech JJ, Hochain P, Leroi AM, Marpeau L (2010) Delayed functional outcomes associated with surgical management of deep rectovaginal endometriosis with rectal involvement: giving patients an informed choice. Hum Reprod 25:890–899
31. Moher D, Cook DJ, Eastwood S, Olkin I, Rennie D, Stroup DF (1999) Improving the quality of reports of meta-analyses of randomised controlled trials: the QUOROM statement. Quality of reporting of meta-analyses. Lancet 354:1896–1900
32. Koh CH, Janik GM (2002) The surgical management of deep rectovaginal endometriosis. Curr Opin Obstet Gynecol 14:357–364
33. Emmanuel KR, Davis C (2005) Outcomes and treatment options in rectovaginal endometriosis. Curr Opin Obstet Gynecol 17:399–402
34. Vercellini P, Barbara G, Abbiati A, Somigliana E, Viganò P, Fedele L (2009) Repetitive surgery for recurrent symptomatic endometriosis: what to do? Eur J Obstet Gynecol Reprod Biol 146:15–21
35. Mohr C, Nezhat FR, Nezhat CH, Seidman DS, Nezhat CR (2005) Fertility considerations in laparoscopic treatment of infiltrative bowel endometriosis. JSLS 9:16–24
36. Vercellini P, Pietropaolo G, De Giorgi O, Daguati R, Pasin R, Crosignani PG (2006) Reproductive performance in infertile women with rectovaginal endometriosis: is surgery worthwhile? Am J Obstet Gynecol 195:1303–1310
37. Brouwer R, Woods RJ (2007) Rectal endometriosis: results of radical excision and review of published work. ANZ J Surg 77:562–571

38. Maytham GD, Dowson HM, Levy B, Kent A, Rockall TA (2009) Laparoscopic excision of rectovaginal endometriosis: report of a prospective study and review of the literature. Colorectal Dis Jul 3 (Epub ahead of print)
39. Fanfani F, Fagotti A, Gagliardi ML, Ruffo G, Ceccaroni M, Scanbia G, Minelli L (2010) Discoid or segmental rectosigmoid resection for deep infiltrating endometriosis: a case-control study. Fertil Steril 94:444–449
40. Redwine DB, Wright JT (2001) Laparoscopic treatment of complete obliteration of the cul-de-sac associated with endometriosis: long-term follow-up of en bloc resection. Fertil Steril 76:358–365
41. Fedele L, Bianchi S, Zanconato G, Bettoni G, Gotsch F (2004) Long term follow up after conservative surgery for rectovaginal endometriosis. Am J Obstet Gynecol 190:1020–1024
42. Ford J, English J, Miles WA, Giannopoulos T (2004) Pain, quality of life and complications following the radical resection of rectovaginal endometriosis. BJOG 111:353–356
43. Thomassin I, Bazot M, Detchev R, Barranger E, Cortez A, Darai E (2004) Symptoms before and after surgical removal of colorectal endometriosis that are assessed by magnetic resonance imaging and rectal endoscopic sonography. Am J Obstet Gynecol 190:1264–1271
44. Darai E, Marpeau O, Thomassin I, Dubernard G, Barranger E, Bazot M (2005) Fertility after laparoscopic colorectal resection for endometriosis: preliminary results. Fertil Steril 84:945–950
45. Darai E, Thomassin I, Barranger E, Detchev R, Cortez A, Houry S, Bazot M (2005) Feasibility and clinical outcome of laparoscopic colorectal resection for endometriosis. Am J Obstet Gynecol 192:394–400
46. Fleisch MC, Xafis D, De Bruyne F, Hucke J, Bender HG, Dall P (2005) Radical resection of invasive endometriosis with bowel or bladder involvement—long-term results. Eur J Obstet Gynecol Reprod Biol 123:224–229
47. Dubernard G, Piketty M, Rouzier R, Houry S, Bazot M, Darai E (2006) Quality of life after laparoscopic colorectal resection for endometriosis. Hum Reprod 21:1243–1247
48. Lyons SD, Chew SS, Thomson AJ, Lenart M, Camaris C, Vancaillie TG et al (2006) Clinical and quality-of-life outcomes after fertility-sparing laparoscopic surgery with bowel resection for severe endometriosis. J Minim Invasive Gynecol 13:436–441
49. Ribeiro PA, Rodrigues FC, Kehdi IP, Rossini L, Abdalla HS, Donadio N et al (2006) Laparoscopic resection of intestinal endometriosis: a 5-year experience. J Minim Invasive Gynecol 13:442–446
50. Langebrekke A, Istre O, Busund B, Johannessen HO, Qvigstad E (2006) Endoscopic treatment of deep infiltrating endometriosis (DIE) involving the bladder and rectosigmoid colon. Acta Obstet Gynecol Scand 85:712–715
51. Seracchioli R, Poggioli G, Pierangeli F, Manuzzi L, Gualerzi B, Savelli L et al (2007) Surgical outcome and long-term follow up after laparoscopic rectosigmoid resection in women with deep infiltrating endometriosis. BJOG 114:889–895
52. Mereu L, Ruffo G, Landi S, Barbieri F, Zaccoletti R, Fiaccavento A et al (2007) Laparoscopic treatment of deep endometriosis with segmental colorectal resection: short-term morbidity. J Minim Invasive Gynecol 14:463–469
53. Zanetti-Dällenbach R, Bartley J, Müller C, Schneider A, Köhler C (2008) Combined vaginal–laparoscopic–abdominal approach for the surgical treatment of rectovaginal endometriosis with bowel resection: a comparison of this new technique with various established approaches by laparoscopy and laparotomy. Surg Endosc 22:995–1001
54. Pereira RM, Zanatta A, Preti CD, de Paula FJ, da Motta EL, Serafini PC (2009) Should the gynecologist perform laparoscopic bowel resection to treat endometriosis? Results over 7 years in 168 patients. J Minim Invasive Gynecol 16:472–479
55. Stepniewska A, Pomini P, Scioscia M, Mereu L, Ruffo G, Minelli L (2010) Fertility and clinical outcome after bowel resection in infertile women with endometriosis. Reprod Biomed Online 20:602–609
56. Ruffo G, Scopelliti F, Scioscia M, Ceccaroni M, Mainardi P, Minelli L (2010) Laparoscopic colorectal resection for deep infiltrating endometriosis: analysis of 436 cases. Surg Endosc 24:63–67
57. Chapron C, Jacob S, Dubuisson JB, Vieira M, Liaras E, Fauconnier A (2001) Laparoscopically assisted vaginal management of deep endometriosis infiltrating the rectovaginal septum. Acta Obstet Gynecol Scand 80:349–354
58. Hollett-Caines J, Vilos GA, Penava DA (2003) Laparoscopic mobilization of the rectosigmoid and excision of the obliterated cul-de-sac. J Am Assoc Gynecol Laparosc 10:190–194
59. Remorgida V, Ragni N, Ferrero S, Anserini P, Torelli P, Fulcheri E (2005) How complete is full thickness disc resection of bowel endometriotic lesions? A prospective surgical and histological study. Hum Reprod 20:2317–2320
60. Angioni S, Peiretti M, Zirone M, Palomba M, Mais V, Gomel V et al (2006) Laparoscopic excision of posterior vaginal fornix in the treatment of patients with deep endometriosis without rectum involvement: surgical treatment and long-term follow-up. Hum Reprod 21:1629–1634
61. Kristensen J, Kjer JJ (2007) Laparoscopic laser resection of rectovaginal pouch and rectovaginal septum endometriosis: the impact on pelvic pain and quality of life. Acta Obstet Gynecol Scand 86:1467–1471
62. Matsuzaki S, Houlle C, Botchorishvili R, Pouly JL, Mage G, Canis M (2009) Excision of the posterior vaginal fornix is necessary to ensure complete resection of rectovaginal endometriotic nodules of more than 2 cm in size. Fertil Steril 91(4 Suppl):1314–1315
63. Donnez J, Squifflet J (2010) Complications, pregnancy and recurrence in a prospective series of 500 patients operated on by the shaving technique for deep rectovaginal endometriotic nodules. Hum Reprod 25:1949–1958
64. Reich H, McGlynn F, Salvat J (1991) Laparoscopic treatment of cul-de-sac obliteration secondary to retrocervical deep fibrotic endometriosis. J Reprod Med 36:516–522
65. Donnez J, Nisolle M, Casanas-Roux F, Bassil S, Anaf V (1995) Rectovaginal septum, endometriosis or adenomyosis: laparoscopic management in a series of 231 patients. Hum Reprod 10:630–635
66. Crosignani PG, Vercellini P, Biffignandi F, Costantini W, Cortesi I, Imparato E (1996) Laparoscopy versus laparotomy in conservative surgical treatment for severe endometriosis. Fertil Steril 66:706–711
67. Donnez J, Nisolle M, Gillerot S, Smets M, Bassil S, Casanas-Roux F (1997) Rectovaginal septum adenomyotic nodules: a series of 500 cases. Br J Obstet Gynaecol 104:1014–1018
68. Bailey HR (1992) Colorectal endometriosis. Perspect Colon Rectal Surg 5:251–259
69. Roman H, Puscasiu L, Kouteich K, Gromez A, Resch B, Marouteau-Pasquier N, Hochain P, Tuech JJ, Scotte M, Marpeau L (2007) Laparoscopic management of deep endometriosis with rectal affect. Chirurgia 102:421–428
70. Anaf V, El Nakadi I, De Moor V, Coppens E, Zalcman M, Noel JC (2009) Anatomic significance of a positive barium enema in deep infiltrating endometriosis of the large bowel. World J Surg 33:822–827

30

Predictors of intra-abdominal adhesions

Fady Shehata · Afsoon Zarei · Einat Shalom-Paz ·
Togas Tulandi

Abstract The objective of this study is to evaluate the prevalence and predicting factors for intra-abdominal adhesions among 1,050 consecutive cases of laparoscopy. This study is designed as a retrospective cohort study. Multivariate linear regression model was constructed to determine factors associated with increased intra-abdominal adhesions including age, number of previous abdominal operations, and endometriosis. Adhesions were graded using a modified (ASRM) classification for adnexal adhesions. Factors affecting the development of intra-abdominal adhesions were number of previous abdominal operations (P<0.0001, 95% CI 0.18–0.30) and degree of endometriosis (P<0.0001, 95% CI 0.25–0.35). Endometriosis had more influence on adhesion formation than number of previous operations as demonstrated by the standardized coefficients beta in endometriosis (0.32) versus previous abdominal operations (0.21). Age, BMI, and PID were not associated with increased abdominal adhesions. Endometriosis and abdominal operations play an important role in development of intra-abdominal adhesions. However, endometriosis has more influence on adhesions than previous operations.

F. Shehata (✉) · E. Shalom-Paz · T. Tulandi
Department of Obstetrics and Gynecology,
McGill University Health Center,
687 Pine Avenue West,
Montreal, QC, Canada H3A 1A1
e-mail: fady.shehata@mail.mcgill.ca

A. Zarei
Department of Obstetrics and Gynecology,
Shiraz University of Medical Sciences,
Shiraz, Iran

Keywords Adhesions · Endometriosis · Laparotomy · Abdominal surgery

Background

Adhesions are fibrous tissues formed as a response to injury during surgical operations. Intra-abdominal adhesions are the most common complication of abdominal operations [1]. Adhesions might cause pelvic pain, infertility, and small bowel obstruction (SBO). In fact, intra-abdominal adhesions are the most common cause of SBO [2–6]. These complications may occur shortly or many years after the operations [7].

Factors contributing to intra-abdominal adhesions include abdominal operations (either laparotomy or laparoscopy), endometriosis, or intra-abdominal infection. Studies of adhesions related readmission showed that 30% of patients would be readmitted at least once after an abdominal surgery [8, 9]. In neonates, the percentage was 8.3% [10]. Although causes of adhesions are well established, the extent and association between these predisposing factors and the formation of adhesions remain unclear.

The purpose of our study was to evaluate predicting factors of intra-abdominal adhesions in a large population of women who underwent a laparoscopy by a single surgeon.

Methods

We evaluated 1,050 consecutive cases of laparoscopy between May 1982 and August 2009. All laparoscopies were performed by the senior author in two McGill University teaching hospitals, the Royal Victoria Hospital and the Sir Mortimer B. Davis, Jewish General Hospital. The study was approved by the director of professional services.

Data were collected directly from patients' charts by two physicians (FS and AZ) and entered in a Microsoft Excel database. All data were obtained from hospital records and cross-checked with office files.

Variables included patient's demography, number and description of previous abdominal operations, history and classification of endometriosis, presence or absence of pelvic inflammatory disease, main presenting symptom, type of operation, and postoperative diagnosis. The senior author routinely drew a diagram using a modified American Society of Reproductive Medicine (ASRM) classification for adnexal adhesions after each surgical procedure. Adhesions, if any, were graded as 0 (no adhesions), 1 (mild), 2 (moderate), and 3 (severe). Endometriosis was classified using ASRM classification for endometriosis as 0 (no endometriosis), 1 (minimal), 2 (mild), 3 (moderate), and 4 (severe).

Statistical analysis

Normality of data distribution was examined using Shapiro–Wilk test. We used multiple linear logistic regression analysis to construct a model for predicting the presence of intra-abdominal adhesions (dependant variable) from other parameters (independent variables). ANOVA was used to determine the usefulness of our model variables to predict the outcome ($P<0.0001$, degrees of freedom=278). The differences were considered statistically significant if P was less than 0.05.

Findings

The mean age and the body mass index of the patients were 38.6±9.2 and 24.0±4.9 years, respectively. Among 1,050 women, 559 women (53.2%) had had no previous abdominal operation, 27% had one previous abdominal surgery, and the remainders had two or more abdominal operations (Table 1). Intra-abdominal adhesions were found in 343 patients (32.6%). These included women who had never undergone any previous abdominal surgery, women who had had previous surgeries and/or endometriosis. Indications for surgery included ovarian cyst removal (27.8%), fibroids (21.7%), and infertility (16.8%, Table 2).

Table 1 Distribution of patients by number of previous abdominal operation

No. of previous surgery	No. of patients	Percentage (%)
0	559	53.2
1	283	27.0
2	131	12.5
3	44	4.2
4	23	2.2
5	6	0.6
6	4	0.4
Total	1,050	100.0

Table 2 Indications for surgery in study population

Indications for surgery	Total
Ovarian cyst	282
Fibroids	220
Infertility	171
Endometriosis	117
Menorrhagia	74
Others	62
Tubal condition	34
Cancer	34
Pelvic pain	22

In a subgroup of patients (subgroup A) who had at least one previous surgery and no endometriosis (n=352), adhesions were found in 140 women (40%). In another subgroup of patients (subgroup B) who had history of endometriosis and no previous operations (n=138), adhesions were found in 61 women (44.2%). In a third subgroup of patients (subgroup C) who had never had any operations, or endometriosis (n=413), adhesions were found in 60 women (14.5%, Fig. 1).

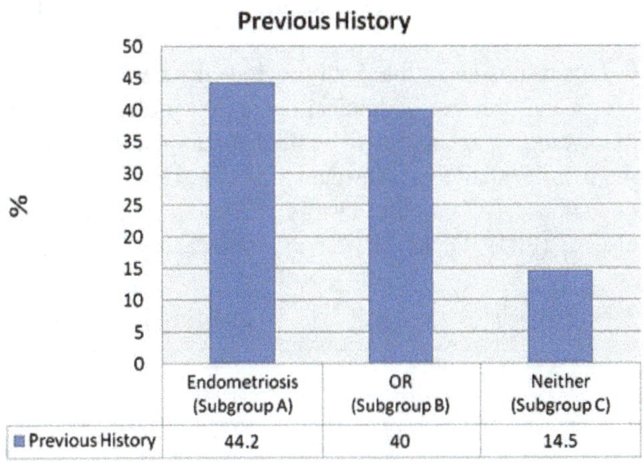

Fig. 1 Prevalence of adhesions in patients with endometriosis, previous abdominal surgery, or neither

Table 3 Multiple linear regression analysis for predictors of intra-abdominal adhesions using age, history of PID, endometriosis, and previous abdominal operation

	B	SE	Beta	*P* value	95% CI
Age	0.005	0.004	0.039	NS	(0.00–0.01)
PID	0.045	0.240	0.005	NS	(−0.43–0.52)
Endometriosis	0.298	0.027	0.325	<0.0001	(0.25–0.35)
Previous abdominal operation	0.238	0.032	0.217	<0.0001	(0.18–0.30)

NS not significant

To evaluate the relationship between the intra-abdominal adhesions (dependent variable) and independent variables, we constructed a multiple linear regression model (Table 3). Both endometriosis and history of previous abdominal operation were significantly associated with the presence of intra-abdominal adhesions ($P<0.0001$). We then examined the standard coefficient beta to determine the variable with more influence. Endometriosis had a stronger influential role than previous abdominal operation (beta 0.27 and 0.17) respectively.

We also evaluated a subgroup of patients who had had only one previous laparoscopy ($n=107$) or laparotomy ($n=59$) and another subgroup of patients who had had clean surgery (not involving intestine, $n=188$) or dirty surgery (involving intestine, $n=59$) (Table 4). Patients who had had a laparotomy were more likely to have intra-abdominal adhesions than those who had had a previous laparoscopy ($P<0.0001$, 95%CI=1.02–1.99). The type of operation (whether clean or dirty) did not affect adhesion formation.

Conclusions

Intra-abdominal adhesions are a major complication of abdominal operations. The presence of adhesions leads to increased operating time [11–13], increased risk of abdominal injury in subsequent surgery [14], and increased health care expenditure to treat subsequent complications [15].

Our results show that both previous history of endometriosis and previous abdominal operations increase the risk of developing adhesions. In addition, endometriosis plays a more influential role than number of previous abdominal operations. Of interest, history of pelvic inflammatory disease (PID) did not appear to increase intra-abdominal adhesions. However, it is possible that some patients in our population had had subclinical PID which was undiagnosed and not reported in the charts.

We found the prevalence of adhesions in patients who only had previous surgeries to be 40%. In a postmortem study, Weibel and Majno reported a 67% adhesion rate in individuals who had a history of previous operations [16]. Dubuisson et al. in 2010 showed 21.1% adhesions rate in a similar population [17]. Whether the patients in their study had endometriosis is not clear. In our study the influential role of endometriosis was reflected in the highest adhesions rate.

In agreement with previous studies, we found that patients who had a previous laparotomy are more likely to develop adhesions than patients with previous laparoscopies. In a randomised trial, Lundorff et al. studied 105 patients who had ectopic pregnancies and were randomised to surgery by either laparoscopy or laparotomy [18]. They found that the laparotomy group had significantly higher density of adhesions than the laparoscopy group [18].

Both types of operations (clean or dirty) were not found to increase the density of adhesions. This may suggest that bowel injury during abdominal operations does not increase the risk of adhesions. This information is useful in consulting patients following gynecological operations complicated with bowel injuries. The limitations of our study included lack of information regarding the type of incision in previous operations and of adhesion site in the laparoscopy report.

We conclude that the risk factors of intra-abdominal adhesions are mainly endometriosis and the number of previous abdominal operations. The incidence of adhesions in patients with previous history of endometriosis is the highest. Patients with previous laparotomy are more likely to develop adhesions than laparoscopy.

Table 4 Multiple regression analysis for predictors of intra-abdominal adhesions in a subgroup of patients with only one previous abdominal operation by laparoscopy or laparotomy, and clean versus dirty operations

	B	SE	Beta	*P* value	95% CI
Laparoscopy versus laparotomy	1.23	0.22	0.47	<0.0001	(0.79–1.68)
Clean versus dirty	0.03	0.44	−0.01	NS	(−0.91–0.84)

NS not significant

Acknowledgments None

Declaration of interest The authors report no conflicts of interest. The authors alone are responsible for the content and writing of the paper.

References

1. DeWilde RL, Trew G (2007) Postoperative abdominal adhesions and their prevention in gynaecological surgery. Expert consensus position. Part 2—steps to reduce adhesions. Gynecol Surg 4 (4):243–253
2. Krebs HB, Goplerud DR (1987) Mechanical intestinal obstruction in patients with gynecologic disease: a review of 368 patients. Am J Obstet Gynecol 157(3):577–583
3. Perry JF Jr, Smith GA, Yonehiro EG (1955) Intestinal obstruction caused by adhesions: a review of 388 cases. Ann Surg 142 (5):810–816
4. Ratcliff JB, Kapernick P, Brooks GG, Dunnihoo DR (1983) Small bowel obstruction and previous gynecologic surgery. South Med J 76(11):1349–1350, 1360
5. Nappi C, Di Spiezio SA, Greco E, Guida M, Bettocchi S, Bifulco G (2007) Prevention of adhesions in gynaecological endoscopy. Hum Reprod Update 13(4):379–394. doi:10.1093/humupd/dml061
6. Vrijland WW, Jeekel J, van Geldorp HJ, Swank DJ, Bonjer HJ (2003) Abdominal adhesions: intestinal obstruction, pain, and infertility. Surg Endosc 17(7):1017–1022. doi:10.1007/s00464-002-9208-9
7. Al-Sunaidi M, Tulandi T (2006) Adhesion-related bowel obstruction after hysterectomy for benign conditions. Obstet Gynecol 108 (5):1162–1166. doi:10.1097/01.AOG.0000239098.33320.c4
8. Ellis H, Moran BJ, Thompson JN, Parker MC, Wilson MS, Menzies D, McGuire A, Lower AM, Hawthorn RJ, O'Brien F, Buchan S, Crowe AM (1999) Adhesion-related hospital readmissions after abdominal and pelvic surgery: a retrospective cohort study. Lancet 353(9163):1476–1480. doi:10.1016/S0140-6736(98)09337-4
9. Parker MC, Ellis H, Moran BJ, Thompson JN, Wilson MS, Menzies D, McGuire A, Lower AM, Hawthorn RJ, O'Briena F, Buchan S, Crowe AM (2001) Postoperative adhesions: ten-year follow-up of 12,584 patients undergoing lower abdominal surgery. Dis Colon Rectum 44(6):822–829, discussion 829–830
10. Wilkins BM, Spitz L (1986) Incidence of postoperative adhesion obstruction following neonatal laparotomy. Br J Surg 73(9):762–764
11. Sot KC, Davidson T, Parker M (1998) Intestinal obstruction in patients with gynaecological malignancies. Ann Acad Med 17:72–75
12. Beck DE, Ferguson MA, Opelka FG, Fleshman JW, Gervaz P, Wexner SD (2000) Effect of previous surgery on abdominal opening time. Dis Colon Rectum 43(12):1749–1753
13. Coleman MG, McLain AD, Moran BJ (2000) Impact of previous surgery on time taken for incision and division of adhesions during laparotomy. Dis Colon Rectum 43(9):1297–1299
14. Van Der Krabben AA, Dijkstra FR, Nieuwenhuijzen M, Reijnen MMPJ, Schaapveld M, Van Goor H (2000) Morbidity and mortality of inadvertent enterotomy during adhesiotomy. Br J Surg 87(4):467–471
15. Al-Fozan H, Dufort J, Kaplow M, Tulandi T (2003) Cost analysis of adhesion-related admissions in a Canadian teaching hospital. Int J Gynaecol Obstet 82(2):227–228
16. Weibel MA, Majno G (1973) Peritoneal adhesions and their relation to abdominal surgery. A postmortem study. Am J Surg 126(3):345–353
17. Dubuisson J, Botchorishvili R, Perrette S, Bourdel N, Jardon K, Rabischong B, Canis M, Mage G (2010) Incidence of intra-abdominal adhesions in a continuous series of 1000 laparoscopic procedures. Am J Obstet Gynecol 203(2):111.e111–111.e113. doi:10.1016/j.ajog.2010.03.031
18. Lundorff P, Hahlin M, Kallfelt B, Thorburn J, Lindblom B (1991) Adhesion formation after laparoscopic surgery in tubal pregnancy: a randomized trial versus laparotomy. Fertil Steril 55(5):911–915

31

Short-term safety and effectiveness of tension-free vaginal tape (TVT) sling insertion for urodynamic stress incontinence alongside other gynaecological operations

Sharif I. M. F. Ismail · Seumas Eckford

Abstract The aim of this study was to assess the safety, effectiveness and pattern of inserting tension-free vaginal tape (TVT) slings alongside other gynaecological operations. It was a retrospective case note review of 116 patients who had a range of minor and major vaginal, laparoscopic and abdominal procedures at the same time as having TVT sling insertion at five district general hospitals in the UK. It showed an overall incidence of complications of 22.4% and laparotomy was not required. A patient had bladder perforation, another had blood transfusion, a third had infection at the site of needle passing, and three patients had urinary tract infection. The overall incidence of complications in this series was significantly higher in those having major concomitant surgery than in the total group. Although 9.5% of patients had catheters for more than a week, only two patients (1.7%) required prolonged intermittent self-catheterisation. Development of overactive bladder symptoms was reported by 8.5% of those who had pure urodynamic stress incontinence prior to surgery. Ninety-four per cent of patients were dry at 6 weeks. All major abdominal procedures were carried out under general anaesthesia prior to TVT sling insertion. A considerable variation was observed in operative and anaesthetic technique with all other concomitant procedures. These results demonstrated that TVT sling insertion alongside other minor and major gynaecological procedures did not undermine the safety or effectiveness of TVT sling insertion. Operative and anaesthetic practice varied considerably, calling for randomised controlled trials to provide evidence for best practice.

S. I. M. F. Ismail
Department of Obstetrics and Gynaecology, Singleton Hospital, Swansea, South Wales, UK

S. I. M. F. Ismail
Department of Obstetrics and Gynaecology, Wrexham Maelor Hospital, Wrexham, North Wales, UK

S. I. M. F. Ismail
Department of Obstetrics and Gynaecology, Royal Bournemouth Hospital, Dorset, UK

S. I. M. F. Ismail · S. Eckford
Department of Obstetrics and Gynaecology, North Devon District Hospital, Barnstaple, Devon, UK

S. I. M. F. Ismail
Department of Obstetrics and Gynaecology, Yeovil District Hospital, Somerset, UK

S. I. M. F. Ismail (✉)
Department of Obstetrics and Gynaecology, Royal Sussex County Hospital, Brighton BN2 5BE, UK
e-mail: sharif212121@yahoo.co.uk

Keywords Concomitant surgery · Effectiveness · Safety · Short term · Subjective · Tension-free vaginal tape (TVT) sling

Background

Patients having tension-free vaginal tape (TVT) sling insertion for urodynamic stress incontinence may also have other gynaecological condition(s) that necessitate additional gynaecological surgery. This particularly applies to pelvic organ prolapse as there is a recognised association between the two conditions [1]. Less commonly, patients may have other problems that require surgical management, such as abdominal hysterectomy for heavy periods [2]. In such situations, there is a choice between performing both procedures at the same time or in two separate settings. Although there are published reports on TVT sling insertions alongside other gynaecological procedures, all of these reports are limited to vaginal management of pelvic organ prolapse and vaginal or laparoscopic-assisted vaginal hysterectomy [3–14]. Of these studies, one looked at prophylactic insertion of TVT sling insertion for occult stress incontinence at the same time as having vaginal surgery for severe (grade 3 or more) pelvic organ prolapse [3] and two included patients with urodynamic as well as occult stress incontinence [10, 13].

This limitation was highlighted by the National Institute of Clinical Excellence in its guidance on the use of the TVT sling [15]. This means that clinicians do not have clear guidance as to how best to manage urodynamic stress incontinence of urine in the era of mid-urethral tape slings at the same time as dealing with other gynaecological problems. It also means that there is no account of current practice under these circumstances. The aim of this study was to look at the safety and short-term effectiveness of TVT sling insertions alongside other gynaecological procedures and provide an account on how such concomitant procedures are carried out.

Method

The primary outcome measure for this study was the incidence of operative or immediate postoperative complications, including voiding dysfunction, during and/or following TVT sling insertion alongside other gynaecological procedures. Subjective outcome at the 6-week follow-up visit was considered as the secondary outcome measure. The nature and order of concomitant gynaecological surgery, type of anaesthesia used and hospital stay were noted.

Sample size calculation was based on noting 39% complication rate when TVT sling insertion was performed alone [16]. To detect a 20% increase in this rate to 59%, with 80% power and 95% confidence (0.05 significance), required 107 cases.

In view of the limited number of such procedures carried out in individual hospitals, it was necessary to get cases from several hospitals, and it was possible to obtain data from five placements. Data were collected from patient notes using data collection sheets and downloaded onto Microsoft Works 5.0 for Windows database (www.msn.com). Statistical tests were carried out on Stata 6.0 for Windows (www.stata.com). Normally distributed continuous data were described using the mean and standard deviation, resorting to the median and interquartile range for those not fitting a normal distribution. Categorical data were described using numbers and percentage and compared using χ^2 test.

Insertions were made according to the technique described by Ulmsten et al. [17]. Patients were followed up at 6 weeks and outcome was assessed subjectively, cure being defined as no leakage, improvement when there was significant reduction in leakage such that patients did not need further management and failure when there was inadequate improvement. The development of overactive bladder symptoms in those with pure urodynamic stress incontinence was noted.

Findings

A total of 116 patients were identified from theatre information systems in the five hospitals since the start of using the TVT sling in 1999 until 2007, and all the notes were available. The number of patients included from each hospital is shown in Table 1. Patients' background features are shown in Table 2. Operations were performed by different consultants or under their direct supervision. Two cases had a combination of general and regional anaesthesia: One had spinal until the TVT sling was inserted and the other was woken up after completion of vaginal hysterectomy and posterior repair for cough test adjustment of the TVT tension. The nature of concomitant surgery is shown in Table 3 and the order in which surgery was performed shown in Table 4. Operative and postoperative complications are shown in Table 5. Subjective outcome at 6 weeks of follow-up is shown in Table 6.

Discussion

This study looked at concomitant gynaecological surgery alongside TVT sling insertion, taking complications as its primary outcome measure. The overall incidence of complications in this study was 22.4%. There was one bladder perforation and no one required laparotomy, which is better than encountered in the randomised trial that

Table 1 Number of patients from individual hospitals

Hospital	Number (%)
Singleton Hospital	15 (12.9)
Wrexham Maelor Hospital	14 (12.1)
North Devon District Hospital	21 (18.1)
Royal Bournemouth Hospital	35 (30.2)
Yeovil District Hospital	31 (26.7)
Total	116

Table 2 Background features

Feature	Statistical test	Result
Age (years)	Mean±SD	57.3±12.8
Previous hysterectomy	Number (%)	41 (35.3)
Previous continence surgery	Number (%)	13 (11.2)
Previous prolapse surgery	Number (%)	23 (19.8)
Medical problems	Number (%)	59 (50.9)
Cardiopulmonary		33 (28.4)
Bone and joint		16 (13.8)
Mixed incontinence (urodynamic)	Number (%)	10 (8.6)
Type of anaesthesia	Number (%)	
Spinal/epidural		68 (58.6)
General		46 (39.7)
Combination		2 (1.7)
Postoperative stay (days)	Median (interquartile range)	3 (2–5)

compared TVT to Burch colposuspension [16]. One patient required blood transfusion and another had infection at the site of passing the needle holding the TVT sling. Urinary tract infection developed in three cases (2.6%). Whilst these are less than that reported in the randomised controlled trial which compared TVT sling to Burch colposuspension [16], one must bear in mind that prospective studies may have better recording of complications.

The low incidence of complications in this series matches most of the published studies [3, 4, 7–9, 12, 13]. On the other hand, one study [5] showed an increased incidence of bladder perforation in those having sling insertion alongside vaginal hysterectomy, mostly in those with previous continence surgery. Another study reported significantly more blood loss in patients having vaginal surgery for pelvic organ prolapse alongside TVT sling insertion in comparison to those having TVT sling insertion alone [11]. However, the study did not indicate whether this was the result of TVT sling insertion or surgery for pelvic organ prolapse. A bladder perforation rate of 6.7% was reported by one study [9] which included 45 patients, of whom eight had sling insertion alone, and the results were grouped together, making it difficult to establish the incidence in patients having concomitant surgery. Another one, which only involved surgery for pelvic organ prolapse, reported a complication rate of 29.7% [6]. This study, however, grouped all complications, including anaesthetic ones, together without providing much detail, making it difficult to make a proper comparison of individual complications.

Table 3 Type of concomitant procedures

Type of concomitant procedure	Number[a]	Percentage
Minor surgery	37	31.9
Hysteroscopy	6	5.2
Mirena insertion/change	9	7.8
Laparoscopic sterilisation	6	5.2
Bladder biopsy	2	1.7
Vulval procedure	9	7.8
Major vaginal surgery	75	64.7
Anterior repair	28	24.1
Posterior repair	33	28.4
Anterior and posterior repair	14	12.1
Sacrospinous fixation	1	0.9
Vaginal hysterectomy	12	10.3
Major abdominal surgery	5	4.3
Hysterectomy	4	3.4
Salpingo-oophorectomy	4	3.4
Sacrocolpopexy	1	0.9

[a] Some patients had more than one concomitant procedure

The incidence of complications in this series was significantly higher in those having major concomitant surgery than in the total group. However, this applied only to all complications grouped together rather than individual complications. The rate was still lower than the rate of complications encountered in the randomised controlled trial that compared TVT sling to Burch colposuspension [16]. Whilst it is logical that major surgery would be associated with more incidence of complications than minor surgery, a similar observation was not reported by any of the published studies that looked at TVT sling insertion alongside other gynaecological procedures [4–14]. Nonetheless, published studies looked at a much smaller range of concomitant gynaecological procedures, whereas this series included the full range of concomitant gynaecological operations. The rate was not significantly higher in those who had previous continence surgery. It is important to bear in mind that neither this series nor the published studies were powered to compare the safety of concomitant surgery in different subgroups of patients.

Table 4 Order of performing concomitant gynaecological surgery

Type of concomitant surgery	Number	Before TVT	After TVT
Laparoscopic surgery	8	6 (75.0%)	2 (25.0%)
Major abdominal surgery	5	4 (80.0%)	1 (20.0%)
Vaginal hysterectomy	12	12 (100.0%)	0 (0.0%)
Anterior repair	42	29 (69.0%)	13 (31.0%)
Posterior repair	47	24 (51.1%)	23 (48.9%)
Minor vaginal surgery	30	11 (36.7%)	19 (63.3%)

The link between bladder perforation and previous continence surgery is controversial. For TVT sling insertion without concomitant surgery, one study showed a significant association [18], though another did not [19]. The patient who had bladder perforation in this series did not have previous continence surgery and did not have a major concomitant gynaecological operation. An association was noted in one of the studies that compared TVT sling insertion with and without vaginal hysterectomy [5]. Two studies reported at least half their bladder perforations in patients with prior continence surgery during TVT sling insertion alongside vaginal surgery for pelvic organ prolapse [4, 11] as well as without concomitant surgery [12]. It is important to bear in mind that none of these studies, including the series outlined here, was powered to detect an association between previous continence surgery and bladder perforation.

Almost a tenth of patients had catheters for more than a week, which is higher than reported in the randomised trial [16]. On the other hand, only two patients (1.7%) required intermittent self-catheterisation for months, which is lower than in the randomised trial [16]. The different ways of bladder management in published studies precludes direct comparison. No catheters were inserted in one study [4] and all the catheters were removed within 9 days in another [9]. Three non-comparative studies showed a higher incidence of voiding dysfunction than encountered in this series. In the first one [8], where no catheter was left more than 5 days irrespective of the post-void residual volume, five patients (9.1%) required intermittent self-catheterisation. In the second one [13], where suprapubic catheters were checked for residual urine volume after 72 h before removal, 12% of patients had dysfunctional voiding and 3% of patients required clean intermittent self-catheterisation for up to 3 weeks postoperatively, which is higher than in this series. In the third [6], 43% of patients required catheterisation more than 3 days, which is more than that encountered in this series. The author noted an association between voiding dysfunction and concomitant posterior vaginal wall repair as well as previous continence surgery. On the other hand, 6.7% of patients had a suprapubic catheter inserted on the tenth postoperative day for up to 2 weeks in a study that entailed prophylactic TVT sling insertion for occult stress incontinence at the time of having vaginal surgery for severe pelvic organ prolapse [3].

Evidence from comparative studies is equally conflicting. On one hand, a study [5] indicated that 7.5%

Table 5 Complications of TVT sling insertions alongside other gynaecological procedures

Complication	All patients (N=116)	Previous continence surgery (n=13)	Major concomitant surgery (n=80)
All cases	22 (19.0%)	4 (30.8%)	25 (31.3%)[a]
Bladder perforation	1 (0.9%)	0 (0%)	0 (0%)
Bleeding ≥500 ml	2 (1.7%)	1 (7.7%)	1 (1.3%)
Blood transfusion	1 (0.9%)	0 (0%)	1 (1.3%)
Urinary tract infection	3 (2.6%)	1 (7.7%)	3 (3.8%)
Suprapubic infection	1 (0.9%)	0 (0%)	0 (0%)
Vaginal infection	1 (0.9%)	0 (0%)	1 (1.3%)
Vaginal haematoma	1 (0.9%)	1 (0.9%)	1 (1.3%)
Catheter >7 days	11 (9.5%)	0 (0%)	6 (7.5%)
Tape stretch under general anaesthesia	7 (6.0%)	2 (15.4%)	7 (8.8%)
Intermittent self-catheterisation	2 (1.7%)	0(0%)	1 (1.3%)
Tape erosion	1 (0.9%)	0 (0%)	1 (1.3%)
Sexual dysfunction	1 (0.9%)	0 (0%)	1 (1.3%)

[a] Significant difference (p=0.048), χ^2 test

Table 6 Outcome at 6 weeks of follow-up

Outcome	Number	Percentage
Cure from stress incontinence	109	94
Improved stress incontinence	5	4.3
Failure, repeat TVT sling insertion	2	1.7
De novo overactive bladder symptoms[a]	9	8.5

[a] Out of the 106 patients who had pure urodynamic stress incontinence

of patients had voiding difficulties lasting more than 15 days when TVT sling was inserted alongside vaginal hysterectomy and there was no significant increase with concomitant surgery; another showed a significant increase in urinary retention in patients having mesh repair for pelvic organ prolapse with TVT sling insertion only up to 7 days after surgery, but no significant difference beyond that [10]. On the other hand, patients having TVT sling insertion alongside vaginal hysterectomy with or without posterior vaginal wall repair required a significantly longer duration of catheterisation than TVT sling insertion alone [5], and another study reported more cases of transient urinary retention in patients having TVT sling insertion alongside vaginal surgery for pelvic organ prolapse [11]. It is worth bearing in mind that neither this series nor published studies were powered to assess the impact of concomitant surgery on retention of urine following TVT sling insertion.

Seven patients (6%) required stretching the sling under general anaesthesia. No such practice was described in the randomised controlled trial that compared TVT sling to Burch colposuspension [16], and it is to be noted that sling stretching was carried out only in three of the five hospitals included in this study, which again shows variation in bladder management. Stretching was needed in 10.4% of cases in one study that included patients having vaginal surgery for pelvic organ prolapse or laparoscopic-assisted vaginal hysterectomy, though no information was provided about the type of anaesthesia used for sling stretching [6]. Sling incision was performed in 2 out of 26 (7.7%) patients after TVT sling insertion alongside mesh repair for pelvic organ prolapse [10]. Notwithstanding the variation in bladder management and conflicting evidence, the overall impression of the results of this series as well as available evidence is that voiding dysfunction can be a temporary problem following TVT sling insertion alongside concomitant gynaecological surgery, but only a minority of patients may need sling stretching/incision or long-term intermittent self-catheterisation.

It is worth looking at voiding dysfunction when concomitant surgery was carried out without TVT sling insertion. It was difficult to do this in all five hospitals included in this series, in view of the distance and number of cases involved. Looking at published studies is fraught with difficulties due to considerable variation in bladder management as well as the criteria used to define voiding dysfunction [20]. In addition, there are no studies comparing non-continence gynaecological surgery with or without TVT sling insertion. One study [21] reported voiding dysfunction in 8.7% 72 h after vaginal surgery for pelvic organ prolapse, dropping to 1.1% after 6 days, with no patients needing intermittent self-catheterisation at 2 months of follow-up. Eight per cent of the patients included in the study had Kelley's sutures (bladder neck buttressing), as a continence procedure, carried out at the same time. The study showed large cystocele (grade ≥3), excessive intra-operative blood loss and levator plication, in addition to Kelley's sutures (bladder neck buttressing), to be independent predictors of short-term retention of urine. With respect to more general gynaecological surgery, one study reported an overall retention of urine incidence of 9.2% following a variety of gynaecological procedures, including surgery for pelvic organ prolapse in 10.2% of cases [20]. This was based on ultrasound post-void bladder volume exceeding preoperative bladder capacity, which in turn was estimated by adding voided volume at spontaneous uroflowmetry to ultrasound post-voided bladder volume. The highest rate was following laparotomy and abdominal hysterectomy, reaching 55.6% and 13.7%, respectively. Regarding vaginal vault surgery, one study reported 15.6% and 8.3% urinary retention beyond 5 days following abdominal sacrocolpopexy and sacropsinous fixation, respectively [22] and another reported spontaneous voiding within 7 days in 75% patients following sacrospinous fixation, with seven patients (11.1%) continuing to have voiding dysfunction at follow-up which resolved within 3 months.

Whilst these studies report higher as well as lower rates of early voiding dysfunction than encountered in this series, long-term voiding dysfunction was lower than those encountered in this series. However, these studies did not focus on continence surgery. It is pertinent to bear in mind that voiding dysfunction can be affected by a multitude of factors, including patient age, nature of surgery, type of anaesthesia, postoperative pain and its management, hydration and ambulation even in surgery not involving the abdomen or the pelvis [23]. This is not to undervalue the observation that inserting TVT slings alongside other gynaecological operations may increase the incidence of early voiding dysfunction as this can potentially have long-term complications [24], but rather shows the complexity of assessing the possible link, which in turn highlights the need for further studies into this area as part of assessing the safety and effectiveness of this combined approach.

Nine out of the 106 patients (8.5%) who had pure urodynamic stress incontinence prior to TVT sling insertion reported new-onset overactive bladder symptoms at 6 weeks of follow-up. The randomised controlled trial that compared TVT sling to Burch colposuspension [16] and one of the studies that reported TVT sling insertion alongside other gynaecological surgery [7] gave no information about overactive bladder symptoms or the incidence of de novo detrusor overactivity. The lowest reported rate was 1.7% in a study that looked at insertions alongside vaginal surgery for pelvic organ prolapse [8]. One study reported an incidence of 6% in a mixed group of patients having TVT sling insertion with as well as without concomitant vaginal surgery for pelvic organ prolapse and was not significantly different between the two groups [11]. The incidence was 6.7% in one study that included patients having laparoscopic-assisted vaginal hysterectomy [14] and 8% after TVT sling insertion alongside vaginal surgery for pelvic organ prolapse [13]. The highest rate was 13.3% following prophylactic TVT sling insertion for occult stress incontinence at the time of having vaginal surgery for severe pelvic organ prolapse [3]. The rate found in this study is therefore within the reported range in published studies.

Ninety-four per cent of patients were dry at 6 weeks, and two patients (1.7%) had failures that required repeat sling insertion. Whilst this is better than the randomised trial that compared TVT sling to Burch colposuspension [16], the outcome in this series was based on subjective evaluation at 6 weeks of follow-up rather than urodynamic assessment at 6 months, which was the case in the randomised trial. It is also higher than in other studies that reported objective outcome at longer duration of follow-up. In one study that involved 45 patients having vaginal surgery for pelvic organ prolapse at the time of sling insertion [9], the objective cure rate was 42.5%, on the basis of urodynamic assessment at 1-year follow-up, bearing in mind that only 40 (88.9%) patients had this assessment. Another study [13] reported an objective failure rate of 8% at a median follow-up duration of 25 months. In one study [3], 10% of patients had positive stress test 3–6 months after surgery, though none reported stress incontinence. This study, however, entailed prophylactic TVT sling insertion for occult stress incontinence at the time of having vaginal surgery for severe pelvic organ prolapse. On the other hand, the cure rate in this series matches the rates in most of the published studies that looked at TVT sling insertions alongside vaginal surgery for pelvic organ prolapse and vaginal as well as laparoscopic-assisted vaginal hysterectomy [4–6, 8, 12, 14].

All major abdominal procedures were performed under general anaesthesia before the insertion of the TVT sling. However, there was considerable variation in surgical as well as anaesthetic technique with all other procedures. This was the case even in the same hospital and sometimes for the same surgeon, as reported in some of the published reports [3–8, 10–14], and simply illustrates the lack of evidence to support one form of anaesthesia or a particular order in doing concomitant surgery over another. Whilst it could be argued that TVT sling prior to vaginal surgery for pelvic organ prolapse may be inappropriate, as prolapse surgery may affect the position, and thus tension, of the tape [11], larger prospective randomised controlled trials will help in clarifying these aspects. This is particularly important to avoid styles like waking patients up for cough test to adjust the tension of the TVT sling after general anaesthesia for major surgery.

The results of this series should be considered in light of its limitations. There was no control arm as it was not easy to identify patients who had their surgery on two sittings. Several published studies did not include a control arm [4, 6–8, 13], and even the ones that included a control arm did not actually have a proper one. Some compared patients having TVT sling insertion alongside concomitant surgery to those having TVT sling insertion alone [3, 9, 11, 12, 14], and one compared them to those having the concomitant surgery without TVT sling insertion [10]. A proper comparison would be comparing single-sitting versus two-sitting approach to those in need of TVT sling insertion alongside other gynaecological procedures. The series, as well most published studies [3–14], only looked at the safety and effectiveness of the TVT sling complications and outcome rather than those of the other gynaecological procedure(s) carried out at the same time. The other side of the comparison, for example looking at hysterectomy alone versus hysterectomy and TVT sling insertion, is also needed to complete the picture. Only one study looked at mesh repair for pelvic organ prolapse with or without concomitant tension-free vaginal tape sling insertion [10].

Other limitations of the study include its retrospective nature and the fact that it only provided short-term outcome. These limitations also mark available studies. Some studies were retrospective [10, 12] and none of the published prospective studies were randomised [4, 5, 8, 11, 13]. It is true that most studies included long follow-up ranging from 1 year [4, 6, 7, 13] to 2 years [12] and 3 years [11]. However, this longer term follow-up did not include all patients [6] and over a third of patients had <6 months of follow-up in one study [12], and long-term data were amalgamated together for those who had TVT sling insertion alone and those who had the insertion alongside other gynaecological operations in another [11]. The series here focused on perioperative complications and subjective short-term outcome, usually when patients are discharged to their general practitioners at British hospitals. This reduces the limitation of the short-term nature of the follow-up.

The study relied on subjective outcome and entailed a relatively small number of cases from each hospital.

Several published studies relied on subjective outcome [3, 11, 12]. Some of the studies that included objective assessment did not include a full urodynamic assessment [4, 6, 8, 13], and not all patients had full urodynamic assessment when it was included [7, 9, 10]. Although the number of cases included in this series exceeded that required by power calculation, cases came from a number of hospitals. This meant that small numbers were obtained from individual hospitals, let alone individual consultants. However, this reflects the frequency with which such concomitant surgery was carried out at the same time as having TVT sling insertion. Whilst it is difficult to identify how many cases had surgery in separate sittings, addressing this area may encourage others to look at it further. All these features underline the limitations of available evidence in this area.

Despite these limitations, the series has a number of features not matched in published studies. It represents the largest series looking at TVT sling alongside concomitant gynaecological surgery. Numbers included in published studies ranged from 26 [10] and 28 [12] to 75 [11, 13]. The series was based on power calculation, which was not carried out in any of the published studies [3, 4, 6–14]. The series included the full range of minor and major abdominal, vaginal and laparoscopic operations for prolapse as well as other gynaecological problems carried out alongside TVT sling, providing a real-life account of current UK practice. It involved those who had previous continence and prolapse surgery as well as those with mixed incontinence.

Although the grade of evidence provided in this series is reduced by its limitations, it is the best available evidence that reflects real life in British Hospitals. It provides reassurance that concomitant surgery alongside TVT sling insertion does not increase its risk or reduce its effectiveness, apart from a possible rise in short-term retention of urine. Its main value, however, is showing the significant variation in practice, therefore highlighting the need for more and better research into this area. Such a detailed look would require looking at far greater number of hospitals. Whilst the availability of a national register (www.BSUG.net) should enhance access to larger cases, all relevant factors are better addressed in a randomised study with provision for long-term follow-up.

Conclusion

From examining the notes of the 116 cases included in this study, it possible to conclude that having TVT sling insertion for urodynamic stress incontinence alongside other gynaecological operations does not increase the incidence of operative or early postoperative complications associated with TVT sling insertion or reduce its subjective short-term effectiveness. It is likely that concomitant surgery effects an increase in short-term voiding dysfunction, though this needs further evaluation. A considerable variation in anaesthetic as well as surgical technique was observed, reflecting the lack of evidence to support one approach over another and calling for randomised studies to inform best practice.

Acknowledgment The authors are grateful to Lorna Keyes and Lesley Stroud at Singleton Hospital, Julie Jones at Wrexham Maelor Hospital, Jennifer Allo, Amanda Kenchington and Martin Poore at the Royal Bournemouth Hospital, Elizabeth Cummins at North Devon District Hospital and Suan Phipps and Charlotte Mitchell at Yeovil District Hospital for their help in getting patient notes.

Declaration of interest The authors report no conflicts of interest. The authors alone are responsible for the content and writing of the paper.

References

1. Chaikin DC, Groutz A, Blaivas JG (2000) Predicting the need for anti-incontinence surgery in women undergoing repair of severe urogenital prolapse. J Urol 163:531–534
2. Sze EH, Milkos JR, Karram MM (1996) Voiding after Burch colposuspension and effects of concomitant pelvic surgery: correlation with pre-operative voiding mechanism. Obstet Gynecol 88:564–567
3. Gordon D, Gold RS, Pauzner D, Lessing JB, Groutz A (2001) Combined genitourinary prolapse repair and prophylactic tension-free vaginal tape in women with severe prolapse and occult stress urinary incontinence: preliminary results. Urol 58:547–550
4. Jomaa M (2001) Combined tension-free vaginal tape and prolapse repair under local anaesthesia in patients with symptoms of both urinary incontinence and prolapse. Gynecol Obstet Investig 51:184–186
5. Darai E, Jeffry L, Deval A, Birsan A, Kadoch O, Soriano D (2002) Results of tension-free vaginal tape in patients with or without vaginal hysterectomy. Eur J Obstet Gynecol 103:163–167
6. Patrol LM (2002) Efficacy of tension-free vaginal tape with other pelvic reconstructive surgery. J Obstet Gynaecol 186:1292–1298
7. Huang KH, Kung FT, Liang HM, Huang LY, Chang SY (2003) Concomitant surgery with tension-free vaginal tape. Act Obstet Gynecol Scand 82:948–953
8. Lo TS, Chang TC, Chao AS, Chou HH, Tseng LH, Liang CC (2003) Tension-free vaginal tape procedure on genuine stress incontinent women with coexisting genital prolapse. Act Obstet Gynecol Scand 82:1049–1053
9. Pang MW, Chan LW, Yip SK (2003) One-year urodynamic outcome and quality of life in patients with concomitant tension-free vaginal tape during pelvic floor reconstruction surgery for genitourinary prolapse and urodynamic stress incontinence. Int Urogynecol J 14:256–260
10. de Tayrac R, Gervaise A, Chauveaud-Lambling A, Fernandez H (2004) Combined genital prolapse repair reinforced with a polypropylene mesh and tension-free vaginal tape in women with genital prolapse and stress incontinence: a retrospective case-control study with short-term follow up. Act Obstet Gynecol Scand 83:950–954

11. Meltomaa S, Backman T, Haarala M (2004) Concomitant vaginal surgery did not affect the outcome of the tension-free vaginal tape operation during a prospective 3-year follow up study. J Urol 172:222–226
12. Yalcin O, Isikoglu M, Beji NK (2004) Results of TVT operations alone and combined with other vaginal surgical procedures. Arch Gynecol Obstet 269:96–98
13. Huang KH, Kung FT, Liang HM, Chen CW, Chang SY, Hwang LL (2005) Concomitant pelvic organ prolapse surgery with TVT procedure. Int Urogynecol J 17:60–65
14. Lin YH, Llang CC, Soong YK, Soong YK, Chang SD, Chang YL (2005) Concomitant tension-free vaginal tape for urinary incontinence during laparoscopic hysterectomy. Aust NZ J Obstet Gynaecol 45:304–307
15. National Institute for Clinical Excellence (2003) Guidance of the use of tension-free vaginal tape (Gynecare TVT) for stress incontinence, Technology Appraisal Guidance No. 56. National Institute for Clinical Excellence, London, UK
16. Ward K, Hilton P, UK and Ireland TVT Trial Group (2002) Prospective multicentre randomised trial of tension-free vaginal tape and colposuspension as primary treatment for stress incontinence. BMJ 325:67–73
17. Ulmsten U, Henriksson L, Johnson P, Varhos G (1996) An ambulatory surgical procedure under local anaesthesia for treatment of female urinary incontinence. Int Urogynecol J 7:81–86
18. Haab F, Sananes S, Amarenco G, Ciofu C, Uzan S, Gattegno B, Thibault P (2001) Results of the tension-free vaginal tape procedure for the treatment of type II stress urinary incontinence at a minimum follow-up of 1 year. J Urol 165:159–162
19. Mazouni C, Karsenty G, Bretelle F, Bladou F, Gamerre M, Serment G (2004) Urinary complications and sexual function after the tension-free vaginal tape procedure. Act Obstet Gynecol Scand 83:955–961
20. Bødker B, Lose G (2003) Postoperative urinary retention in gynecologic patients. Int Urogynecol J 14:94–97
21. Hakvoort RA, Dijkgraaf MG, Burger MP, Emanuel MH, Roovers JP (2009) Predicting short-term urinary retention after vaginal prolapse surgery. Neurourol Urodyn 28:225–228
22. Demirci F, Ozdemir I, Somunkiran A, Topuz S, Iyibozkurt C, Duras Doyran G, Kemik Gul O, Gul B (2007) Perioperative complications in abdominal sacrocolpopexy and vaginal sacrospinous ligament fixation procedures. Int Urogynecol J 18:257–261
23. Tammela T, Kontturi M, Lukkarinen O (1986) Postoperative urinary retention. I. Incidence and predisposing factors. Scand J Urol Nephrol 20:197–201
24. Tammela T, Kontturi M, Lukkarinen O (1986) Postoperative urinary retention. II. Micturition problems after the first catheterization. Scand J Urol Nephrol 20:257–260

32

Relation of high CA125 and CA19-9 levels with recent rupture of endometrioma

Murat Gözüküçük · Salih Taşkın · Tolga Taşcı · Murat Sönmezer · Cem Atabekoğlu

Abstract Most of endometriomas with CA125 level over 1,000 IU/mL have related with rupture. This is important in differential diagnosis from malign ovarian disease. However, the mechanism of elevation of CA125 in patients with endometrioma is not clear. We reviewed elevation of CA125 level over 1,000 IU/mL in endometriomas and attempted to explore possible mechanisms of this elevation together with presentation of our current case. A review of the literature suggests that extremely elevated CA125 level combined with high CA19-9 level may indicate a recent rupture of endometrioma.

Keywords Endometrioma · Laparoscopy · Rupture · CA125 · CA19-9

Introduction

CA125, recognized by the monoclonal antibody OC 125, is an antigen marker of a high molecular weight glycoprotein and it is the most eligible tumor marker for epithelial ovarian carcinomas of coelomic cell origin. Serum CA125 concentration may also be moderately elevated in advanced endometrial and cervical adenocarcinomas and several benign conditions such as pelvic inflammatory disease, uterine fibroids, and especially in endometriosis [1].

Although there has been an increasing number of case reports that ovarian endometrioma and advanced endometriosis may be associated with extremely elevated serum CA125 levels, patients with endometriosis have rarely CA125 concentrations >100 U/mL [2]. The American College of Obstetricians and Gynecologists suggested that patients with a pelvic mass and CA125 level above the 200 IU/mL should be considered for referral or consultation with a gynecological oncologist [3]. However, in the last two decades, there is an increase in the number of reports associating unusually high CA125 level over 1,000 IU/mL in patients with endometriosis (Tables 1 and 2). Another tumor marker, CA19-9, is essentially elevated in gastrointestinal system malignancies. Although malignant and benign ovarian disorders may cause elevation, it rarely increases above 1,000 U/mL in endometriosis [4]. In this review, endometrioma cases with high levels of CA125 and CA19-9 were evaluated and the relation between the rupture of endometriomas and these markers was discussed.

Clinical presentation

A 25-year-old nulligravida was referred to the emergency department with a history of intense lower abdominal pain accompanied by nausea and vomiting. She was observed in emergency service due to suspicion of acute abdominal pain. She was transferred to our clinic on the second day of admission. Her menstrual cycles were regular and she was on tenth day of her 30-day cycle. There was no gynecological disorder in her past medical history. Physical examination upon admission revealed bilateral lower quadrant tenderness, and ultrasound showed a large loculated 5×4×4.5 cm cyst in

M. Gözüküçük · S. Taşkın · T. Taşcı · M. Sönmezer · C. Atabekoğlu
Department of Obstetrics and Gynecology, Ankara University Medical Faculty, Ankara, Turkey

M. Gözüküçük (✉)
Ankara Universitesi Tip Fak, Kadin Dog, AD 06100 Cebeci, Ankara, Turkey
e-mail: muratgozukucuk@gmail.com

Table 1 Reported ruptured cases with endometriosis with CA125 level over 1,000 IU/mL

Author	Patient age	CA125 (IU/mL)	CA19-9 (IU/mL)	Ovarian endometrioma (size)	Presenting symptoms	Day of referral	Treatment approach
Johansson et al. [1]	45	9,300	ND	7×10 cm	Acute abdominal pain	Day 2	Laparotomy
Kashyap[14]	28	6,114	ND	11 cm	Acute abdominal pain, lower abdominal tenderness	Day 7	Laparotomy
Caroline et al. [15]	40	6,291	ND	20×10 cm	Intense lower abdominal pain associated with sweating,nausea and vomiting	Day 25	Laparotomy
Kurata et al. [9]	23	9,537	15,653	8×10 and 7×7 cm, bilateral	Intermittent abdominal pain	Day 3	Laparoscopy
Göçmen et al. [16]	24	5,674	56	7×8 cm, at the left site and ruptured at the right site	Abdominal pain	Day 2	Laparoscopy
Rettenmaier et al. [17]	43	2,275	ND	5.8×6.4 cm	Abdominal pain	ND	Laparotomy
Uharcek et al. [18]	53	2,650	In the normal range	7×8 cm	Acute abdominal pain, tender palpable adnexal mass	Day 5	Laparoscopy
Present case	25	11,834	2,257	5×4×5.5 and 4×3×3 cm bilateral	Acute abdominal pain	Day 10	Laparoscopy

ND no data

Table 2 Reported unruptured cases with endometriosis with CA125 level over 1,000 IU/mL

Author	Patient age	CA125 (IU/mL)	CA19-9 (IU/mL)	Ovarian endometrioma (size)	Presenting symptoms	Day of referral	Treatment approach
Takemori et al. [4]	39	380	2,380	12×8 cm	Acute abdominal pain	Day 2	Laparotomy
Yılmazer et al. [19]	22	1,742	171	4.4×3.5 and 5.6×4.2 cm, bilateral	Abdominal pain and bilateral adnexal mass	Day 2	Laparoscopy
Atabekoğlu et al. [20]	41	3,890	289	12×10 cm	Abdominal pain and dysmenorrhea	Day 3	Laparotomy
Goumenou et al. [21]	46	3,504	1,010	Enlarged right ovary (12.8−6.5−5.8 cm) contained both solid and cystic areas	Abdominal pain, menorrhagia and severe dysmenorrhea, severe dyspnea, increasing abdominal distension, nausea, and 7 kg of weight loss	ND	Laparotomy
Kahraman et al. [22]	25	7,900	ND	5×5×4 cm	Adnexal mass	Day 2	Laparoscopy
Ghaemmaghami et al. [23]	26	1,138	ND	5.9×3.8 cm	Secondary dysmenorrhea, pain, and pelvic discomfort	ND	Laparotomy

ND no data

the left adnexal region and a 4×3×3 cm hypoechoic mass with diffuse low-level internal echoes in the right adnexal region. Abdominopelvic computed tomography confirmed the findings of ultrasonography. A full blood count, renal and liver function tests, as well as beta hCG, CA125, and CA19-9 were ordered. Urine analysis and chest X-rays were also ordered. All the blood works were within the normal limits except for an elevated white cell count of 15,900 cells/μL, serum CA125 of 11,834 IU/mL, and serum CA19-9 of 2,257 IU/mL. CA125 and CA19-9 levels were measured by using appropriate chemiluminescent micro particle immunoassay kits (Abbott Diagnostics, Abbott Park, IL)

The patient was observed for 6 days because of the regression of symptoms. There was no difference in ultrasonographic findings between the first visit and preoperative evaluation. Ca125 and Ca19-9 levels were 5,273 and 737 IU/mL, respectively, before the surgery. Laparoscopic surgery was performed on day 8 of admission. It revealed a ruptured endometrioma on the right ovary and an intact cyst on the left ovary. Thick brown fluid from the right ruptured cyst entirely covered the peritoneum. Additionally, most parts of the intestinal and peritoneal surfaces, as well as omentum, were covered by diffuse endometriotic implants. Bilateral ovarian cystectomy and partial omentectomy were performed and peritoneal washings were taken. Histopathology confirmed the diagnosis of endometrioma. The patient was discharged uneventfully on the third postoperative day. Depot GnRH analogue goserelin acetate, (Zoladex, Astra Zeneca, Istanbul, Turkey) was started 3.6 mg/month postoperatively for 2 months. CA125 and CA19-9 levels reduced to 28.95 IU/mL and 33.31 IU/mL, respectively, in 2 months and the treatment was continued with combined oral contraceptives.

Discussion

Endometiromas are rarely seen with extremely high level of CA125. Rupture presence in most of the cases with CA125 level over 1,000 IU/mL suggested the relation between extremely high level of this marker and rupture of endometiroma. In addition to CA125 level, CA19-9 level could also be found high.

One immunohistochemical study has shown that although the degree of positive staining showed considerable variation, all of the endometriotic lesions were positive for CA125 [5]. Another immunohistochemical study demonstrated that the glandular epithelial cells in the ovarian chocolate cyst were stained intensely with the anti-CA19-9 antibody in almost three quarters of the specimens [6]. This difference may explain why some cases presented only an extremely high level of CA125 without high levels of CA19-9.

What is the mechanism of elevation of CA125 and CA19-9 in ruptured endometriomas?

The fluid of endometrioma may contain high level of CA125 and CA19-9 molecules and diffusion of this fluid through the peritoneal surface into the circulation may cause extremely elevated serum CA125 and CA19-9 concentrations. Koninckx et al. reported that the CA125 concentration in the cyst fluid of an ovarian endometrioma may exceed 1×10^6 IU/mL [7]. According to the authors, the thick wall of the endometriotic cyst prevents the large CA125 glycoprotein molecules from reaching the peripheral circulation [8]. Kurata et al. reported the highest CA125 serum level of 9,537 IU/mL in a ruptured endometrioma, which was confirmed by histological analysis as well [9]. In that case, the serum CA19-9 level was 15,653 IU/mL and CA125 and CA19-9 levels in the peritoneal fluid were 160,000 and 208,192 IU/mL, respectively. Kurata et al. proposed that after the rupture of the endometrioma, the cyst fluid spilled into the peritoneum and ascites–serum exchange may cause extremely elevated serum levels of CA125 and CA19-9. An enlarged surface area of endometrial tissue may contribute to the elevated levels of CA125 [10]. We speculated that measuring CA125 and/or CA19-9 in the peritoneal fluid could be offered for the confirmation or differential diagnosis of a ruptured endometrioma in cases with very high serum levels of CA125 or CA19-9. Table 1 summarizes ruptured endometriomas with CA125 level up to 1,000 IU/mL.

Mesothelial cells as a CA125 source

There is evidence that peritoneal mesothelial cells are even more potent than ovarian cancer cells in producing CA125 [11]. The irritation of the peritoneal surface as a result of the rupture of the endometriotic cyst probably causes a major part of excess CA125 in the circulation [12, 13]. Johansson et al. presented a case with extremely elevated CA125 levels whose highest level was seen 4 days after the onset of the symptoms, but persistence of pathological CA125 levels for 4–5 months support the concept that mesothelial cells of the peritoneum were the most important source of CA125 in that case [1].

The CA125 level in our case was 11,834 IU/mL, which is the highest value reported thus far in a ruptured endometrioma. In the current case, we measured serum CA125 3 days after symptoms appeared, and we think that associated inflammatory reaction of the mesothelial cells of the peritoneum due to endometrioma rupture may be a strong contributing factor to this highest value.

CA19-9 is localized in the glandular epithelial cells in endometriotic cysts in many patients with endometriosis [6]. CA19-9 level was also found extremely high as 2,257 IU/mL in presented case. Because no evidence exists regarding the production of CA19-9 by peritoneal mesothelial cells, the same hypothesis cannot be put forward to explain high CA19-9 level. We believe that an increase in serum CA19-9 levels is caused by the spillage of chocolate cyst fluid along with rupture or diffusion of this molecule through a thin-walled cyst to the peritoneum.

Unruptured endometriomas and high CA125 levels

Although extremely high levels of serum CA125 were reported in patients with unruptured endometriomas, initial symptoms and intraoperative findings of these patients resemble each other; we assume that high level of CA125 in unruptured endometriomas is pointing out a previous rupture. Almost in all cases, patients had abdominal pain at the time of hospital admittance, and the pelvic peritoneal surfaces, omentum, and uterus were covered with diffused endometriotic foci at the time of the laparoscopy. All of these cases presented in the follicular phase, especially during the menstruation. Unruptured endometriomas with CA125 level up to 1,000 IU/mL is demonstrated in Table 2.

Conclusion

Endometriomas may be with extraordinary high CA125 and/or CA19-9 levels. Rupture of endometriomas has been demonstrated in most of these cases. Although it required more number of data, endometiromas should be kept in mind in differential diagnosis from malignancy in the cases with very high level of CA125 and CA19-9.

Conflicts of interest The authors report no conflicts of interest. The authors alone are responsible for the content and writing of the paper.

References

1. Johansson J, Santala M, Kauppila A (1998) Explosive rise of serum CA125 following the rupture of ovarian endometrioma. Hum Reprod 13:3503–3504
2. Kauppila A, Telimaa S, Rönnberg L, Vuori J (1988) Placebo-controlled study on serum concentrations of CA-125 before and after treatment of endometriosis with danazol or high-dose medroxyprogesterone acetate alone or after surgery. Fertil Steril 49:37–41
3. ACOG Committee on Gynecologic Practice (2003) The role of the generalist obstetrician-gynecologist in the early detection of ovarian cancer. Int J Gynaecol Obstet 80:235–238
4. Takemori M, Sugimura K (1991) Ovarian chocolate cyst with markedly elevated serum CA19-9 level: a case report. Eur J Obstet Gynecol Reprod Biol 42:241–244
5. Toki T, Kubota J, Lu X, Nakayama K (2000) Immunohistochemical analysis of CA125, CA19-9, and Ki-67 in stage III or IV endometriosis: positive correlation between serum CA125 level and endometriotic epithelial cell proliferation. Acta Obstet Gynecol Scand 79:771–776
6. Harada T, Kubota T, Aso T (2002) Usefulness of CA19-9 versus CA125 for the diagnosis of endometriosis. Fertil Steril 78:733–739
7. Koninckx PR, Muyldermans M, Moerman P, Meuleman C, Deprest J, Cornillie F (1992) CA125 concentrations in ovarian 'chocolate' cyst fluid can differentiate an endometriotic cyst from a cystic corpus luteum. Hum Reprod 7:1314–1317
8. Koninckx PR, Riittinen L, Seppala M, Cornillie FJ (1992) CA125 and placental protein 14 concentrations in plasma and peritoneal fluid of women with deeply infiltrating pelvic endometriosis. Fertil Steril 57:523–530
9. Kurata H, Sasaki M, Kase H, Yamamato Y, Aoki Y, Tanaka K (2002) Elevated serum CA125 and CA19-9 due to spontaneous rupture of endometrioma. Eur J Obstet Gynecol Reprod Biol 105:75–76
10. Barbieri RL (1987) CA125 and endometriosis. Contracept Gynecol Obstet 16:103–108
11. Zeimet AG, Marth C, Offner FA et al (1996) Human peritoneal mesothelial cells are more potent than ovarian cancer cells in producing tumor marker CA125. Gynecol Oncol 62:384–389
12. Barbieri RL, Niloff JM, Bast RC Jr, Scaetzl E, Kistner RW, Knapp RC (1986) Elevated serum concentrations of CA125 in patients with advanced endometriosis. Fertil Steril 45:630–634
13. Bouquet de Jolinière J, Validire P, Canis M, Doussau M, Levardon M, Gogusev J (1997) Human endometriosis-derived permanent cell line (FbEM-1): establishment and characterization. Hum Reprod Update 3:117–123
14. Kashyap RJ (1999) Extremely elevated serum CA125 due to endometriosis. Aust NZ J Obstet Gynaecol 39:269–270
15. Caroline C, Bashir T (2002) Exceptionally high levels of CA125 due to endometriosis. J Obstet Gynaecol 22:329–330
16. Göçmen A, Karaca M, Tarakçioğlu M (2003) A ruptured ovarian endometrioma mimicking ovarian malignancy: case report. Eur J Gynaecol Oncol 24:445–446
17. Rettenmaier MA, Goldstein BH, Stallman JM, Brown JV, Micha JP (2005) Greatly elevated serum CA125 Level in a patient with a ruptured endometrioma. J Gynecol Surg 21:117–120
18. Uharcek P, Mlyncek M, Ravinger J (2007) Elevation of serum CA125 and D-dimer levels associated with rupture of ovarian endometrioma. Int J Biol Markers 22:203–205
19. Yılmazer M, Sonmezer M, Gungor M, Fenkci V, Cevrioglu S (2003) Unusually elevated serum carbohydrate antigen 125 (CA125) and CA19-9 levels as a result of unruptured bilateral endometrioma. Aust N Z J Obstet Gynaecol 43:329–330
20. Atabekoglu CS, Sönmezer M, Aydinuraz B, Dünder I (2003) Extremely elevated CA125 level due to an unruptured large endometrioma. Eur J Obstet Gynecol Reprod Biol 110:105–106
21. Goumenou A, Matalliotakis I, Mahutte N, Koumantakis E (2006) Endometriosis mimicking advanced ovarian cancer. Fertil Steril 86(219):e23–e25
22. Kahraman K, Ozguven I, Gungor M, Atabekoglu CS (2007) Extremely elevated serum CA125 level as a result of unruptured unilateral endometrioma: the highest value reported. Fertil Steril 88(968):e15–e17
23. Ghaemmaghami F, Karimi Zarchi M, Hamedi B (2007) High levels of CA125 (over 1,000 IU/mL) in patients with gynecologic disease and no malignant conditions: three cases and literature review. Arch Gynecol Obstet 276:559–561

33

How to improve the optimal cytoreductive surgery in advanced ovarian carcinoma

Santiago Domingo • Marta Gurrea • Antonio Pellicer

Abstract Advanced ovarian carcinoma is a lethal tumour, and its standard treatment is consists of aggressive primary cytoreductive surgery followed by a chemoadjuvance based on platinum agents. We searched the Cochrane Gynaecological Cancer Group Trials Register of 2010, Cochrane Central Register of Controlled Trials, MEDLINE and EMBASE of 2010. We also searched registers of clinical trials, abstracts of scientific meetings, and reference lists of included studies. One of the goals of its management is to achieve the longest overall survival possible, and the most important survival factor is the residual tumour after cytoreductive surgery, obtaining the best surveillance in the cases where no tumour is left in the abdomen. To improve the cytoreductive rates in the actual management strategy, a change is necessary, selecting the cases not suitable for primary debulking surgery and adding, if necessary, procedures different than the ovarian tumour resection, like bowel resections, peritonectomies (particularly diaphragmatic ones) and splenectomies. This review pretends to understand why advanced ovarian carcinoma should be treated with primary surgery whenever possible and to rationate the use of extrapelvic surgical procedures. The improvement of surgical rates with these manoeuvres can determine the best management of our patients, without clinical complications.

Keywords Ovarian cancer · Cytoreduction · Debulking · Upper abdominal · Survival

S. Domingo (✉) · M. Gurrea · A. Pellicer
Gynecology Oncology Service, Department of Obstetrics and Gynecology, Hospital Universitario La Fe,
Avda Campanar, 21,
46009 Valencia, Spain
e-mail: santiago.domingo@ono.com

Background

Ovarian carcinoma is the second most common gynaecological cancer in developed countries, but the most mortal of them. The American Cancer Society estimated 21,550 new cases in the USA in 2009, and 14,600 women (more than half) will die of this disease [1]. These figures can be explained by the fact that most of these patients will be diagnosed with advanced disease, this is, stages III–IV. These data have not changed, and although standard treatment has improved the average overall survival from 1 year in the 1970s to nearly 5 years in the last decade [2], even in the best circumstances, only a third part of the patients will have a long-term cure rate. The best option for our patients is to improve the interval-free disease with an optimal management. Standard treatment consists in debulking surgery and adjuvant chemotherapy (ADJ). This ADJ is standard, and it is based in six cycles of a combination of platinum agents and paclitaxel, with a significant improvement when platinum agents are administrated intraperitoneally [3]. So, the factor we can modify is surgery. A debulking procedure may not be enough: the goal is to achieve a complete cytoreduction. In this review, we will study the rationality of advanced ovarian cancer surgery and the abdominal procedures the oncologist gynaecologist should be familiarized to improve the complete cytoreduction rates.

Surgery in advanced ovarian carcinoma

The optimal concept of cytoreduction in ovarian carcinoma surgery was stated with Griffith's report in the 1970s, when he observed that overall survival was inversely proportional to residual mass under 1.6 cm [4]. From then on, many authors have discussed the optimal size of residual disease in advanced ovarian cancer to be limiting in surveillance [2, 5–9].

Historically, this threshold of optimal cytoreduction was defined in a 2-cm residual burden disease, and any smaller dimensions of residual disease were considered to have a favourable 5-year survival [10]. This definition was subsequently revised by the GOG, and in Protocol 97, which opened in 1986, the definition was set as≤1-cm residual tumour [11]. But even when a clinical benefit was observed with this definition in several GOG trials (52, 158, and 172), it could be associated to a more favourable prognosis if the tumour left was <1 cm, or even more, if a complete absence of macroscopic disease was achieved [2, 3].

This relationship between surveillance and tumour left in the abdomen was demonstrated in a meta-analysis by Bristow et al. who reported a consistent 5.5% increase in median survival associated with each 10% increase in "maximal" cytoreduction among series with various fractions (median, 41.9%; range, 0–100%) undergoing "maximal" cytoreduction [8]. To establish the optimal threshold of residual disease is mandatory, as the transcendent end point is to get a potential survival benefit with the surgery approach, and do not harm unnecessarily with futility surgeries that will not give any benefit to the patient and potentially, can decrease her quality of life.

Why is primary surgery so determinant in ovarian carcinoma surveillance? Thigpen hypothesized the next reasons [12]:

1. Surgery is able to remove resistant clones of tumour cells and thus decreases the likelihood of the early onset of drug resistance.
2. The removal of large masses likely to be associated with poorly vascularized areas of tumour purportedly improved the probability of delivering adequate drug doses to the remaining cancer cells.
3. The higher growth fraction in better vascularized small masses enhanced the effect of chemotherapy.
4. In principle, smaller masses require fewer cycles of chemotherapy and thus decrease the likelihood of drug resistance.
5. Removal of bulky disease theoretically enhanced the immune system.
6. The patients feel better after removal of ascites and large tumour masses, particularly from the omentum.
7. Surgery alleviates the associated nausea and satiety these patients feel.

By reviewing the literature, some authors question the real role of surgery in advanced epithelial ovarian carcinoma [13]. Up to date, primary cytoreductive surgery has not been shown to be beneficial in any randomized controlled trial. Several retrospective studies have shown that the quantity of tumour remaining is a major determinant of prognosis, but some authors assume that this may have more to do with tumour biology than the cytoreductive surgery per se. More on, the criteria by which surgical success is marked is inaccurate, with tumour residual underestimated more likely than overestimated. The concept of residual maximum largest diameter does not always reflect the residual disease, as one lesion of 1.5 cm is supposed to have better prognose than multiple widespread 0.5-cm miliar lesions. In addition, the morbidity of the procedures employed to achieve a complete surgery can be unacceptably high, delaying the initiation of chemotherapy and diminishing quality of life. So, for women in whom residual disease is inevitable, primary chemotherapy could be an alternative.

Although the concept of biological aggressiveness of the tumour is not well defined in the literature, it tries to explain those ovarian carcinomas whose natural history present in an abdominal cavity with a technical impossibility of achieving a complete cytoreduction. It is long-time discussed whether it is the surgical procedure itself that is responsible for the superior outcome associated with smaller disease or whether the ability to achieve an optimal debulking simply identifies a biologically more favourable patient group. This relationship between the extent of disease and the aggressive tumour biology has been long-time studied, and many variables have been tried to be correlated: the CA 125 levels, the ascites volume, the largest size of metastasis observed in a scanner, the disease affection of retroperitoneum or abdominal organs, etc., but no one has showed a practical consistent relationship [6, 7, 14–16].

More on, no clinical/laboratory/image technique has shown to be a determinant variable in survival, being always the absence of macroscopic residual disease the only variable related to the survival improve [9]. All the trials that have been initiated to answer this question were prematurely closed because of the bias favouring surgery [17, 18].

Optimal debulking rate

Studying the literature, a large account of different rates in optimal debulking, and therefore, in survival outcome can be observed. That suggests that it is necessary to have adequate systems to quantify the extent of abdominal disease and, somehow, standardize the surgical procedures, to achieve a complete cytoreductive surgery. Median and estimated 5-year survivals exceeding 75 months and 50% have been reproduced within multiple phase III trials and large primary surgical series for patients with optimal debulked stage III disease, with the prognosis uninfluenced by inclusion of patients with stage IIIA/B disease (Table 1) [2, 7, 9, 20, 22, 25].

While a randomized trial to confirm the effect of cytoreductive surgery on long-term survival is near impossible because of ethical and practical considerations, description of surgical procedures should be studied and used to increase the possibility of this optimal debulking [26].

One of the institutions which has more deeply studied the relationship between overall survival and advanced ovarian cancer surgery is the Memorial Sloan-Kettering Cancer Center. In their study, analysed various residual disease sizes, they could observe that patients with no-gross residual disease had the longest survival (106 months), but when the residual disease was less of 0.5 mm the survival went down to 66 months and to 48 months when the tumour left was 0.6–1 cm. The worst prognosis was observed when the tumour left was greater than 1 cm: the patient's survival was 33 months [22]. Similar long-term survival has been reported by other authors when no-gross disease is left in the abdomen [3, 27].

One of the most determinant situations in this surgery in order to achieve an optimal cytoreduction is the presence of upper abdominal metastasis. The Memorial Center has recently reported in a series of 474 EOC stage IIIC that only 24% had no upper abdominal disease; meanwhile, a 42% rate of patients had metastasis of >1 cm involving the upper abdomen above the greater omentum. In particular, these metastases were present in the diaphragm, especially in the right hemi-diaphragm, and up to 40% of them with bulky metastatic diaphragmatic disease [28].

Chi, from this institution [22], has reported the surgical abdominal procedures needed to achieve its rate of optimal cytoreductive surgery. Up to 46 out of 465 patients had extension to the diaphragm peritoneum and needed a resection of it to achieve an optimal debulking. Large bowel resection was even more usual to be done (78/645). Less frequent were the next procedures: splenectomy (6/465), distal pancreatectomy (2/465), cholecystectomy (9/465), and liver resection (6/465). If we thoroughly study the extra procedures, different than the ones performed during

Table 1 Cytoreductive rates and overall survival with a primary surgery approach in the management of advanced ovarian carcinoma published by different authors

Article	Year	Number	FIGO stage	Cytoreduction rate	OS (months)
Eisenkop [19]	1992	250	IIIC–IV	Complete, 11.2%	>60
				<1 cm, 43.6%	32
				>1 cm, 42.5%	16
Makar [6]	1995	455	IIIA, B, C	Complete, 9.9%	75
				<2 cm, 17%	45
				>2 cm, 73%	18
Le [20]	1997	330	IIIA, B, C	Complete, 15.4%	54
				<2 cm, 27.0%	21
				>2 cm, 57%	16
Ozols [2]	2003	792	IIIA, B, C	Complete, 35.5%	60
				≤1 cm, 64.5%	38
Eisenkop [21]	2003	408	IIIC	Complete, 86.0%	76
				≤1 cm, 10.0%	32
				>1 cm, 4%	16
Aletti [9]	2006	194	IIIC	Complete, 23.7%	80
				<1 cm, 43%	38
				1–2 cm, 11.3%	22
				>2 cm, 21.1%	16
Chi [22]	2006	465	IIIC	Complete, 14.7%	106
				<0.5 cm, 15.1%	66
				0.6–1 cm, 21.3%	48
				1–2 cm, 11.4%	33
				>2 cm, 37.8%	34
Du Bois [23]	2009	3126	IIIC	Complete, 33.4%	99
				<1 cm, 31.2%	36
				>1 cm, 35.4%	29
Vergote [24]	2010	310	IIIC–IV	Complete	45
				<1 cm	32
				>1 cm	26

OS overall survival

staging (bilateral salpingo-ophorectomy, hysterectomy, omentectomy, appendicectomy, and pelvic/aortic lymphadenectomy), bowel resection, and diaphragm stripping/resection account the 74% of them. So, most of the surgery in case of affection of the upper abdomen is removing peritoneal tissue. With this attitude, the median survival time for the entire cohort (optimal and suboptimal result) was 48 months. Probably, these figures have gone up in this institution, as this retrospective study included patients from the period 1998–2003, and they only performed upper abdominal procedures since 2000. So, as they improved the surgical skills in new surgical procedures in upper abdomen, they moved to different figures. In a series of 141 cases with bulky upper abdominal disease (2001–2006) presented at SGO meeting in 2009 [29], this institution gets a 90% of optimal debulking (<1 cm) with a major complication rate of 29% and a 1.4% mortality. For obtaining 57 months overall survival, they reached an 86% rate of procedures in the diaphragm area and 32% splenectomies. It can be concluded that the more surgery is done, the better survival you get: near 10 months changing surgical strategy. Their experience suggests that incorporation of extensive upper abdominal debulking procedures may increase the optimal cytoreduction rate of primary surgery by 50%. As they have reported, this implantation of new procedures can dramatically change favourably the rates of an institution. And so, employing new approaches in the upper abdomen and extrapelvic anatomic spaces during the last decade, their optimal (<1 cm residual disease) and complete cytoreductive rates have improved in 26% and 17%, respectively, and more interesting, without increasing the complications rate [30].

Eisenkop et al. conclude the same idea finding that cytoreduction has more significant influence on survival that the extent of metastatic disease observed before surgery [21]. Incorporating extensive upper abdominal debulking procedures with standard pelvic cytoreduction (rectosigmoid resection, peritoneal stripping, diaphragm stripping, extensive bowel resection, splenectomy, partial gastrectomy, resection of liver and kidney) not only improved significantly the disease-free survival rate of patients left with optimal residual disease (85%), but also lead to a significant improvement in overall survival, with a median and estimated 5-year survival for this cohort of 54 months and 48%, respectively.

When studying deeply the multivisceral cytoreductive surgery procedures employed by different authors, it can be observed a different rate of bowel resection, splenectomy and peritonectomy needed to achieve an optimal debulking. This can indicate the different surgical criteria and, maybe, the "different concept" of complete cytoreduction. Scholz reports a median survival of 47 months and a 33% survival rate in a 5-year follow-up in a cohort of 101 patients affected of stage IIIC ovarian carcinoma with a high rate of extra procedures [31]. With a high rate of bowel procedures (81% modified posterior exenteration and 19% ileocoecal resection), 56% splenectomies, 39% Glisson's capsule resection and 22% cholecystectomies, and >80% rate of complete debulking, this institution gets 3 months of difference of mean time to disease recurrence (29 vs 26 months) between patients without gross residual disease and patients with post-operative residual disease. Studying these results, 10% of the patients died within the first 6 months after surgery in the no-gross residual disease group, and although it is a one-center experience, that sets out if so much surgery is needed. Near a half of the cohort received neoadjuvant therapy, with a significant worse survival and time to progression in this group. This implies, somehow, that primary surgery should be the first patient's option. We should consider that ovarian carcinoma is a celomic disease, with no near infiltration of solid viscera, and with superficial affection of the bowel serosa; so, the superficial resection should always be the first attempt whenever possible.

Two particular situations deserve some considerations: stage IV ovarian carcinoma and the primary peritoneal carcinoma. Stage IV disease presents an obstacle toward maximal surgical cytoreduction in primary ovarian cancer. Early reports suggested that even with stage IV disease, optimal cytoreduction may be associated with improved outcome [32]. However, many of these reports defined "optimal" cytoreduction as residual disease of less than 2 cm. Furthermore, these early reports identified pleural cavity disease by positive cytology alone. The optimal method to evaluate disease in the pleural cavity is with video-assisted thoracic surgery (VATS). Recent reports suggest the utilization of VATS to guide management of primary ovarian cancer [33]. Findings with VATS can quantify intrathoracic disease and allow intrathoracic cytoreduction achieving maximal cytoreduction.

Near 10% of supposed advanced ovarian carcinomatosis are really peritoneum papillary serous carcinomas [34]. Most of the patients (about 98%) present stages III or IV [35] and that explains its worse prognosis, with a median survival of near 2 years (21–26 months). Although the cornerstone of treatment is surgery, the suboptimal debulking rate is higher than in ovarian carcinoma, as it usually presents with extensive nodular infiltration of the mesenteric, visceral and peritoneal surfaces, and involvement of the porta hepatis, liver, stomach, and retroperitoneal nodes [36].

It would be a simple statement that optimal surgery by itself is the most important surveillance prognosis factor. Surgery and chemotherapy are hand with hand along the time life of the disease. So, when we are pointing that optimal debulking to no disease in the abdomen is the most important prognosis factor, we suggest that chemotherapy is in its best moment to adjuvant the therapy. And this can be observed in the significant improvement in long-term survival with the maximum benefit of intraperitoneal chemotherapy schedules when an optimal surgery has been achieved [3].

Interestingly, one of the “historically” criticisms to primary surgery has been that aggressive surgery often dilates in time the starting of the chemotherapy treatment. The common and intuitive belief that chemotherapy should start as soon as possible after surgery, and especially after suboptimal surgery, has never been demonstrated in the literature. On the contrary, the few published studies [37, 38] in the literature indicate that the time interval has little or no importance, and it may even be disadvantageous to start the chemotherapy too early after surgery.

In light of the above considerations, the cornerstone of management for patients with a diagnosis of ovarian cancer is surgical intervention. Surgery plays an essential role in any stage because establishes a diagnosis and determine the extent of disease and, of course, tries to achieve a complete debulking of abdominal metastasis. This surgery should be done by an experienced gynaecologist oncologist team as it has been shown to improve the patients’ outcome and result in a more favourable cost-effective analysis [39]. Probably this is one of the more real prognosis factors in these patients, and there should not be any excuse to refer an advanced ovarian cancer patient to an expertise surgical team. Recently, a study of the National Cancer Data Base established in≥21 cases/year the ovarian cancer surgical volume in hospital to be associated with a higher likelihood of patients with advanced disease to be treated correctly with standard treatment, being a prognostic factor for overall survival. But in this study, only 61% of all the patients studied had a recommended treatment (surgery plus adjuvant treatment), identifying the above mentioned problem: how many patients are not correctly managed by non expertise specialist [40].

Strategies to improve surgical management

The first intention when attempting a cytoreductive surgery should be to achieve a complete debulking surgery. Different procedures than the staging ones should be considered. Upper abdominal surgery procedures and bowel surgery, the most employed, should be included in the knowledge of the gynaecological oncologist surgeon. But prior to surgery, correct selection and diagnosis of the real extension of disease should be properly done, being the laparoscopic exploration probably the best tool. It is important to describe the most important considerations of these procedures to know the real impact on the disease and to be aware of the potential complications.

Laparoscopic exploration

Laparotomy constitutes the most accurate way to evaluate tumour burden and establish whether or not a patient is suitable of optimal surgery, but it is an aggressive approach if used only to explore the abdomen and to consider tumor resectability. In the last decade, some institutions have matched the laparoscopic exploration in order to assess resectability in advanced disease [24, 41–43]. Advantages of laparoscopy include magnification of pelvic and abdominal anatomy and enhanced visualization of the peritoneum surface of the upper abdomen, particularly diaphragm. It also allows exploring de “traditional” places of surgical contraindications: hepatic hilio, bowel serosa, and small bowel mesenterium. Its short operative time permit an out day patient surgery and a correct strategy of a future surgery or, otherwise, a neoadjuvant surgery. With this more comprehensive approach, we avoid a hypothetic incomplete debulking during an initial laparotomy, improving the proportion of patients achieving an optimal residual disease. And so, with the use of a diagnostic open laparoscopy, Anglioli et al. have reported a 96% rate of complete cytoreduction [42].

A disadvantage with the use of open laparoscopy is the magnification of the disease, increasing the number of patients treated with neoADJ. The laparoscopic exploration can lead the surgeon to believe there is more extensive disease than there really is, creating doubts on a successful cytoreduction. When studying deeply Anglioli’s results, about 10–15% of patients submitted to neoADJ after open laparoscopy could probably be optimally cytoreducted.

Bowel resection

Near 25% of women with advanced ovarian carcinoma needs a bowel resection as part of their primary cytoreductive operation [44–46].

The data regarding colon resection for the purpose of surgical cytoreduction of ovarian cancer and the potential benefit that can be achieved are all retrospective, but all the information published supports a benefit in terms of survival when cytoreduction is clearly optimal, confirming the benefit of complete debulking of the disease.

The most frequent bowel segment involved in surgery is the rectum-sigmoid. Bulky disease involving the cul-de-sac can require an en-bloc resection with low-anterior resection in order to achieve a complete gross resection of the pelvic disease [45, 47–49]. Most women undergo a primary colorectal anastomosis without a protective colostomy. The most important complication is the fail of a low-anterior rectal anastomosis, but usually it is presented with a low rate, less than 5% [44, 48, 50].

The second most frequent bowel resection in cytoreductive surgery is the terminal ileum and the ceccum, because their proximity to the pelvis and usual affection of the appendix [51]. Other important part of the bowel than can be considered to be removed is the transverse colon, because the high incidence of bulky omental metastasis than can infiltrate the bowel wall/mesentery. So many times this resection can be avoided because superficial affection, with an easy finding of a surgical plane for dissection between the fatty tissue and the colon serosa. When this situation is not possible, omentectomy en bloc with transverse colectomy has to be considered.

Whenever possible, it is important to avoid large bowel resections and multiple anastomoses. And also, it has a great impact on quality of life to avoid estomas, as they have not shown to protect a leaking in the anastomosis [46, 52].

The impact on quality of life of large bowel resections is not as important as it can be thought, with a median frequency of two bowel movements per day 6 months after surgery, although the patients should be aware of dehydrations problems, mostly the first weeks after surgery and during chemotherapy treatment [50]. Antimotility medications have to be considered, and also resincolestiramine agents whenever the ileocecum valve is removed.

Diaphragm surgery

The Morrison pouch is, because of gravity, one of the most frequent places of disease affection in advanced ovarian cancer, and, negatively, one of the most usual related places of residual disease in cases of cytoreductive surgery [53]. Diaphragmatic disease can be optimally debulked with several procedures described in the literature, as ablation techniques, peritonectomy and diaphragm resection [54, 55]. The procedures in this part of the upper abdomen should be included in the surgical oncology training programs, as they are determinant in achieving an optimal cytoreduction. As in other procedures, it is necessary a deep knowledge of the liver and diaphragmatic anatomy, basically to avoid any injury of major vessels (retro-hepatic cava vein, hepatic hilio, supra-hepatic veins, and diaphragmatic vessels). Technically, it is determinant to do a complete liver mobilization at the beginning of the surgical procedure in order to avoid difficulties in the diaphragm suturing in case that a closure of a defect is needed. Even if part of the muscle is removed, there are not usually problems in making a closure without tension. Although rarely needed, a permanent mesh can be used.

The most important complication is pleural effusion, presented in near a half of the patients, and correlates with liver mobilization, size of diaphragmatic resection and the diaphragmatic perforation that can be present in near 50% of the cases [56]. Intra- and post-operative management of this complication varies between authors, but the low rate of thoracocentesis or pleural drainage really needed does not support the routinely use of prophylactic chest tube placement, saving it for patients with a complete liver mobilization and large diaphragmatic peritoneal/muscle resection, situation that can be presented in 7–30% of the cases [56–60]. It is important to teach the patient preoperatively breathing exercises and to have a strict early post-operative pulmonary follow-up. Less frequent complications are pulmonary embolism, hemothorax and pneumothorax.

Ablation systems can be employed to facilitate a complete cytoreduction of the diaphragm peritoneum. And so, the argon beam coagulation can achieve homogeneous and consistent tissue destruction [61]. Using a combination of the argon beam coagulation and the cavitron ultrasonic surgical aspirator with radical surgical techniques, Eisenkop et al. [7] reported removal of all visible tumour in 85.3% of 163 consecutive patients with advanced ovarian cancer presented for primary cytoreductive surgery. This study demonstrated that complete surgical elimination of all macroscopic disease was feasible and associated with prolonged survival.

Splenectomy

To perform optimal cytoreductive surgery in patients with advanced ovarian cancer, it is often necessary to perform a splenectomy, many times because of the extension of the omentum invasion. The surgical technique is well described in the literature [62, 63]. When splenic lesions are macroscopically suspected during cytoreductive surgery for an ovarian cancer, up to 80% of the cases the disease is confirmed by histology, justifying the splenectomy [64].

Up to 13% of the splenectomy indications can be due to intra-operative trauma, frequently observed during omentum debulking, omentum manoeuvres and large bowel dissection [65].

After a splenectomy, a number of considerations should be taken into account. Changes typically occur in the blood composition, and frequently leukocytosis, trombocytosis and Howell–Jolly bodies in blood analysis can be observed temporally. More serious are pulmonary complications, (lower lobe atelectasis that can derivate to pneumonia and pleural effusions) and subphrenic abscess, many times aggravated with a pancreatic leakage, that can be diagnosed because a pseudocyst [66].

Because the immunological impact promotes a decrease of serum immunoglobulin M, the administration of pneumococcus vaccine, meningococcus vaccine, and a vaccine against haemophilus influenzae are mandatory. And because of the increase rate of sepsis, antibiotic prophylaxis is recommended [62].

Lymph nodes debulking

Retroperitoneal lymph node dissection is well described in the literature [67]. Whether systematic removal of retroperitoneal lymph nodes should be part of maximal cytoreductive surgery or not is still unclear. Retroperitoneal lymph node involvement occurs in approximately 50–80% of women with advanced ovarian cancer, but not always in a bulky fashion [68]. An association between lymph node involvement and clinical outcome has been long established, with a worse prognosis when they are involved. In a randomized trial considering systematic pelvic and aortic lymphadenectomy versus only selected bulky nodes dissection, it could be observed a 25% improvement in progression-free survival in the systematic lymphadenectomy arm, although this did not translate into an improvement in overall survival [69].

Neoadjuvant chemotherapy in advanced ovarian carcinoma

NeoADJ is an "attractive" strategy for patients considered to be suboptimal debulked. Table 2 shows different overall survivals published in the literature when a neoADJ approach is employed. Reasons for suboptimal debulking in ovarian carcinoma surgery may be due to several causes. Probably, surgery related ones are important: surgeon skills, the surgeon "believing" in cytoreductive surgery, the institution and its facilities. But more important are the disease dependent factors, like abdominal and retroperitoneal extension, with affection of the upper abdomen, the small bowel mesenterium, the hepatic hileo, etc., and the comorbidity of the patient (age, other medical disease, and medical status). Indicate a neoadjuvant therapy should be done with caution, cause taking directly this option is potentially worsening the patient vital prognosis. Disease factors associated with suboptimal debulking have a big amount of false positives, and they should not be taken into account only when making up the clinical decision. As it has been discussed above, many reports in the literature have showed the limitations of this clinical criteria (CA 125, computed tomography), with a false-positive rate as high as 62–86% predicting an optimal cytoreduction [75, 76].

The "optimal" rate of patients that should be managed with neoADJ may be "patients whom a primary surgery would result in an incomplete cytoreduction". Identify these patients is difficult, as it depends on so many factors above related. Probably, the rate should keep in a wide range around 20%, as the best figures of optimal cytoreductive surgery are actually around 80%. The problem probably is not the rate of neoadjuvant therapy but the proper identification of patients not suitable for surgery. Nowadays, we have to play with all the tools we can offer the patient in our institutions: the clinical data, including CA 125, the radiographic findings and the laparoscopic exploration.

Recently it has been published an EORTC-GCG/NCIC-CTG randomized trial lead by Vergote [24], comparing primary debulking surgery with neoADJ. They demonstrated similar PFS and overall survival when compared with patients undergoing primary cytoreductive surgery. The median overall survival was 29 months in the primary surgery group and 30 months in the neoADJ group, with a median progression-free survival in both groups of 12 months. It has to be stand out the low optimal debulking rate in the primary debulking surgery arm they published (41.6%), being the most frequent sites of residual disease the diaphragm, the abdominal peritoneum and pelvis (pouch of Douglas, uterus, bladder, rectum, and sigma), anatomical places that have been long discussed above that are technically and safely removable. Again, the strongest independent predictor of prolonged survival was the absence of residual tumour after surgery, situation that confronts with their low optimal debulking rate. The median overall survival for women with no residual tumour (optimal result), those with residual tumours that measured 1–10 mm in diameter (suboptimal result), and those with residual tumours larger than 10 mm (other result) was 45, 32, and 26 months, respectively, in the group that underwent primary debulking surgery and 38, 27, and 25 months, respectively, in the group that underwent neoADJ. Additionally, they did not observe significant advantages between these approaches in adverse effects, quality of life or post-operative morbidity or mortality.

Table 2 Cytoreductive rates and median overall survival with a neo-adjuvant chemotherapy protocol in the management of advanced ovarian carcinoma published by different authors

Article	Year	Number	FIGO stage	Cytoreduction rate	Median OS (months)
Vergote [70]	1998	75	IIIC–IV	36%	24
Schwartz [71]	1999	59	IIIC–IV	67.8%	12.8
Ushijima [72]	2002	65	IIIC–IV	41.5%	21
Fanfani [73]	2003	73	IIIC–IV	71.2%	27
Le [74]	2005	61	IIIC	80%	41.7
Vergote [24]	2010	322	IIIC–IV	80.6%	30

OS overall survival

One fact when performing surgery after neoADJ is that gross disease is sometimes difficult to identify, with the original tumour extension frequently not visible. We can hypothesize that the microscopic tumour burden left is bigger, with more possible tumour resistance clones and so, more facilities for tumour recurrence. Also, after chemotherapy and after a failed attempt of primary surgery, the abdominal procedures (peritoneal stripping and cytoreductive procedures) are more difficult, as tissue characteristics change to fibrosis and neovascularization [31].

Impact on quality of life and morbimortality

Quality of life of patients with advanced ovarian carcinoma should be, with the cure rate and progression-free survival, end points of treatment. Which negative impacts have standard treatment in quality of life patients? We have to consider separately surgery and chemotherapy impact. Surgical menopause, infertility, sexual dysfunction and bowel obstruction are the most frequent observed because of surgery [77]. Population-based reports on post-operative mortality after primary cytoreductive surgery for advanced stage EOC vary with rates from 2.5% to 4.8%, with a mean of 3.7% [78]. This low-operative risk corroborates the current treatment strategy of primary cytoreductive surgery followed by platinum-based chemotherapy in patients with advanced stage EOC. But this figures move to 5.4% till 11.7% in patients older than 80 years, and we should consider to change the management to a neoADJ schedule in this group of patients [79].

But optimal debulking with a more aggressive surgery not necessarily implies more comorbidity or mortality. And so, Soegaard [80] and Marx [81] have reported similar post-operative mortality (4.8% and 4.4%, respectively) with very different surgical outcomes (79% vs 39% optimal cytoreduction rates, respectively).

Conclusions

Actual surgical management goal of advanced ovarian cancer is to achieve a complete cytoreduction of the tumour. This is constantly reported in the literature as the most important factor in patient's surveillance. It is our responsibility to employ different procedures than the tumoral ovarian and uterus removal, mainly outside the pelvis. These new procedures should be trained in any institution specialized in the surgical management of this tumour.

Conflicts of interest The authors report no conflicts of interest. The authors alone are responsible for the content and writing of the paper.

References

1. Jemal A, Siegel R, Ward E, Hao Y, Xu J, Thun MJ (2008) Cancer statistics 2009. CA Cancer J Clin 59:225–249
2. Ozols RF, Bundy BN, Greer BE et al (2003) Phase III trial of carboplatin and paclitaxel in patients with optimally resected stage III ovarian cancer: a Gynecological Oncology Group study. J Clin Oncol 21(17):3194–3200
3. Armstrong DK, Bundy B, Wenzel L, Huang HQ, Baergen R, Lele S et al (2006) Intraperitoneal cisplatin and paclitaxel ovarian cancer. N Engl J Med 354:34–43
4. Griffiths CT (1978) Surgical resection of tumor bulk in the primary treatment of ovarian cancer. Natl Cancer Inst Monogr 42:131–136
5. Hoskins WJ, McGuire WP, Brandy MF, Homsley HD, Creasman WT, Berman M et al (1994) The effect of diameter oflartgest residual disease on survival after primary cytoreductive surgery in patients with suboptimal residual epithelial ovarian carcinoma. Am J Obstet Gynecol 170(4):974–979
6. Makar AP, Baekelandt M, Trope' CG, Kristensen GB (1995) The Prognostic significance of residual disease, FIGO substage, tumor histology, and grade in patients with FIGO stage III ovarian cancer. Gynecol Oncol 56:175–180
7. Eisenkop SM, Friedman RL, Wang H (1998) Complete cytoreductive surgery is feasible and maximizes survival in patients with advanced epithelial ovarian cancer: a prospective study. Gynecol Oncol 69:103–106
8. Bristow RE, Tomacruz RS, Armstrong DK, Trimble ELS, Montz FJ (2002) Survival effect of maximal cytoreductive surgery for advanced ovarian carcinoma during the platinum era: a meta-analysis. J Clin Oncol 20:1248–1259
9. Aletti G, Dowdy SC, Gostout BS, Jones MB, Stanhope RC, Wilson TO et al (2006) Aggressive surgical effort and improved survival in advanced-stage ovarian cancer. Obstet Gynecol 107:77–85
10. Hacker NF, Berek JS, Lagasse LD, Nieberg RK, Elashoff RM (1983) Primary cytoreductive surgery for ovarian cancer. Obstet Gynecol 61:413–420
11. Omura GA, Blessing J, Ehrlich C et al (1991) Long follow-up and prognostic factor analysis in advanced ovarian carcinoma: the gynecologic oncology group experience. J Clin Oncol 9:1138–1150
12. Thigpen T (2004) The if and when of surgical debulking for ovarian carcinoma. N Engl J Med 351(24):2544–2546
13. Carter J (2004) Primary surgery for ovarian cancer. In: Gershenson DM, McGuire WP, Gore M, Quinn MA, Thomas G (eds) Gynecologic cancer: controversies in management. Elsevier, pp 399–409
14. Gemer O, Lurian M, Gdalevich M, Kapustian V, Piura E, Schneider D et al (2005) A multicenter study of CA-125 level as a predictor of non-optimal cytoreduction of advanced epithelial ovarian cancer. Eur J Surg Oncol 31:1006–1010
15. von Georgi R, Franke FE, Munstedt K (2003) Influence of surgery and postoperative therapy and tumor characteristics on patient prognosis in advanced ovarian carcinomas. Eur J Obstet Gynecol Reprod Biol 111:189–196
16. Naik R, Nordin A, Cross PA, Hemming D, Lopes AB, Monaghan JM (2000) Complete cytoreduction: is epithelial ovarian cancer confined to the pelvis biologically different from bulky abdominal disease? Gynecol Oncol 78:176–180
17. Covens AL (2000) A critique of surgical cytoreduction in advanced ovarian cancer. Gynecol Oncol 78(3):269–274
18. Markman M (2007) Conceptr of optimal cytoreduction in advanced ovarian cancer: a brief critique and a call for action. J Clin Oncol 25(27):4168–4170

19. Alberts DS, Liu PY, Hannigan EV, O'Tolle R, Williams SD, Young JA et al (1996) Intraperitoneal cisplatin plus intravenous cyclophosphamide versus intravenous cisplatin plus intravenous cyclophosphamide for stage III ovarian cancer. N Engl J Med 335:1950–1955
20. Le T, Krepart GV, Lotocki RJ, Heywood MS (1997) Does debulking surgery improve survival in biologically aggressive ovarian cancer. Gynecol Oncol 67:208–214
21. Chi DS, Eisenhauer EL, Lang J, Huh J, Haddad L, Abu-Rustum NR, Sonoda Y, Levine DA, Hensley M, Barakat RR (2006) What is the optimal goal of primary cytoreductive surgery for bulky stage IIIC epithelial ovarian carcinoma (EOC)? Gynecol Oncol 103:559–564
22. Eisenkop S, Spirtos NM, Lin WM (2006) "Optimal" cytoreduction for advanced epithelial ovarian cancer: a commentary. Gynecol Oncol 103:329–335
23. Benedetti Panici P, Maggioni A, Hacker N, Landoni F, Ackermann S, Campagnutta E et al (2005) Systematic aortic and pelvic lymphadenectomy versus resection of bulky nodes only in optimally debulked advanced ovarian cancer: a randomized clinical trial. J Natl Cancer Inst 97:560–566
24. Zivanovic O, Eisenhauer EL, Zhou Q, Iasonos A, Sabbatini P, Sonoda Y et al (2008) The impact of bulky upper abdominal disease cephalad to the greater omentum on surgical outcome for stage IIIC epithelial ovarian, fallopian tube, and primary peritoneal cancer. Gynecol Oncol 108:287–292
25. Zivanovic O et al (2009) Upper abdominal disease chephalad to the greater omentum and the impact on progression-free survival in patients with stage IIIC ovarian cancer. SGO 112(Suppl) abstract 1
26. Chi DS, Franlkin CC, Levine D, Akselrod F, Sabbatini P, Jarnigan WR et al (2004) Improved optimal cytoreduction rates for stages IIIC and IV epithelial ovarian, fallopian tube, and primary peritoneal cancer: a change in surgical approach. Gynecol Oncol 94:650–654
27. Eisenkop SM, Spirtos NM, Friedman RL, Lin WC, Pisani AL, Perticucci S (2003) Relative influences of tumor volume before surgery and the cytoreductive outcome on survival for patients with advanced ovarian cancer: a prospective study. Gynecol Oncol 90:390–394
28. Scholz HS, Tasdemir H, Hunlich T, Turnwald W, Both A, Egger H (2007) Multivisceral cytoreductive surgery in FIGO stages IIIC and IV epithelialovarian cancer: results and 5-year follow-up. Gynecol Oncol 106:591–595
29. Curtin JP, Malik R, Venkatraman ES, Barakat RR, Hoskins WJ (1997) Stage IV ovarian cancer: impact of surgical debulking. Gynecol Oncol 64:9–12
30. Diaz JP, Abu-Rustum NR, Sonoda Y, Downey RJ, Park BJ, Flores RM et al (2010) Video-assisted thoracic surgery (VATS) evaluation of pleural effusions in patients with newly diagnosed advanced ovarian carcinoma can influence the primary management choice for these patients. Gynecol Oncol 116:483–488
31. Fromme GL, Gershenson DM, Silva E (1990) Papillary serous carcinoma of the peritoneum. Obstet Gynecol 75:89–95
32. Ben-Baruch G, Sivan E, Moran O, Rizel S, Menczer J, Seidman D (1996) Primary peritoneal serous papillary carcinoma: a study of 25 cases and comparison with Stage III–IV ovarian papillary serous carcinoma. Gynecol Oncol 60:393–396
33. Killackey MA, Davis AR (1993) Papillary serous carcinoma of the peritoneal surface: matched-comparison with papillary serous ovarian carcinoma. Gynecol Oncol 51:171–174
34. Flynn PM, Paul J, Cruickshank DJ (2002) Does the interval from primary surgery to chemotherapy influence progression-free survival in ovarian cancer? Gynecol Oncol 86:354–357
35. Sorbe B (2004) Prognostic importance of the time interval from surgery to chemotherapy in treatment of ovarian carcinoma. Int J Gynecol Cancer 14:788–793
36. Bristow RE, SAntillan A, Diaz-Montes TP et al (2007) Centralization of care for patients with advanced-stage ovarian cancer: a cost-effectiveness analysis. Cancer 109(8):1513–1522
37. Bristow R, Palis BE, Chi DS, Cliby WA (2010) The National Cancer Database report on advanced-stage epithelial ovarian cancer: impact of hospital surgical case volume on overall survival and surgical treatment paradigm. Gynecol Oncol 118(3):262–267
38. Vergote I, Tropé CG, Amant F et al (2010) NeoADJ or primary surgery in stage IIIC or IV ovarian cancer. NEJM 363:943–953
39. Fagotti A, Fanfani F, Ludovisi M, Lo Voi R, Bifulco G, Testa A et al (2005) Role of laparoscopy to assess the chance of optimal cytoreductive surgery in advanced ovarian cancer: a pilot study. Gynecol Oncol 96:729–735
40. Angioli R, Palaia I, Zullo MA, Muzii L, Manci N, Calcagno M, Panici PB (2006) Diagnostic Panici open laparoscopy in the anagement of advanced ovarian cancer. Gynecol Oncol 100 (3):455–461
41. Fagotti A, Fanfani F, Vizzielli G, Gallotta V, Ercoli A, Paglia A, Costantini B, Vigliotta M, Scambia G, Ferrandina G (2010) Should laparoscopy be included in the work-up of advanced ovarian cancer patients attempting interval debulking surgery? Gynecol Oncol 116:72–77
42. Scarabelli C, Gallo A, Franceschi S, Campagnutta E, De Piero G, Giorda G (2000) Primary cytoreductive surgery with rectosigmoid colon resection for patients with advanced epithelial ovarian carcinoma. Cancer 88:389–397
43. Aletti GD, Podratz KC, Jones MB, Cliby WA (2006) Role of rectosigmoidectomy and stripping of pelvic peritoneum in outcomes of patients with advanced ovarian cancer. J Am Coll Surg 203:521–526
44. Hoffman MS, Griffin D, Tebes S, Cardosi RJ, Martino MA, Fiorica JV et al (2005) Sites of bowel resected to achieve optimal ovarian cancer cytoreduction: implications regarding surgical management. Am J Obstet Gynecol 193:582–586
45. Gillette-Cloven N, Burger RA, Monk BJ, McMeekin DS, Vasilev S, DiSaia PJ et al (2001) Bowel resection at the time of primary cytoreduction for epithelial ovarian cancer. J Am Coll Surg 193:626–632
46. Mourton SM, Temple LK, Abu-Rustum NR, Gemignani ML, Sonoda Y, Bochner BH et al (2005) Morbidity of rectosigmoid resection and primary anastomosis in patients undergoing primary cytoreductive surgery for advanced epithelial ovarian cancer. Gynecol Oncol 99:608–614
47. Estes JM, Leath CA 3rd, Straughn JM Jr, Rocconi RP, Kirby TO, Huh WK et al (2006) Bowel resection at the time of primary debulking for epithelial ovarian carcinoma: outcomes in patients treated with platinum and taxane-based chemotherapy. J Am Coll Surg 203:527–532
48. Silver DF, Zgheib NB (2009) Extended left colon resections as part of complete cytoreduction for ovarian cancer: tips and considerations. Gynecol Oncol 114:427–430
49. Hoffman MS, Zervose E (2008) Colon resection for ovarian cancer: intraoperative decisions. Gynecol Oncol 111:S56–S65
50. Konishi T, Watanabe T, Kishimoto J, Nagawa H (2006) Risk factors of anastomotic leakage after surgery for colorectal cancer: results of prospective surveillance. J Am Coll Surg 202:439–444
51. Tangjitgamol S, Manusirivithaya S, Laopaiboon M, Lumbiganon P (2009) Interval debulking surgery for advanced epithelial ovarian cancer: a Cochrane systematic review. Gynecol Oncol 112:257–264
52. Cliby W, Dowdy S, Feitoza SS, Gostout BS, Podratz KC (2004) Diaphragm resection for ovarian cancer: technique and short-term complications. Gynecol Oncol 94:655–660
53. Kehoe SM, Eisenhauer EL, Chi DS (2008) Upper abdominal surgical procedures: liver mobilization and diaphragm peritonectomy/resection, splenectomy, and distal pancreatectomy. Gynecol Oncol 111:S51–S55

54. Fanfani F, Fagotti A, Gallotta V, Ercoli A, Pacelli F, Costantini B, Vizzielli G, Margariti PA, Garganese G, Scambia G (2010) Upper abdominal surgery in advanced and recurrent ovarian cancer: role of diaphragmatic surgery. Gynecol Oncol 116:497–501
55. Dowdy SC, Loewen RT, Aletti G et al (2008) Assessment of outcomes and morbidity following diaphragmatic peritonectomy for women with ovarian carcinoma. Gynecol Oncol 109:303–307
56. Devolder K, Amant F, Neven P et al (2008) Role of diaphragmatic surgery in 69 patients with ovarian carcinoma. Int J Gynecol Cancer 18:363–368
57. Gouy S, Chereau E, Custodio AS, Uzan C, Pautier P, Haie-Meder C, Duvillard P, Morice P (2010) Surgical procedures and morbidities of diaphragmatic surgery in patients undergoing initial or interval debulking surgery for advanced-stage ovarian cancer. J Am Coll Surg 210(4):509–514
58. Einenkel J, Ott R, Handzel R et al (2009) Characteristics and management of diaphragm involvement in patients with primary advanced-stage ovarian, fallopian tube, or peritoneal cancer. Int J Gynecol Cancer 19:1288–1297
59. Bristow RE, Smith Sehdev AE, Kaufman HS et al (2001) Ablation of metastatic ovarian carcinoma with the argon beam coagulator: pathologic analysis of tumor destruction. Gynecol Oncol 83(1):49–55
60. Poulin EC, Schlachta CM, Mamazza J (2005) Splenectomy. Gastrointestinal tract and abdomen. In: Souba WW, Fink MJ, Jurkovich GJ et al (eds) ACS surgery. WebMd, New York
61. Ramirez PT, Dos Reis R (2007) Splenectomy in patients with advanced or recurrent ovarian cancer: open and laparoscopic surgical techniques and clinical outcomes. Gynecol Oncol 104: S29–S32
62. Uzan C, Bontoux LM, Gouy S, Duvillard P, Pautier P, Lhommé C, Morice P (2010) Correlation between macroscopic and microscopic diseases on splenectomies performed in the surgical management of ovarian cancer. Int J Gynecol Cancer 20(6):965–970
63. Magtibay PM, Adams PB, Silverman MB, Cha SS, Podratz KC (2006) Splenectomy as part of cytoreductive surgery in ovarian cancer. Gynecol Oncol 102:369–374
64. Eisenkop SM, Spirtos NM, Lin WM (2006) Splenectomy in the context of primary cytoreductive operations for advanced epithelial ovarian cancer. Gynecol Oncol 100:344–348
65. Chi DS, Roberts CA, Abu-Rustum NR (2007) Retroperitoneal lymph node dissection. Gynecol Oncol 104:S37–S39
66. Burghardt E, Girardi F, Lahousen M, Tamussino K, Stettner H (1991) Patterns of pelvic and paraaortic lymph node involvement in ovarian cancer. Gynecol Oncol 40:103–106
67. Panici PB, Maggioni A, Hacker N et al (2005) Systematic aortic and pelvic lymphadenectomy versus resection of bulky nodes only in optimally debulked advanced ovarian cancer: a randomized clinical trial. J Natl Cancer Inst 8:560–566
68. Salani R, Axtell A, Gerardi M, Holschneider C, Bristow RE (2008) Limited utility of conventional criteria for predicting unresectable disease in patients with advanced stage epithelial ovarian cancer. Gynecol Oncol 108:271–275
69. Axtell AE, Lee MH, Bristow RE et al (2007) Multi-institutional reciprocal validation study of computed tomography predictors of suboptimal primary cytoreduction in patients with advanced ovarian cancer. J Clin Oncol 25(4):384–389
70. Sun CC, Ramirez P, Bodurka DC (2007) Quality of life for patients with epithelial ovarian cancer. Nat Clin Pract Oncol 4 (1):18–29
71. Gerestein CG, Damhuis RAM, Burger CW, Kooi GS (2009) Postoperative mortality after primary cytoreductive surgery for advanced stage epithelial ovarian cancer: a systematic review. Gynecol Oncol 114:523–527
72. Alphs HH, Zahurak ML, Bristow RE, Diaz-Montes TP (2006) Predictors of surgical outcome and survival among elderly women diagnosed with ovarian and primary peritoneal cancer. Gynecol Oncol 103(3):1048–1053
73. Soegaard Andersen E, Knudsen A, Svarrer T, Lund B, Nielsen K, Grove A et al (2005) The results of treatment of epithelial ovarian cancer after centralisation of primary surgery. Results from North Jutland, Denmark. Gynecol Oncol 99(3):552–556
74. Marx C, Bendixen A, Hogdall C, Ottosen C, Kehlet H, Ottesen B (2007) Organisation and quality of primary surgical intervention for ovarian cancer in Denmark. Acta Obstet Gynecol Scand 86 (12):1496–1502
75. Eisenkop SM, Spirtos NM, Montag TW, Nalick RH, Wang H (1992) The impact of subspecialty training on the management of advanced ovarian cancer. Gynecol Oncol 47:203–209
76. du Bois A, Reuss A, Pujade-Lauraine E, Harter P, Ray-Coquard I, Pfisterer J (2009) Role of surgical outcome as prognostic factor in advanced epithelial ovarian cancer: a combined exploratory analysis of 3 prospectively randomized phase 3 multicenter trials: by the Arbeitsgemeinschaft Gynaekologische Onkologie Studiengruppe Ovarialkarzinom (AGO-OVAR) and the Groupe d'Investigateurs Nationaux Pour les Etudes des Cancers de l'Ovaire (GINECO). Cancer 115:1234–1244
77. Vergote I, DeWever I, Tjalma W, Van Gramberen M, Decloedt J, van Dam P (1998) Neoadjuvant chemotherapy or primary debulking surgery in advanced ovarian carcinoma: a retrospective analysis of 285 patients. Gynecol Oncol 71:431–436
78. Schwartz PE, Rutherford TJ, Chambers JT, Kohorn EI, Thiel PR (1999) Neoadjuvant chemotherapy for advanced ovarian cancer: long-term survival. Gynecol Oncol 72:93–99
79. Ushijima K, Ota S, Komai K, Matsuo G, Motoshima S, Honda S et al (2002) Clinical assessment of neoadjuvant chemotherapy and interval cytoreductive surgery for unresectable advanced ovarian cancer. Int Surg 87:185–190
80. Fanfani F, Ferrandina G, Corrado G, Fagotti A, Zakut HV, Mancuso S et al (2003) Impact of interval debulking surgery on clinical outcome in primary unresectable FIGO Stage IIIc ovarian cancer patients. Oncology 65:316–322
81. Le T, Faught W, Hopkins L, Fung MFK (2005) Primary chemotherapy and adjuvant tumor debulking in the management of advanced-stage epithelial ovarian cancer. Int J Gynecol Cancer 15:770–775

34

Is the presence of endometrioma always associated with more severe disease?

M. Setälä · P. Härkki · P. Suvitie · J. Fraser · J. Jalkanen · J. Kössi · A. Perheentupa · J. Mäkinen

Abstract The aim of this prospective study was to estimate whether the presence of endometrioma was associated with more severe disease, and with operative findings that were considered to make surgery more demanding in patients with deeply infiltrating endometriosis located in the posterior fornix of the vagina. Ninety-eight patients scheduled for primary surgery underwent complete excision of all visible endometriotic lesions and adhesions by laparoscopy (86 patients, 87.8%) or by laparotomy (12 patients, 12.2%) in four hospitals specialized in the surgical treatment of endometriosis. Endometrioma was detected in 46 patients (47.0%). No statistically significant difference was detected between patients with and without an endometrioma, in the presence of six studied operative findings: total obstruction of the pouch of Douglas (28% vs. 27%, p=0.88), attachment of a posterior deep lesion to the ureter (52% vs. 44%, p=0.43), peritoneal endometriotic lesions (80% vs. 75%, p=0.52), other deep lesions (24% vs. 33%, p=0.34), attachment of bowel to the uterosacral ligament deep lesion (65% vs. 69%, p=0.71), and attachment of the rectum to a rectovaginal deep lesion (81% vs. 84%, p>0.99). Endometrioma did not seem to be associated with operative findings that were considered to represent more severe disease, and make surgery more demanding in patients with deep endometriotic lesions in the posterior fornix of the vagina and with no previous pelvic surgery.

Keywords Endometriosis · Endometrioma · Deeply infiltrating endometriosis · Surgery

M. Setälä
Department of Obstetrics and Gynecology,
Päijät-Häme Central Hospital,
Lahti, Finland

M. Setälä (✉) · P. Suvitie · A. Perheentupa · J. Mäkinen
Department of Obstetrics and Gynecology,
Turku University Hospital,
P0 BOX 52, 20521 Turku, Finland
e-mail: marjaleena.setala@fimnet.fi

P. Härkki · J. Jalkanen
Department of Obstetrics and Gynecology,
Helsinki University Hospital,
Helsinki, Finland

J. Fraser
Department of Obstetrics and Gynecology,
North Karelian Central Hospital,
Joensuu, Finland

J. Kössi
Department of Surgery, Päijät-Häme Central Hospital,
Lahti, Finland

Abbreviations

DIE	Deeply infiltrating endometriosis
RVE	Rectovaginal endometriosis
rASRM	Revised American Society of Reproductive Medicine
BMI	Body mass index

Background

Endometrioma, an ovarian cyst caused by endometriosis, is one of the most commonly found endometriotic lesions. Endometrioma may be present in 30–40% of surgically treated endometriosis patients [1, 2]. It has been estimated earlier that endometrioma could be a marker for more severe endometriotic disease [1, 3, 4]. Among surgically treated endometriosis patients, its presence has been associated with an increased risk of intestinal and posterior cul-de-sac involvement [1, 3]. In patients with deeply infiltrating disease, the presence of endometrioma has been shown to be associated with multifocality of deep lesions and increased risk of intestinal and ureteral involvement [4].

Deeply infiltrating endometriotic (DIE) lesions located in the posterior fornix of the vagina, i.e., lesions in the uterosacral ligaments and rectovaginal space, represent the most common form of deeply infiltrating endometriotic disease [5, 6]. These lesions are among the few endometriotic lesions that can be clinically diagnosed before the operation [7, 8]. Although they are usually quite easy to detect, it is often difficult to know how demanding the surgical procedures will be and how much operating time will be needed to operate on these patients. Isolated deeply infiltrating lesions in the uterosacral ligaments or in the posterior fornix of the vagina are not necessary associated with severe adhesion formation and can often be treated with a relatively easy and short surgical procedure [9, 10]. However, technically more demanding and time-consuming surgery is needed when lesions infiltrate to the ureters or when the bowel is adherent to the lesion, causing obstruction of the pouch of Douglas, or when the lesion infiltrates to the wall of the bowel, causing a possible need for bowel surgery [10–14].

Between 23% and 50% of patients with deeply infiltrating endometriosis have endometriomas [4, 15]. Even though endometrioma is often detected in connection with DIE lesions, severe cases of deep disease can also be found without an endometrioma [3, 15]. We performed this prospective study to find out whether the presence of endometrioma is associated with intraoperative findings that were considered to represent more severe endometriotic disease, and make surgery more demanding in patients with DIE lesions located in the posterior fornix of the vagina.

Materials and methods

Consecutive premenopausal patients who were scheduled to undergo endometriosis surgery for DIE lesions located in the posterior fornix of the vagina were enrolled to this study in four Finnish hospitals between January 2005 and December 2008. This study was performed as a part of a larger prospective multicenter trial investigating the presence of different types of endometriotic lesions and other endometriosis related findings in surgically treated endometriosis patients. Patients were considered eligible for this study if they had not undergone previous endometriosis surgery, oophorectomy, salpingectomy, hysterectomy, tubal sterilization, gastrointestinal tract surgery, or urinary tract surgery. All operations were performed by gynecologists experienced in laparoscopic endometriosis surgery. Patients requiring bowel resection were operated by multidisciplinary approach. Patients received written and verbal information on the purpose of the study and were required to give signed informed consent before being enrolled. The study was approved by the ethics committees of all participating hospitals.

Preoperative evaluation included clinical gynecological examination and transvaginal ultrasound examination in all cases. Patients completed a questionnaire concerning pain symptoms, fertility history, and medical treatment before the surgery. During the operation, location and size of all endometriotic lesions (DIE lesions, endometrioma, and peritoneal lesions), location of adhesions, and attachment of DIE lesions to the ureters were recorded in the study database. DIE was defined as an endometriotic nodule ≥0.5 cm of size that infiltrated to the retroperitoneal space [16]. The size of the lesion was visually detected after lesion was excised. The infiltration of endometriosis was confirmed histologically. Uterosacral ligament DIE was defined as a lesion infiltrating to one or both uterosacral ligaments. Rectovaginal endometriosis (RVE) was defined as a nodular lesion that was located in the posterior fornix of the vagina and that had infiltrated through the vaginal wall to the retroperitoneal space. The stage of the endometriosis was classified according to the revised classification of the American Society of Reproductive Medicine (rASRM) [17]. Only patients with histologically confirmed diagnosis of deeply infiltrating endometriosis and endometrioma were included.

The presence of six operative findings that were considered to represent more severe disease and make surgery more demanding: (1) total obstruction of the pouch of Douglas, (2) attachment of a DIE lesion to the ureter, (3) presence of peritoneal lesions, (4) presence of other DIE lesions, (5) attachment of bowel to uterosacral ligament DIE lesion (with or without infiltration of endometriosis to the bowel wall), and (6) attachment of the rectum to a RVE lesion (with or without infiltration of endometriosis to the bowel wall) was compared between patients with and without an endometrioma. Categorical variables were analyzed using chi-square test or Fisher's exact test, as appropriate. These associations were further quantified by odds ratios (OR) with 95% confidence intervals (CI). Differences in means of continuous variables were compared using the independent-samples t test. Statistical analyses were performed using SAS for Windows version 9.2 (SAS Institute Inc., Cary, NC, USA). Differences were considered statistically significant if the p value was <0.05.

Findings

A total of 205 premenopausal patients with no previous pelvic surgery were operated on suspected endometriosis in four study hospitals during the recruitment time. Of these, 98 patients (47.8%) had DIE lesions located in the posterior fornix of the vagina. All patients participated to this study.

Indication for surgery was pain in 69 patients (70.4%), pain and infertility in 26 patients (26.5%), and infertility in three patients (3.1%). At the time of surgery, 27 patients (27.6%) were using contraceptive pills, two patients (2.0%) were using progestins, and two patients (2.0%) had levonorgestrel-releasing intrauterine device. Surgical procedures performed on study patients are presented in Table 1.

Uterosacral ligament DIE lesions were detected in 88 patients (89.8%), and 47 patients (48.0%) had rectovaginal DIE lesions. Thirty-seven patients (37.8%) had both rectovaginal and uterosacral ligament DIE lesions. The mean of the largest diameter of the uterosacral ligament DIE lesions and of the RVE lesions was 1.4 cm (SD 1.4, range 0.5–4.0) and 2.4 cm (SD 1.0, range 0.8–4.0), respectively.

Endometrioma was detected in 46 patients (47.0%). Comparison of clinical characteristics, rASRM scores, and surgical characteristics, between patients with and without an endometrioma is presented in Table 2. Of 46 patients with an endometrioma, 16 patients (35%) had bilateral endometriomas, 22 patients (48%) had endometrioma on the left ovary, and eight patients (17%) on the right ovary. Five patients had more than one endometrioma per ovary. The mean of the largest diameter of the endometriomas was 3.6 cm (SD 2.4, range 0.5–10 cm).

Peritoneal lesions were detected in 76 patients (78%). Twenty-eight patients (28.6%) had 36 other DIE lesions: 19 patients (19%) in the sigmoid colon, seven patients (7%) in the appendix, seven patients (7%) in the urinary bladder, and three patients (3%) in the cecum. The mean number of DIE lesions per patient was 2.0 (SD 1.1, range 1–5) in patients with an endometrioma, and 2.2 (SD 1.1, range 1–5) in patients without an endometrioma (p=0.33). The association between the presence of endometrioma, and the total obstruction of the pouch of Douglas, the attachment of posterior DIE lesion to the ureter, and the presence of other endometriotic lesions is presented in Table 3.

Of 88 patients with uterosacral DIE lesions, 43 patients (49%) had an endometrioma. Bowel was attached to the uterosacral ligament DIE lesion in 28 of 43 patients (65%) with an endometrioma and in 31 of 45 patients (69%) without an endometrioma (p=0.71, OR 0.83, CI 0.35–2.05).

Of 47 patients with RVE lesions, 16 patients (34%) had an endometrioma. The rectum was attached to the RVE lesion in 13 of 16 patients (81%) with an endometrioma and in 26 of 31 patients (84%) without an endometrioma (p> 0.99, OR 0.83, CI 0.17–4.14).

Table 1 Surgical procedures performed on 98 study patients

Surgical procedure	Number of patients
Division of adhesions	97
Excision of peritoneal endometriosis	76
Resection of uterosacral ligament, unilateral	48
Resection of uterosacral ligament, bilateral	40
Vaginal resection	40
Rectal resection	28
Extirpation of endometrioma, unilateral	27
Rectal shaving	19
Hysterectomy	15
Salpingectomy, unilateral	14
Appendectomy	13
Extirpation of endometrioma, bilateral	9
Salpingectomy, bilateral	8
Bladder resection	7
Oophorectomy, unilateral	7
Oophorectomy, bilateral	6
Sigmoid resection	5
Extirpation of benign ovarian tumor	4
Ileocecal resection	3
Enucleation of myoma	2
Cecal resection	1
Disk excision of rectum	1
Ureteroneocystostomy, unilateral	1
Ureteral resection and reanastomosis, bilateral	1

Discussion

Endometriosis, and especially deeply infiltrating endometriosis, is a disease with very different clinical presentations, and it is often difficult to know how demanding surgical procedures will be needed when operating patients with suspected endometriosis. Any preoperative marker associated with the severity of the disease would be helpful in clinical practice.

Current data suggests that endometrioma could be a marker for more severe disease [1, 3, 4]. It seems to be a common finding in patients with DIE lesions located in the posterior fornix of the vagina, as 47% of our study patients had an endometrioma. However, although mean total rASRM score was significantly higher in patients with an endometrioma, our results revealed no statistically significant association between the presence of endometrioma and the six studied operative findings.

These six operative findings were chosen because they were considered to represent more severe disease and make surgery more demanding. The presence of other endometri-

Table 2 Comparison of clinical characteristics, rASRM scores, and surgical characteristics between patients with and without an endometrioma

	Patients with endometrioma (*n*=46)			Patients without endometrioma (*n*=52)			
	Mean	SD	Range	Mean	SD	Range	*p* Value
Age (years)	33.5	6.9	20–52	29.5	5.6	19–43	0.002
BMI	23.7	5.0	15.6–40.6	23.7	3.5	17.5–34.2	0.97
Total rASRM score	60	31	9–128	24	26	3–114	<0.001
rASRM adnexal adhesion score	17	15	0–64	6	14	0–64	<0.001
Total operating time (min)	157	85	40–520	160	102	30–450	0.85
Laparoscopy[a]	41 (89%)			45 (87%)			0.69

[a] Data presented as *n* (%)

otic lesions was considered to represent the overall severity of the disease. The goal of contemporary endometriosis surgery is to remove all endometriosis which can be very complex especially in cases with multiple deep lesions. Totally obstructed pouch of Douglas, attachment of bowel to the DIE lesion and attachment of DIE lesion to the ureter are often detected in patients with posterior DIE lesions, but not all gynecologists are used to perform demanding adhesiolysis or ureterolysis needed in these cases. If it could be demonstrated that the presence of endometrioma is associated with this kind of findings and surgery, it could help gynecologists to decide, where and by whom these patients should be operated.

In previous studies, patients with superficial ovarian endometriosis and endometriomas had more pelvic areas involved by endometriosis, and endometrioma was a good preoperative marker for pouch of Douglas obliteration [1, 3]. Furthermore, the presence of endometrioma was associated with multifocality, and ureteral involvement of the deeply infiltrating lesions [4]. We also did expect to find out that endometrioma would be associated with studied findings, but although patients with an endometrioma had significantly more adnexal adhesions compared to the patients without an endometrioma, no other significant association was detected.

The most important factor influencing our results is probably the fact that we included only patients with no previous pelvic surgery. For that, we had two reasons. Firstly, postoperative adhesions are often difficult to differentiate from adhesions caused by endometriosis, which would probably greatly alter the detected results. We now observed, that the presence of totally obstructed pouch of Douglas was not very frequent finding in patients without previous pelvic surgery. It was detected in 28% of the patients with an endometrioma and in 27% without an endometrioma.

Second reason to include only patients without previous pelvic surgery was the knowledge that the probability of recurrence seems to differ according to the type of operated endometriotic lesion. The recurrence of DIE lesions seems to be very rare if complete excision has been performed in the first operation, while the recurrence of endometrioma seems to be quite common, even after complete excision of the capsule [18–22]. If patients with previous endometriosis surgery had been included, the detected findings would have been largely dependent on the type of previous surgery.

There is very little previous knowledge of the prevalence of these six studied operative findings in patients with no previous pelvic surgery. Based on our findings, it seems that in general, DIE lesions in the posterior fornix of the vagina have a considerable ability to provoke adhesion formation by themselves, although the total obstruction of the pouch of Douglas was not very frequent finding. Even without an endometrioma, bowel was attached to the uterosacral ligament DIE lesion in 69%, and to the rectovaginal lesion in 84% of the patients. Associated endometrioma probably does not have a significant addi-

Table 3 Four studied operative findings in patients with and without an endometrioma

Operative finding	Endometrioma (*n*=46)		No endometrioma (*n*=52)				
	n	%	*n*	%	*p* Value	OR	95% CI
Total obstruction of the pouch of Douglas	13	28	14	27	0.88	1.1	0.44–2.60
Attachment of DIE lesion to the ureter	24	52	23	44	0.43	1.4	0.62–3.05
Presence of peritoneal lesions	37	80	39	75	0.52	1.4	0.52–3.58
Presence of other DIE lesions	11	24	17	33	0.34	0.6	0.26–1.58

tional effect on adhesion formation in these patients. The attachment of DIE lesion to the ureter was also a common finding, as it was detected in 48% of the patients. Additionally, 29% had other DIE lesions located in the bladder, or in the intestine. When present, these findings represent the most severe forms of the endometriotic disease, and gynecologists who operate these patients, should have the technical skills to perform needed surgical procedures. We believe that the knowledge of the prevalence of these findings could help to plan surgical treatment.

The fact that we included only patients with no previous surgery is also a reflection of the small number of study patients. A large number of endometriosis patients undergo repeated surgery for endometriosis, and therefore it is very difficult to obtain a large enough study population, especially if only certain types of endometriosis patients are studied. Due to the relatively small sample size, our result needs to be interpreted with caution. The nonsignificant p values could reflect either the fact that the true effect is nil or the fact that our study had low power. A larger prospective study with a proper power calculation based on the prevalence of these operative findings in patients with no previous pelvic surgery would be needed to confirm our results.

Conclusions

It would be very useful if it could be demonstrated that endometrioma is also a practical marker for more severe disease in patients with posterior DIE lesions, as that would enable more individually tailored planning of surgical treatment and more detailed patient counseling. However, at least in this cohort of patients with DIE lesions in the posterior fornix of the vagina and with no previous pelvic surgery, the presence of endometrioma did not seem to be associated with operative findings that were considered to make surgery more demanding.

Acknowledgments This study was supported by a grant from the Research Fund of The Joint Authority for Päijät-Häme Social and Health Care. We would wish to thank statistician Jaakko Matomäki for expert help with the statistical analysis, and study nurse Minna Tuuri for her assistance in this study.

Declaration of interest The authors report no conflicts of interest. The authors alone are responsible for the content and writing of the paper.

References

1. Redwine DB (1999) Ovarian endometriosis: a marker for more extensive pelvic and intestinal disease. Fertil Steril 72(2):310–315
2. Vercellini P, Fedele L, Aimi G, De Giorgi O, Consonni D, Crosignani PG (2006) Reproductive performance, pain recurrence and disease relapse after conservative surgical treatment for endometriosis: the predictive value of the current classification system. Hum Reprod 21(10):2679–2685. doi:10.1093/humrep/del230
3. Banerjee SK, Ballard KD, Wright JT (2008) Endometriomas as a marker of disease severity. J Minim Invasive Gynecol 15(5):538–540. doi:10.1016/j.jmig.2008.05.004
4. Chapron C, Pietin-Vialle C, Borghese B, Davy C, Foulot H, Chopin N (2009) Associated ovarian endometrioma is a marker for greater severity of deeply infiltrating endometriosis. Fertil Steril 92(2):453–457. doi:10.1016/j.fertnstert.2008.06.003
5. Chapron C, Fauconnier A, Vieira M, Barakat H, Dousset B, Pansini V, Vacher-Lavenu MC, Dubuisson JB (2003) Anatomical distribution of deeply infiltrating endometriosis: surgical implications and proposition for a classification. Hum Reprod 18(1):157–161
6. Chapron C, Chopin N, Borghese B, Foulot H, Dousset B, Vacher-Lavenu MC, Vieira M, Hasan W, Bricou A (2006) Deeply infiltrating endometriosis: pathogenetic implications of the anatomical distribution. Hum Reprod 21(7):1839–1845. doi:10.1093/humrep/del079
7. Koninckx PR, Oosterlynck D, D'Hooghe T, Meuleman C (1994) Deeply infiltrating endometriosis is a disease whereas mild endometriosis could be considered a non-disease. Ann NY Acad Sci 734:333–341
8. Wright JT (2000) The diagnosis and management of infiltrating nodular recto-vaginal endometriosis. Curr Opin Obstet Gynecol 12(4):283–287
9. Chapron C, Dubuisson JB (1996) Laparoscopic treatment of deep endometriosis located on the uterosacral ligaments. Hum Reprod 11(4):868–873
10. Martin DC, Batt RE (2001) Retrocervical, retrovaginal pouch, and rectovaginal septum endometriosis. J Am Assoc Gynecol Laparosc 8(1):12–17
11. Chapron C, Dubuisson JB, Fritel X, Fernandez B, Poncelet C, Beguin S, Pinelli L (1999) Operative management of deep endometriosis infiltrating the uterosacral ligaments. J Am Assoc Gynecol Laparosc 6(1):31–37
12. Redwine DB, Wright JT (2001) Laparoscopic treatment of complete obliteration of the cul-de-sac associated with endometriosis: long-term follow-up of en bloc resection. Fertil Steril 76 (2):358–365
13. Ford J, English J, Miles WA, Giannopoulos T (2004) Pain, quality of life and complications following the radical resection of rectovaginal endometriosis. BJOG 111(4):353–356
14. Darai E, Marpeau O, Thomassin I, Dubernard G, Barranger E, Bazot M (2005) Fertility after laparoscopic colorectal resection for endometriosis: preliminary results. Fertil Steril 84(4):945–950. doi:10.1016/j.fertnstert.2005.04.037
15. Somigliana E, Infantino M, Candiani M, Vignali M, Chiodini A, Busacca M (2004) Association rate between deep peritoneal endometriosis and other forms of the disease: pathogenetic implications. Hum Reprod 19(1):168–171
16. Cornillie FJ, Oosterlynck D, Lauweryns JM, Koninckx PR (1990) Deeply infiltrating pelvic endometriosis: histology and clinical significance. Fertil Steril 53(6):978–983
17. American Society for Reproductive Medicine (1997) Revised American Society for Reproductive Medicine classification of endometriosis: 1996. Fertil Steril 67(5):817–821
18. Fedele L, Bianchi S, Zanconato G, Bettoni G, Gotsch F (2004) Long-term follow-up after conservative surgery for rectovaginal endometriosis. Am J Obstet Gynecol 190(4):1020–1024. doi:10.1016/j.ajog.2003.10.698
19. Parazzini F, Bertulessi C, Pasini A, Rosati M, Di Stefano F, Shonauer S, Vicino M, Aguzzoli L, Trossarelli GF, Massobrio M,

Bracco G, Perino A, Moroni S, Beretta P (2005) Determinants of short-term recurrence rate of endometriosis. Eur J Obstet Gynecol Reprod Biol 121(2):216–219. doi:10.1016/j.ejogrb.2004.11.033

20. Angioni S, Peiretti M, Zirone M, Palomba M, Mais V, Gomel V, Melis GB (2006) Laparoscopic excision of posterior vaginal fornix in the treatment of patients with deep endometriosis without rectum involvement: surgical treatment and long-term follow-up. Hum Reprod 21(6):1629–1634. doi:10.1093/humrep/del006
21. Fedele L, Bianchi S, Zanconato G, Berlanda N, Raffaelli R, Fontana E (2006) Laparoscopic excision of recurrent endometriomas: long-term outcome and comparison with primary surgery. Fertil Steril 85(3):694–699. doi:10.1016/j.fertnstert.2005.08.028
22. Koga K, Takemura Y, Osuga Y, Yoshino O, Hirota Y, Hirata T, Morimoto C, Harada M, Yano T, Taketani Y (2006) Recurrence of ovarian endometrioma after laparoscopic excision. Hum Reprod 21(8):2171–2174. doi:10.1093/humrep/del125

35

A pragmatic evaluation of sleep patterns before gynecologic surgery

Boaz Sheizaf · Beniamin Almog · Kareemah Salamah · Fady Shehata · Janet Takefman · Togas Tulandi

Abstract The aim of this study was to evaluate preoperative sleep patterns in-patients scheduled for elective endoscopic surgery and to compare sleep characteristics before different types of endoscopic procedures. A prospective survey cohort study (Canadian Task Force classification II-2) was designed to evaluate quantitative and qualitative (score 1–7) sleep parameters. Patients completed sleep-monitoring forms on the baseline (6 weeks before surgery), two nights (night-2), and the night before surgery (night-1). Of a total 119 women, 73 (61%) underwent laparoscopies and 46 (39%) hysteroscopies. Forty-seven (40%) operations involved organ removal and 72 (60%) were reconstructive surgery. The mean overall sleep-quality score on night-1 (3.29±0.15) was higher (worse) than on baseline (2.09±0.10, $P<0.0001$) and night-2 (2.45±0.11, $P<0.001$, respectively). Patients reported more difficulty falling asleep on night-1 (2.53±0.15) than on baseline (1.61±0.09, $P<0.0001$) and night-2 (1.84±0.12, $P=0.001$, respectively). The mean number of nocturnal awaking events was also highest on night-1 (1.52±0.17) than on baseline (0.69±0.09, $P<0.001$) and night-2 (0.87±0.09, $P<0.05$ respectively). Using logistic regression, we found that age, stress level, and time before surgery (baseline, night-2, night-1), were significant predictors of poor sleep. The type of planned surgery did not influence the quality of sleep. Falling asleep on night-1 took longer than on baseline and night-2. There was no difference in the sleep quality measures between the baseline and night-2. Poor sleep quality is common mainly in the night before surgery. The nature and extent of planned surgery do not affect sleep quality variables.

Keywords Sleep · Gynecologic surgery · Surgery · Preoperative

B. Sheizaf · B. Almog · K. Salamah · F. Shehata · J. Takefman · T. Tulandi (✉)
Department of Obstetrics and Gynecology, McGill University, 687 Pine Avenue West,
Montreal, QC, Canada H3A 1A1
e-mail: togas.tulandi@mcgill.ca

Background

Sleep is essential to maintain body energy and for quality of life [1, 2]. The quality of sleep influences health and day time function [3], and it is independently related to various physiological systems [4]. Sleep deprivation is recognized as a stressor [5], but it can also result from stress.

As surgery is one of the most stressful events physically and mentally, it could be associated with sleep disturbances [6, 7]. Murphy et al. [5] performed a survey examining perioperative sleep patterns in 110 in-hospital patients who were admitted for abdominal surgery. They found a reduction in the mean duration of sleep before and up to 10 days after surgery. The deficit was mainly due to early awakening.

In another study, Kavey and Ahshuler [8] evaluated sleep patterns of ten elective herniorrhaphy patients. They used continuous polysomnography from night 1 of hospitalization until discharge on day 4 or 5. The patients showed loss of REM (rapid eye movement) and deep phases of sleep in the first two postoperative nights, with a gradual return toward normal sleep over the hospitalization period.

Gogenur et al. [9] studied 12 patients undergoing laparoscopic cholecystectomy and 15 others undergoing laparotomy. They used a sleep questionnaire starting 4 days before surgery until 4 weeks postoperatively. They concluded that immediately after a laparotomy, total sleep time increased (probably due to the use of opioids) and there was a change in diurnal sleep distribution. These alterations were less pronounced after laparoscopy. Sleep pattern was disturbed for 4 weeks after major abdominal surgery but only for 1 week after laparoscopic cholecystectomy. On the other hand, Rosenberg et al. [10] found that among ten patients undergoing laparoscopic cholecystectomy, there was no significant difference in the sleep between the night before operation and the first night after operation.

Those studies focused mainly on postoperative sleep pattern while that before surgery generally served as a baseline. In fact, sleep quality a few days before surgery has never been thoroughly investigated. The objectives of our study were to evaluate and describe preoperative sleep patterns in women undergoing gynecologic endoscopic surgery. Increased knowledge of this subject may direct therapy of perioperative sleep disturbances, hence improving quality of life and patient's satisfaction.

Methods

We conducted a prospective survey among 119 women scheduled to undergo gynecologic endoscopic surgery for benign condition by a single surgeon over a period of 8 months. Women with a known sleep disorder, psychological or mental illness, or inability to complete the study questionnaire in English or French were excluded from the study. The study was approved by the Institutional Review Board of the Sir Mortimer B. Davis, Jewish General Hospital, Montreal, Quebec.

After recruitment, the participants were asked to complete a baseline Sleep Monitoring Form (SMF) under the direction of one of the investigators (BS or KS). The SMF comprises of three groups of questionnaires:

a) Objective (quantitative) queries consists of estimated time the patient went to bed, time to fall asleep, time of morning waking, and the number of nocturnal waking events. These queries are designed to evaluate the three main types of sleep disturbances: difficulty falling asleep, interrupted sleep, and early morning awaking [11].
b) Subjective queries assesses sleep quality on a visual analog scale and consist of the difficulty of falling asleep, the extent of sleep interruption, overall quality of sleep, and the quality of sleep compared with the typical night-sleep.
c) Subjective queries assessing stress level.

The baseline SMF was completed 6 weeks before surgery in the clinic. The participants were then given the SMF and were asked to complete it at home daily, during morning hours. Initially, we asked the patients to complete the questionnaire starting 6 days before surgery until the morning of surgery. However, our preliminary study in 15 patients showed no difference in the sleep patterns between the baselines and sixth to third preoperative nights. Accordingly, we evaluated only the last two preoperative nights before surgery.

All patients were admitted in the morning of surgery and no patient spent the preoperative nights in the hospital. Surgery was performed by a single primary surgeon (TT).

Statistical analysis Data were analyzed using the StatsDirect software (StatsDirect Ltd, Altrincham, Cheshire, UK) and PASW Statistics v18 (formerly SPSS Statistics, Chicago, IL, USA). We used Shapiro Wilks test to evaluate the distribution of the data. Normally distributed data were analyzed using Student t test, skewed data with Mann–Whitney U test, and proportion with Chi-square test or Fisher's exact test when appropriate. We calculated the means and standard errors for the quantifiable and qualitative sleep variables along the various stages of the preoperative period (defined as "timing"). The second preoperative night was termed night-2 and the last preoperative night was termed night-1. Sleep quality was evaluated by the questionnaires and by a composite poor sleep end point. Sleep was defined as poor if the score of any one of the quality assessing variables (difficulty of falling asleep, extent of sleep interruption, overall sleep quality) was five or higher, and/or more than two events of nocturnal waking were reported.

In addition, we compared the results by three different subgroups: hysteroscopy vs. laparoscopy, organ removal surgery (hysterectomy, oophorectomy, salpingectomy, salpingo-oophorectomy) vs. reconstructive surgery (myomectomy, cystectomy, polypectomy, tubal re-anastomosis, etc.) and major surgery (hysterectomy, laparoscopic myomectomy) vs. non-major surgery. Multivariate logistic regression was constructed to evaluate the effect of various possible predictors on the composite end point of poor sleep throughout the preoperative period. The variables used in the regression included patient age, type of operation (laparoscopy vs. hysteroscopy), nature of operation (organ removal vs. reconstructive surgery), extent of surgery (major vs. minor), and time (baseline night, night -2, and night -1). P value of less than 0.05 was required to reject the null hypothesis.

Findings

The mean age of the patients was 40.3±0.7 years. Of a total 119 women, 73 (61%) underwent laparoscopy and 46 (39%) others underwent hysteroscopy. Forty-seven (40%) of operations involved organ removal and 72 (60%) others were reconstructive surgeries. Thirty-five (29%) of the patients had major procedures (hysterectomy, myomectomy), and 84 (71%) had non-major surgeries. Two candidates for participation in the study were excluded due to language difficulties not allowing completion of the SMF. Two eligible patients denied participation. One patient was excluded from the study after recruitment. This was due to a death in the family (the Haiti earthquake) the day before surgery.

Sleep quality parameters The different sleep quality variables on baseline night, night-2, and night-1 are presented in Table 1. The mean overall sleep-quality scores on baseline, night-2, and night-1 were 2.09±0.10, 2.45±0.11, and 3.29±0.15 respectively. The score on night-1 was significantly higher (worse) when compared with either the baseline night ($P<0.0001$, 95% CI 0 to 1) or night-2 ($P<0.001$, 95% CI 1 to1).

Additional parameters suggested poorer sleep quality on night-1 compared with baseline and night-2 (Table 1). Twenty-two women had poor sleep on baseline as defined by the composite poor sleep end point. More women slept poorly on night-2 (33) and night-1 (60). Of those patients who slept poorly on baseline, all but six also had poor sleep on night-2, and all but four slept poorly on night-1. Poor sleep was significantly more frequent on night-1 than on baseline ($P\leq0.001$, 95% CI 0 to 0) or night-2 ($P\leq0.001$, 95% CI 0 to 0). There was no difference in the sleep quality measures between the baseline and night-2.

Quantitative parameters Quantitative sleep variables were also significantly different when night-1 was compared with night-2 and baseline night (Table 2). Compared with baseline and night-2, the time to fall asleep on night-1 was longer and morning awaking time was earlier.

Predictors of poor sleep Table 3 demonstrates the results of the logistic regression evaluating the impact of possible predictors on sleep quality. Timing, age, and stress level before sleep were all significant predictors of poor sleep. The type of planned surgery did not influence the quality of sleep. The same was applicable when laparoscopy was compared with hysteroscopy, organ removal versus reconstructive operations, and major versus less major surgeries.

Discussion

The results of our study show that sleep quality is only impaired in the very last night before surgery (night-1). The additional main finding is the lack of association between the nature of the planned surgery and preoperative sleep characteristics. When compared to either the baseline or the second pre-operative night (night-2), patients on night-1 reported higher (worse) mean overall sleep-quality score, more difficulty of falling asleep, more interrupted sleep, and higher mean number of nocturnal waking events. Night-1 was also characterized by longer period of falling asleep, earlier awaking, and shorter nightly sleep. The latter could probably be attributed to more frequent use of alarm clocks and to deliberate early rising for preparations before surgery.

To date, there is a paucity of information of pre-operative sleep studies in the surgical literature. The few available publications [5, 8, 10, 12], though generally methodologically fair, cannot be directly compared with our research. None of them directly addresses pre-operative sleep pattern as the main study objective. Fortunately, some data is available on the related subject of preoperative anxiety.

Sleep disturbance likely represents preoperative anxiety. This subject has been previously studied and described primarily in the anesthesiology literature. Significant preoperative anxiety was reported in 45% of in-patients and 38% of day-care patients [13]. Others reported preoperative anxiety in up to 80% of patients [13, 14]. Caumo et al. [15] described risk factors for preoperative anxiety in 592 adults. They found a twofold incidence of preoperative anxiety in female patients when compared with males. Other risk factors included a variety of pre-

Table 1 Sleep quality parameters in the preoperative period of 119 women

	Mean±SE			*P* value		
	Baseline	Night-2	Night-1	Baseline vs. night-2	Baseline vs. night-1	Night -2 vs. night-1
No. of nocturnal waking	0.69±0.09	0.87±0.09	1.52±0.17	0.1	0.0002	0.01
Difficulty falling asleep (1–7)	1.61±0.09	1.84±0.12	2.53±0.15	0.3	<0.0001	0.0005
Interrupted sleep (1–7)	1.73±0.10	1.95±0.11	2.94±0.17	0.2	<0.0001	<0.0001
Overall sleep quality (1–7)	2.09±0.10	2.45±0.11	3.29±0.15	0.06	<0.0001	0.0001
Stress before sleep (1–7)	1.53±0.08	2.17±0.14	3.26±0.18	0.002	<0.0001	< 0.0001

night-1 one night before surgery, *night-2* = two nights before surgery, SE = standard error

Table 2 Quantitative sleep parameters in the preoperative period of 119 women

	Mean±SE			*P* value		
	Baseline	Night-2	Night-1	Baseline vs. night-2	Baseline vs. night-1	Night-2 Vs. night-1
Bed time (hh:mm)	22:47±00:04	23:12±00:06	22:34±00:16	0.002	0.3	0.07
Falling asleep (hh:mm)	23:07±00:04	23:36±00:05	23:24±00:13	0.0009	0.01	0.51
Time to fall asleep (min)	20±2	24±2	38±5	0.3	0.0004	0.01
Waking time (hh:mm)	06:40±00:05	08:34±12:46	05:31±00:14	<0.0001	<0.0001	<0.0001
Sleep duration (min)	453±6	465±7	367±8	0.11	<0.0001	<0.0001

Night-1 one night before surgery, *Night-2* two nights before surgery, *SE* standard error. *hh* hours; mm minutes

existing psychiatric disorders, high education, and poor general health state. A previous surgery decreased the risk for preoperative anxiety.

Contrary to our findings, one study showed that the risk of having anxiety was highest in-patients scheduled to medium surgeries [15]. Whether this discrepancy is related to hospitalization before surgery or the type of surgery is unclear. All our patients underwent minimally invasive operations. Besides hysterectomized patients, others were discharged the day of surgery. Perhaps, the patient's background, personality, and individual perceptions play more important roles than the type of planned surgery. Furthermore, our patients underwent surgery for benign condition. Accordingly, cancer phobia, an important contributor to preoperative stress, was probably non-existent.

The significantly poor sleep only in the very last preoperative night suggests a late psychological change when the threat of surgery becomes imminent. Whether deterioration in sleep quality begins earlier in the preoperative period and gradually becomes more severe remain to be examined in a larger study or using more sensitive testing method such as polysomnography. However, this test has an inherent limit of the sample size, and it is not applicable to the patient's natural environment. Furthermore, it is expensive, time-consuming, and requires skilled personnel for testing and interpretation of data [16]. Polysomnography is suitable for evaluation of patients with certain pathologies such as obstructive sleep apnea or chronic sleeping disorders. It is not the tool of choice for large-scale studies with healthy population like ours. Our study is a pragmatic way to evaluate sleep pattern.

Pre operative sleep disturbances are probably triggered by the same factors producing preoperative anxiety including fear of surgery, anesthesia and death, anticipation of postoperative pain, temporary separation from family or friends, incapacitation, and loss of independence [17]. Poor sleep as a marker of anxiety can possibly predict reactions such as increased intraoperative anesthetic requirements [14, 18], more difficult control of postoperative pain [19, 20] and higher or more frequent requirement of self administered analgesia [18]. Patients, who report poor quality of sleep, may also report lower satisfaction with treatment and overall quality of life.

Sleep may have a direct effect on physiological systems, not as an intermediate of stress. Sufficient sleep may be involved in healing processes. Reports suggesting that sleep deprivation per se adversely affect the postoperative period or surgical outcome is scarce. Wright et al. [21] tested the hypothesis that poor sleep the night before surgery would predict heightened postoperative pain. Patients (n=24) scheduled for routine breast-conserving surgical procedures for the diagnosis or treatment of cancer were recruited and wore an actigraphy device providing objective estimation of sleep duration and disruption. Their findings did support. Our study suggests that patients might need sleeping medication the night before surgery. Effective short-term treatment for sleep disturbances is fairly simple and available. Benzodiazepines and other hypnotic drugs have

Table 3 Logistic regression: impact of various variables on poor sleep

	P value	95% CI
Age	0.005	1.017–1.101
Type of surgery (laparoscopy vs. hysteroscopy)	0.488	0.323–1.714
Nature of surgery (organ removal vs. reconstructive surgery)	0.691	0.357–1.978
Extent of surgery (major vs. minor surgery)	0.535	0.623–2.489
Timing (baseline, night-2, night-1)	0.001	0.260–0.883
Stress level before going to sleep	0.000	1.196–1.644

Night-1 one night before surgery; Night-2 two nights before surgery been shown to relieve preoperative anxiety. Other therapeutic measures like relaxation techniques or acupuncture [22–24] may also be effective.

This study's main limitation is the use of questionnaires. Questionnaire-based studies are susceptible to certain biases [13, 25, 26] and often address quality of life variables which are of subjective nature. The strength of our study is its prospective nature, and it is the first study evaluating preoperative sleep before gynecological operations. To date, there is a paucity of information of preoperative sleep studies in surgical literature.

Conclusions

We conclude that poor sleep quality is frequent in the night before surgery. The nature and extent of the scheduled surgery do not affect sleep quality variables. We advocate increased awareness of both medical staff and patients to this issue. We suggest further research to examine the value of preoperative sleep therapy, in an effort to improve our care to patients undergoing surgery.

Declaration of interest The authors report no conflicts of interest. The authors alone are responsible for the content and writing of the paper.

References

1. Shapiro CM, Flanigan MJ (1993) Abc of sleep disorders. Function of sleep. BMJ 306:383–385, Clinical research ed
2. Iliescu EA, Coo H, McMurray MH, Meers CL, Quinn MM, Singer MA, Hopman WM (2003) Quality of sleep and health-related quality of life in haemodialysis patients. Nephrol Dial Transplant 18:126–132
3. Alapin I, Fichten CS, Libman E, Creti L, Bailes S, Wright J (2000) How is good and poor sleep in older adults and college students related to daytime sleepiness, fatigue, and ability to concentrate? J Psychosom Res 49:381–390
4. Ferin M (1999) Clinical review 105: stress and the reproductive cycle. J Clin Endocrinol Metab 84:1768–1774
5. Murphy F, Bentley S, Ellis BW, Dudley H (1977) Sleep deprivation in patients undergoing operation: a factor in the stress of surgery. BMJ 2:1521–1522
6. Nishiyama T, Yamashita K, Yokoyama T, Imoto A, Manabe M (2007) Effects of quazepam as a preoperative night hypnotic: comparison with brotizolam. J Anesth 21:7–12
7. Kawahara R, Nishimura S, Taenaka N (2005) Actigraphic assessment of the effects of hypnotics on the night before surgery in relation with the severity of surgery. Masui 54:1263–1267
8. Kavey NB, Ahshuler KZ (1979) Sleep in herniorrhaphy patients. Am J Surg 138:683–687
9. Gogenur I, Rosenberg-Adamsen S, Kiil C, Kjaersgaard M, Kehlet H, Rosenberg J (2001) Laparoscopic cholecystectomy causes less sleep disturbance than open abdominal surgery. Surg Endosc 15:1452–1455
10. Rosenberg-Adamsen S, Skarbye M, Wildschiodtz G, Kehlet H, Rosenberg J (1996) Sleep after laparoscopic cholecystectomy. Br J Anaesth 77:572–575
11. Panossian LA, Avidan AY (2009) Review of sleep disorders. Med Clin North Am 93:407–425
12. Gogenur I, Bisgaard T, Burgdorf S, van Someren E, Rosenberg J (2009) Disturbances in the circadian pattern of activity and sleep after laparoscopic versus open abdominal surgery. Surg Endosc 23:1026–1031
13. Wetsch WA, Pircher I, Lederer W, Kinzl JF, Traweger C, Heinz-Erian P, Benzer A (2009) Preoperative stress and anxiety in day-care patients and inpatients undergoing fast-track surgery. Br J Anaesth 103:199–205
14. Maranets I, Kain ZN (1999) Preoperative anxiety and intra-operative anesthetic requirements. Anesth Analg 89:1346–1351
15. Caumo W, Schmidt AP, Schneider CN, Bergmann J, Iwamoto CW, Bandeira D, Ferreira MB (2001) Risk factors for preoperative anxiety in adults. Acta Anaesthesiol Scand 45:298–307
16. Vaughn BV, Giallanza P (2008) Technical review of polysomnography. Chest 134:1310–1319
17. Egan KJ, Ready LB, Nessly M, Greer BE (1992) Self-administration of midazolam for postoperative anxiety: a double blinded study. Pain 49:3–8
18. Wells JK, Howard GS, Nowlin WF, Vargas MJ (1986) Presurgical anxiety and postsurgical pain and adjustment: effects of a stress inoculation procedure. J Consult Clin Psychol 54:831–835
19. Anderson KO, Masur FT 3 rd (1983) Psychological preparation for invasive medical and dental procedures. J Behav Med 6:1–40
20. Thomas V, Heath M, Rose D, Flory P (1995) Psychological characteristics and the effectiveness of patient-controlled analgesia. Br J Anaesth 74:271–276
21. Wright CE, Bovbjerg DH, Montgomery GH, Weltz C, Goldfarb A, Pace B, Silverstein JH (2009) Disrupted sleep the night before breast surgery is associated with increased postoperative pain. J Pain Symptom Manage 37:352–362
22. Hulse RS, Stuart-Shor EM, Russo J (2010) Endoscopic procedure with a modified reiki intervention: a pilot study. Gastroenterol Nurs 33:20–26
23. Pritchard MJ (2009) Managing anxiety in the elective surgical patient. Br J Nurs 18:416–419
24. Movafegh A, Alizadeh R, Hajimohamadi F, Esfehani F, Nejatfar M (2008) Preoperative oral *Passiflora incarnata* reduces anxiety in ambulatory surgery patients: a double-blind, placebo-controlled study. Anesth Analg 106:1728–1732
25. Smyth C (2003) The Pittsburgh sleep quality index. Medsurg Nurs 12:261–262
26. Yi H, Shin K, Shin C (2006) Development of the sleep quality scale. J Sleep Res 15:309–316

36

Treatment options for dysfunctional uterine bleeding: evaluation of clinical results

George Pados · Dimitrios Athanatos ·
Dimitrios Tsolakidis · Panagiotis Stamatopoulos ·
Basil Tarlatzis

Abstract Abnormal uterine bleeding is one of the most common problems in women of reproductive age, and dysfunctional uterine bleeding (DUB) accounts for about half the cases. The aim of this review is to present all treatment options for women suffering from DUB and to evaluate their effectiveness. A detailed search strategy on electronic databases was carried out to identify trials and reviews on management of abnormal uterine bleeding. Tranexamic acid is the most effective medical treatment. A levonorgestrel-releasing intrauterine device is a low-cost, simple, and effective medical method, comparable to hysterectomy in terms of quality of life. In cases of DUB resistant to medical treatment, surgical treatment should be offered. First-generation ablation techniques are effective, but have a long learning curve. Second-generation ablation devices are highly effective and safe alternatives, thoroughly compared to first-generation techniques. Hysterectomy is the only method that guarantees treatment of dysfunctional uterine bleeding, but is a major operation associated with higher morbidity and mortality rates. Proper counseling of each woman with DUB regarding all treatment modalities can provide the best choice for each patient. More prospective randomized trials are needed to establish the effectiveness of these methods

Keywords Dysfunctional uterine bleeding · Ablation · Menorrhagia · Hysteroscopy

G. Pados (✉) · D. Athanatos · D. Tsolakidis · P. Stamatopoulos · B. Tarlatzis
First Department OB-GYN, Aristotle University, Thessaloniki, Greece
e-mail: padosgyn@hol.gr

Background

Abnormal uterine bleeding (AUB) is one of the most common problems in women of reproductive age, with a prevalence of more than 5% in this age group [1]. Women who seek for help from their gynecologists complain of cyclical (menorrhagia) or irregular noncyclic bleeding (metrorrhagia) that may have physical, emotional, and social impacts in their life. It is estimated that AUB affects 10–30% of menstruating women at any time [2], and about 20% of referrals of women to their gynecologists are due to menstrual disorders [3].

Menorrhagia is defined as excessive menstrual loss more than 80 ml per cycle in a cyclical pattern over consecutive cycles [4]. The duration of abnormal menstruation also varies greatly with an average of 7 days, and the heaviest blood loss on the first 2 days. However, an accurate measurement is quite difficult, and studies have shown that up to 60% of women presenting with a complaint of dysfunctional uterine bleeding (DUB), have objectively measured blood loss above the normal range [5, 6], while conversely there is a proportion of women with definite measured excessive blood loss who paradoxically do not seek for help [7].

In clinical studies, objective methods should be used to estimate the menstrual blood loss. However, in clinical practice the discomfort of the patient and the assessment of the hematological status are the basis for considering an appropriate treatment. Since subjective and objective estimates of menstrual loss do not correlate well, the severity of bleeding must be quantified. The gold standard method of measuring blood loss is Hallberg's alkaline hematin technique [8]. Tampons and towels are collected. Hemoglobin is extracted by a 5% NaOH solution and related back to actual blood loss. Although this method has been modified by other researchers to simplify and quicken the procedure [9], all versions require women to collect their used sanitary wear. In order to create a simpler method of estimation of blood loss, Higham [10] developed a semiquantitative measurement using a pictorial blood loss assessment chart. This chart consists of a simple scoring system of the used pads and tampons and the degree of staining of each item in a way that results in a score. According to Higham, a score above 100 correlates with menstrual loss of more than 80 ml, while Janssen [11] slightly modified the chart and recommended a cutoff score of 185 for menorrhagia. Although the technique is semiquantitative and there is poor correlation between actual loss and chart score [12], Higham's pictorial chart flow is nowadays the most widely used method of assessing menstrual blood loss, although efforts are done from time to time to make the chart more accurate [13].

AUB may be due to anatomical, endocrine, hematological, and iatrogenic factors, though there are cases without any obvious pathology. The latter is usually referred under the name of DUB. It is a diagnosis of exclusion, wrongly used synonymously from time to time as menorrhagia. Dysfunctional uterine bleeding accounts for about half the cases of excessive menstrual loss [14]. It is recommended that women with AUB should be examined in total by ultrasound scan, or preferably hysteroscopy and blood tests (platelets, coagulation parameters), in order to exclude causes of bleeding that can be treated successfully [15, 16].

Methods and findings

The aim of this review is to present the treatment options and the data on their clinical outcomes for women suffering from DUB.

Medical treatment for dysfunctional uterine bleeding

Medical treatment options for DUB include tranexamic acid, nonsteroidal anti-inflammatory drugs (NSAIDs), combined oral contraception pill, progestogen, danazol and gonadotropin-releasing hormone analogues (GnRH-a). The effectiveness of the reported medical therapy for DUB has been evaluated and reviewed in systematic reviews in the Cochrane Library.

Tranexamic acid

Antifibrinolytic tranexamic acid has proven to be more effective than placebo, NSAIDs, progestogen in the luteal phase of menstrual cycle, or ethamsylate when subscribed to women with DUB, without any serious adverse effects [17]. A reduction in menstrual flow by 34–59% has been reported by Wellington and Wagstaff [18], which is quite impressive. However, this drug is mainly indicated for acute or short-term use and not as a definite treatment for DUB.

The main problem with the administration of tranexamic acid for the treatment of DUB is the potential risk of thromboembolic disease due to its antifibrinolytic effect. Although this is always an issue, especially in cases of severe anemia, it seems that the risk does not reach a statistical significance [19].

Nonsteroidal anti-inflammatory drugs

Prostaglandins are found in high concentrations in the endometrial shedding. Nonsteroidal anti-inflammatory drugs inhibit prostaglandin synthesis and decrease menstrual blood loss. NSAIDs are quite effective in cases of DUB compared to placebo, but they are less effective than either tranexamic acid, danazol, or levonorgestrel intrauterine system [20].

Combined oral contraceptive pill

The combined oral contraceptive pill is another effective alternative treatment for DUB, offering at the same time contraception to women. It reduces menstrual blood loss, but there are not enough data to determine its value in comparison to other drugs [21, 22]. So it seems reasonable to offer a combined oral contraceptive pill (COC) in young women suffering from DUB who also seek for contraception at the same time.

Progestogens

The administration of progestogens for the treatment of anovulatory DUB was always a tempting alternative for physicians, in order to restore the natural cycle of endometrial growth and shedding. The oral luteal phase progestogens do not seem to be more advantageous over other hormonal medical treatments or levonorgestrel-releasing intrauterine device [23, 24]. A long-term administration of progestogen is sometimes followed by severe side effects, such as water retention and hirsutism, depending on the type and dose of progestagen.

Danazol–gonadotropin-releasing hormone analogues

Danazol and the GnRH analogues were found as highly effective agents for DUB compared to other medical treatments [25, 26]. However, the administration of danazol or GnRH-a is limited due to their strong side effects. Long-term administration of danazol may cause hirsutism while GnRH-a is associated with irreversible bone loss when used for more than 6 months. Thus, their utility is restricted mainly for short-term use, especially in cases of severe anemia, until further treatment is decided.

Levonorgestrel-releasing intrauterine device

Another medical method for the treatment of DUB is the levonorgestrel-releasing intrauterine system (Mirena®). It was originally developed as a contraceptive method [27], but it has been proven quite effective in the treatment of DUB, so the device acquired approval for that indication too.

Its efficacy is based on the continuous local release of the progestogen (levonorgestrel) within the uterine cavity, which suppresses endometrial growth. Studies report reduction of blood loss in menstrual cycles up to 97%, with its maximum efficacy 1 year after insertion [24, 28-31]. The majority of women with Mirena® bleed only for 1 day or experience just spotting during their period, while 15% of them become amenorrheic [31].

There are two trials comparing levonorgestrel intrauterine device (IUD) with medical treatment, two trials to transcervical resection of the endometrium and three trials comparing Mirena® with balloon ablation [24]. Mirena® was found superior to cyclical progestogens and mefenamic acid, but is significantly less effective than endometrial ablation in reducing blood loss. Interestingly, levonorgestrel IUD was found more cost effective than hysterectomy in Hurskainen et al.'s trial. [32].

Surgical treatment for dysfunctional uterine bleeding

In cases of DUB resistant to medical treatment, physicians should offer to women an alternative surgical treatment. In such patients, one could choose between endometrial ablation techniques and hysterectomy, taking into consideration patient's age, physical condition, and will.

Dilatation and curettage, which is offered as an alternative treatment option in women with excessive blood loss during menstrual periods, results in a temporary reduction of blood loss for the first month after the procedure, therefore it should not be proposed and performed in women suffering from DUB [33].

Endometrial ablation techniques

Since Ashermann in 1948 [34] described for the first time the association between amenorrhea and dilatation and curettage for termination of pregnancies, several investigators have studied the possibility of a controlled destruction of the basal layer of the endometrium in order to treat abnormal uterine bleeding.

Several methods have been developed from the early 1980s for the ablation of the endometrium and have been studied in cohort studies and randomized controlled trials. Basically, all these methods are divided in two large groups with a criterion, the need of direct visualization of the endometrial cavity.

First-generation endometrial ablation techniques

First-generation endometrial ablation techniques are based on direct visualization of the endometrial cavity with a hysteroscope. Three methods were developed since the late 1980s, and their efficacy were studied and compared to other techniques by many investigators. Before the application of each technique, endometrial thinning was necessary by using GnRH-a or danazol.

Hysteroscopic laser ablation The first laser method was a neodymium-YAG laser, which destroyed the endometrium through a hysteroscope [35]. Observational studies have reported a satisfaction rate up to 97% and amenorrhea rates ranging between 25% and 60% after hysteroscopic laser ablation (HLA) (Table 1) [36-40]. Failure rates varied between 7% and 21% in the same studies. There is only one prospective randomized trial comparing laser ablation with transcervical resection of the endometrium reporting 23% amenorrhea rate and 90% satisfaction rate [41]. Despite the promising results of its use, the equipment's high cost and extended learning curve remain obstacles for its wide application.

Table 1 Results of hysteroscopic laser ablation

Study	Study	No. of patients	Follow-up	Satisfaction rate	Amenorrhea rate	Failure rate
Garry et al., 1991 [36]	Observational	859	6 months	97%	60%	Not reported
Erian, 1994 [37]	Observational	2,342	>12 months	93%	56%	7%
Garry et al., 1995 [38]	Observational	524	6-42 months	Not reported	28.9%	14.3%
Bhattacharya et al., 1997 [41]	RCT	372 (188)	1 year	90%	45%	16%
Philips et al., 1998 [40]	Observational	746	6.5 years	89%	37%	Not reported
Shankar et al., 2003 [39]	Observational	174	1.5–9 years	Not reported	24.7%	20.7%

randomized controlled trials

Transcervical endometrial resection The wide use of a resectoscope in gynecological operations allowed its application as a method for treatment of DUB [42]. Transcervical endometrial resection (TCRE) has been shown to be an effective and safe method for treating DUB [43]. TCRE was tested in nonrandomized prospective studies, which reported a satisfaction rate between 85% and 87% and an amenorrhea rate varying up to 46% (Table 2) [44, 45]. TCRE is comparable to other hysteroscopic endometrial ablation techniques in terms of amenorrhea and satisfaction rates [46, 47]. Direct visualization of the endometrial cavity and the possibility of treating concomitant endometrial pathology at the time of endometrial ablation remain the major advantages of the method.

Rollerball endometrial ablation The technique was developed in 1989 in Australia by Vancaillie [48] and soon became quite popular due to its relative simplicity and excellent results [49] (Table 3). Studies report comparable results from its application to the other two first-generation ablation techniques (satisfaction rate up to 94% and amenorrhea rate varying between 29% and 35%) [46, 47]. Rollerball endometrial ablation requires less operative time and shorter learning curve compared to TCRE and HLA [47].

Studies evaluating first-generation ablation techniques revealed quite impressive results regarding their effectiveness, treating three fourths of the women suffering from DUB, who would otherwise proceed to hysterectomy in terms of definite treatment. They are acknowledged to be the "gold standard" by which other, newer procedures are judged [47].

A large retrospective study, though, that was carried out in United Kingdom, caused great skepticism in the medical community. The Mistletoe study [50] reports on the complications of the application of first-generation endometrial ablation techniques and showed that all three methods are safe procedures for the treatment of DUB, with a complication rate of 4.4%. HLA and rollerball ablation are considered safer methods than TCRE, while resection of the endometrium caused more of the serious and possibly fatal complications, which include uterine perforation and bleeding, bowel injury, visceral burn, and hyponatremic encephalopathy with cerebral edema. In cases of performing any of these techniques by inadequate trained gynecologists, the failure rate rose significantly, while serious complication rates increased dramatically [51, 52].

All these issues reported in the Mistletoe study triggered researchers and companies to offer new methods for the treatment of DUB.

Second-generation endometrial ablation techniques

Many endometrial ablation devices have been developed in the early 1990s for the treatment of DUB and categorized as second-generation ablation techniques. Their application did not require the use of a hysteroscope, so the advantage of a direct visualization of the endometrial cavity no longer existed. Therefore, endometrial biopsy prior to ablation is a mandatory prerequisite.

Every method consists of a different device which, by different means (hot liquid, laser, bipolar energy, ultrasound, microwaves, heating balloons, or cryoablation), causes selective destruction of the endometrial layer. These devices require less skills of the surgeon, as they are very simple to use, so the learning curve is smaller. The operation time is shorter, the anesthesia/analgesia can become minimal, and the complication rate is reduced, as all the devices have a self-control mechanism [53].

In some of these techniques, a preoperative thinning of the endometrium with GnRH-a or danazol is not necessary, in contrast to all first-generation ablation techniques [54].

Table 2 Results of TCRE

Study	Study	No of patients	Follow-up	Satisfaction rate	Amenorrhea Rate	Failure rate
O'Connor and Magos, 1996 [44]	Observational	525	5 years	87%	40%	Not reported
O'Connor et al., 1997 [45]	RCT	172 (116)	1 year	87%	46%	Not reported
			2 years	86%	Not reported	Not reported
			3 years	85%	21%	Not reported
Bhattacharya et al., 1997 [41]	RCT	372 (184)	1 year	91%	49%	20%
Vercelleni et al., 1999 [84]	RCT	91 (44)	1 year	Not reported	48%	5%
Pellicano et al., 2002 [85]	RCT	82	1 year	63%	Not reported	15.7%
			2 years	60.5%	Not reported	24.2%
Perino et al., 2004 [67]	RCT	116 (58)	1 year	Not reported	23%	Not reported
			3 years	Not reported	24%	
	RCT	51	1 year	79%	29%	Not reported

randomized controlled trials

Table 3 Results of rollerball endometrial ablation

Study	Study	No of patients	Follow-up	Satisfaction rate	Amenorrhea rate	Failure rate
Paskowitz, 1995 [49]	Observational	200	2.5 years	90%	Not reported	Not reported
	Observational	142	4.2 years	84%	28%	Not reported
	RCT	255	1 year	87%	23%	Not reported
Vercelleni et al., 1999 [84]	RCT	91 (47)	1 year	Not reported	36%	0%
Corson, 2001 [86]	RCT	276 (89)	1 year	Not reported	51%	Not reported
Cooper et al., 2002 [87]	RCT	265	1 year	94%	35%	Not reported
Cooper J et al., 2004	RCT	322	1 year	Not reported	28.9%	Not reported

randomized controlled trials

Thermal balloon endometrial ablation The technique consists of a balloon for insertion in the endometrial cavity and a generator. After insertion, the balloon is filled with hot liquid that causes a destructive thermal effect to the surrounding endometrium. There are several devices that are commercially available: Thermachoice®, Cavaterm®, Menotreat®, and Thermablate®. A preoperative preparation of the endometrium with GnRH-a is suggested, although this is not necessary.

Thermachoice® was the first of the second-generation ablation technique, and its effectiveness has been evaluated intensively. After the application of Thermachoice®, a satisfaction rate is reported to be up to 90%, while the amenorrhea rate was up to 20% 1 year following treatment [55]. Following clinical evaluation of Thermachoice®, improved devices were introduced in 1998 (Thermachoice® II) and 2004 (Thermachoice® III). The efficacy of Thermachoice® III was evaluated and amenorrhea rates up to 32.6% were reported [56]. Thermachoice® has been compared to first-generation endometrial ablation techniques in several studies. Overall, the existing evidence suggests that success and satisfaction rates are equal, while the duration of surgery was significantly shorter with balloon [47]. Thermachoice® is one of the most safe endometrial ablation devices. According to MEDLINE and MAUDE databases, the complication rate of the method, including minor and major, is reported to be only 0.03% [57, 58].

Cavaterm® is the second most often used device based on thermal balloon. Its application results seem slightly improved compared to Thermachoice® in nonrandomized studies (satisfaction rate varying between 91% and 96%, amenorrhea rate ranging between 15% and 68%, overall success rate of 92–98% and failure rate up to 7%) [55]. There are few randomized trials comparing Cavaterm® with first- and second-generation ablative techniques, showing no evidence of significant differences in the rates of amenorrhea at any follow-up time, from 6 months to 5 years after surgery [54]. There is just one limitation in the application of Cavaterm® in comparison to Thermachoice®; Cavaterm® cannot be used in women whose endometrial cavity length exceeds 10 cm, while Thermachoice® can be used even when endometrial cavity measures 12 cm.

The Menotreat® thermal balloon is similar to the Cavaterm® endometrial ablation system. There is only one small observational study in the literature regarding the effectiveness of this device reporting an amenorrhea rate of 10% at 1 year follow-up [59], and just one small randomized control study comparing Menotreat® and Cavaterm® [60], reporting amenorrhea rates up to 19% in the Menotreat® group and up to 13% in the Cavaterm® group.

The Thermablate® thermal balloon was developed in 2004, and since then, various authors have studied the application results of this device. Amenorrhea rate ranges between 22.2% and 35% with a failure rate varying between 3% and 5.5% [55].

Endometrial ablation by hysteroscopic instillation of hot saline (hydrotherm ablator) This technique, although applied hysteroscopically, is categorized as a second-generation endometrial ablation technique. Externally heated saline of 90°C is infused into the uterine cavity through the external sheath of a diagnostic hysteroscope. The pressure used for the infusion is less than 45 mmHg, thus preventing flow through the fallopian tubes. Under direct hysteroscopic view, the hot saline causes ablation of the endometrium. The application experience of the method is tested in several observational studies and in one randomized controlled trial compared to rollerball. Amenorrhea rates are reported up to 53%, cure rate up to 94%, and satisfaction rate up to 98% [61].

Microwave endometrial ablation (MEA®) Sharp et al. [62] first developed in 1995 the use of microwave energy for the treatment of abnormal uterine bleeding. Microwave energy of 9.2 GHz is generated in a magnetron and is applicated by a probe within the endometrial cavity. The ablation effect is achieved when the temperature in the uterus reaches 95°C. In the meantime, the surgeon moves the probe in all directions within the uterus, and therefore, successful ablation of the endometrial lining is achieved. A pretreatment preparation of the endometrium with GnRH-a or danazol is necessary.

The microwave endometrial ablation system has been compared to first-generation ablative techniques (TCRE and rollerball) in randomized trials with similar results in terms of amenorrhea and satisfaction rates, even 10 years following surgery with low complication rates [47, 53, 63]. There is also one randomized controlled trial comparing MEA and thermal balloon ablation, showing similar results in relation to menstrual scores and satisfaction [64].

Endometrial laser intrauterine thermal therapy (ELITT®) The technique was developed by Donnez et al. in 1996 and causes endometrial ablation by laser photocoagulation [65]. Preparation of the endometrium prior to laser application is considered necessary. The technique has been evaluated in a prospective observational study. Satisfaction rate was reported up to 90% at 12 months after treatment, while amenorrhea rate was 71% [66]. There is only one randomized controlled trial comparing ELITT and TCRE, reporting at 12 months amenorrhea rates of 56% and 23%, respectively [67] .

Cryo-endometrial ablation (Her Option®) Endometrial ablation is achieved by a cooling gas, which achieves a temperature of −90 to −100°C within the endometrial cavity. The treatment has been evaluated in prospective observational studies with encouraging results (amenorrhea 28% and satisfaction up to 91%) [53], while there is only one randomized trial comparing cryoablation and rollerball, showing no significance difference in terms of amenorrhea [47].

Bipolar impedance controlled endometrial ablation (Novasure®) The device consists of a radio frequency generator and a single-use bipolar ablation probe. The probe consists of a three-dimensional expandable bipolar electrode, which comes in touch with the entire endometrial cavity, when opened. There is also a vacuum pump within the generator, which provides continuous suction of the endometrial lining and debris; therefore, preoperative preparation of the endometrium is not generally needed. The generator operates at 500 KHz and has a power cutoff limit of 50 Ω of tissue impedance. Once the myometrial layer is reached, immediately the tissue impedance increases to 50 Ω, and the generator automatically switches off.

This method has been evaluated in prospective observational studies and women reported a satisfaction rate of up to 87%, an amenorrhea rate of up to 58%, and a failure rate of up to 3% 1 year after treatment, while amenorrhea rate at 3 years postablation reported to be 65% [68]. At 5 years following treatment, women report an impressive amenorrhea rate of 75%, while the study reveals an overall success of the method up to 98% [68]. There is one clinical trial comparing Novasure® with combined loop excision plus rollerball ablation, reporting an amenorrhea rate of 41% and a satisfaction rate of 93% in the Novasure® arm, compared with 35% and 94%, respectively in the rollerball arm [69]. Novasure® has been compared in prospective randomized controlled trials with other second-generation ablation techniques. In the Novasure® versus the Cavaterm® trial, at 1 year follow-up, an amenorrhea rate of 43% was reported for Novasure® compared with Cavaterm® [70]. In the Novasure® versus Thermachoice® trial, an amenorrhea rate of 56% in the Novasure® arm was reported 12 months after the ablation [71], while the overall cost, including re-treatment in the balloon ablation group is lower [72].

Despite the safety features of the device, Della Badia et al. [73] reported a high number of complications caused by Novasure® in comparison to other ablation devices, a feature that caused great skepticism in the medical community.

Hysterectomy

Hysterectomy is the only method that guarantees permanent treatment of DUB and 100% amenorrhea rates. It is a major operation, performed either by laparotomy, laparoscopy, or vaginally [74], with associated morbidity and even mortality that requires hospitalization for a few days and several weeks for full recovery. TCRE or ablation is an effective and possibly cheaper alternative to hysterectomy with faster recovery although re-treatment is sometimes needed [75]. The CREST study on the complication rate for minor and major operations, reports a 25% complication rate for vaginal hysterectomy and a 43% for abdominal hysterectomy [76]. The VALUE study confirmed that more than 10% of women treated by hysterectomy for DUB reported immediate or long-term complications [77]. These complication rates are significantly higher than those of first-generation endometrial ablation techniques. Despite this fact, the satisfaction rate remains higher in women treated with hysterectomy, so does quality of life [75].

Conclusions

DUB is a common problem in women of reproductive age with serious impact on their personal and social life. Treatment options vary among medical, levonorgestrel intrauterine device, first- and second-generation endometrial ablation techniques and hysterectomy.

Tranexamic acid is the most effective treatment in cases of DUB. NSAIDs and COC pills may be used as second-line drugs, the latter especially in cases of young women who also seek for contraception. Levonorgestrel releasing intrauterine device is a low-cost, simple, and quite effective medical method for the treatment of DYB, comparable to hysterectomy in terms of quality of life [78]. First-generation endometrial ablation techniques have been evaluated thoroughly in randomized controlled trials and found impressively effective in terms of blood loss and satisfaction, compared to hysterectomy. Second-generation endometrial ablation devices have been compared intensively to first-generation techniques in randomized controlled trials and found to have equivalent results in terms of definite blood loss, satisfaction, and effect on quality of life [47, 53]. Prospective randomized clinical trials comparing hysterectomy to second-generation ablation devices are needed to establish the effectiveness of these two treatment options. Surprisingly, there is a lack of RCTs between second-generation ablation devices. This may be partly due to the differences between the devices regarding their ability to treat women with concomitant uterine pathology and not just DUB. However, it seems more likely that there is a commercial resistance in comparing devices due to the possible effect on the market share that these trials could provoke.

It seems that none of the treatment options is significantly superior to the others, in terms of satisfaction, amenorrhea, failure, and complication rate. The role of the physician in counseling the patient is crucial in order to reach the abovementioned goals. Gynecologists should inform women suffering from DUB regarding all treatment options, published application results, and of course their complication rates. This way, every patient can participate in the decision-making process and provide a definite and mature consent, even accept a possible failure of the method [79-83]. Furthermore, the patient should be informed that contraception should be recommended in cases of not achieving permanent amenorrhea after endometrial ablation.

In conclusion, since none of the treatments for DUB is significantly superior to another, and all methods have their advantages and disadvantages, proper counseling of each woman suffering from DUB regarding all treatment modalities can provide the best choice for each patient. The only way forward is to perform well-designed clinical trials on the subject in order to reach definite conclusions on the effectiveness of all the treatment modalities.

Declaration of interest The authors report no conflicts of interest. The authors alone are responsible for the content and writing of the paper.

References

1. National Statistics Online (2001) Census. http://www.statistics.gov.uk/census2001/pop2001/england_wales.asp.2002 Accessed 21 April 2002
2. Prentice A (1999) Healthcare implications of dysfunctional uterine bleeding. In: Smith SK (ed) dysfunctional uterine bleeding. Bailliere Tindal, London, pp 325–341
3. Coulter A, Bradlow J, Agass M et al (1991) Outcomes of referrals to gynaecology out-patients clinics for menstrual problems: an audit of general practice records. Br J Obstet Gynaecol 98:789–796
4. Royal College of Obstetricians and Gynaecologists (1998) The initial management of menorrhagia. Evidence based guidelines no. 1. Royal College of Obstetricans and Gynaecologists, London
5. Chimbira TH, Anderson ABN, Turnbull AC (1980) Study of menstrual blood loss. Br J Obstet Gynaecol 87:603–609
6. Fraser IS, McCarron G, Markham R (1984) A preliminary study of factors infuencing perception of menstrual blood loss volume. Am J Obstet Gynecol 149:788–793
7. Hallberg L, Hogdahl A, Nilsson L, Rybo G (1966) Menstrual blood loss—a population study. Acta Obstet Gynecol Scand 45:320–351
8. Hallberg L, Nilsson L (1964) Determination of menstrual blood loss. Scand J Clin Lab Invest 16:244–248
9. Cannon MJ, Day P, Hammaddieh N, Johnson N (1996) A new method for measuring menstrual blood loss and its use in screening women before endometrial ablation. Br J Obstet Gynaecol 103:1029–1033
10. Higham JM, O' Brien PM, Shaw RW (1990) Assessment of menstrual blood loss using a pictorial chart. Br J Obstet Gynaecol 97:734–739
11. Janssen CA, Scholten PC, Heintz AP (1995) A simple visual assessment technique to discrimitate between menorrhagia an normal menstrual blood loss. Obstet Gynaecol 85:977–982
12. Reid PC, Coker A, Coltart R (2000) Assessment of menstrual blood loss using a pictorial chart: a validation study. Br J Obstet Gynaecol 107:320–322
13. Wyatt KM, Dimmock PW, Walker TJ, O'Brien PMS (2001) Determination of total menstrual blood loss. Fertil Steril 76:125–131
14. Beazley JM (1972) Dysfunctional uterine haemorrhage. Br J Hosp Med 7:573–578
15. Vercellini P, Cortesi I, Oldani S et al (1997) The role of transvaginal ultrasonography and outpatient diagnostic hysteroscopy in the evaluation of patients with menorrhagia. Hum Reprod 12:1768–1771
16. Dijkuizen FPHLJ, De Vries LID, Mol BWJ (2000) Comparison of transvaginal ultrasonography and saline infusion sonography for the detection of intracavitary abnormalities. Ultrasound Obstet Gynecol 15:372–376
17. Lethaby A, Farquhar C, Cooke I (2000) Antifibrinolytics for heavy menstrual bleeding. Cochrane Database Syst Rev (4): CD000249
18. Wellington K, Wagstaff AJ (2003) Tranexamic acid: a review of its use in the management of menorrhagia. Drugs 63(13):1417–1433
19. Sundstrom A, Seaman H et al (2009) The risk of venous thromboembolism associated with the use of tranexamic acid and other drugs used to treat menorrhagia: a case-control study using the General Practice Research Database. BJOG 116 (1):91–97
20. Lethaby A, Augood C, Duckitt K, Farquhar C (2007) Nonsteroidal anti-inflammatory drugs for heavy menstrual bleeding. Cochrane Database Syst Rev (4):CD000400

21. Farquhar C, Brown J (2009) Oral contraceptive pill for heavy menstrual bleeding. Cochrane Database Syst Rev(4): CD000154
22. Fraser IS, McCarron G (1991) Randomized trial of 2 hormonal and 2 prostaglandin-inhibiting agents in women with a complaint of menorrhagia. Aust NZ J Obstet Gynaecol 31:66–70
23. Hickey M, Higham JM, Fraser I (2007) Progestogens versus oestrogens and progestogens for irregular uterine bleeding associated with anovulation. Cochrane Database Syst Rev (4): CD001895
24. Lethaby A, Cooke I, Rees MC (2005) Progesterone or progestogen-releasing intrauterine systems for heavy menstrual bleeding. Cochrane Database Syst Rev (4):CD002126
25. Beaumont HH, Augood C, Duckitt K, Lethaby A (2007) Danazol for heavy menstrual bleeding. Cochrane Database Syst Rev (3): CD001017
26. Duckitt K (2007) Medical management of perimenopausal menorrhagia: an evidence-based approach. Menopause Int 13 (1):14–18
27. French RS, Cowan FM, Mansour D et al (2000) Levonorgestrel-releasing (20 ug/day) intrauterine systems (Mirena) compared with other methods of reversible contraceptives. Br J Obstet Gynaecol 107:1218–1225
28. Irvine GA, Campbell-Brown MB, Lumsden MA et al (1998) Randomised comparative study of the levonorgestrel itrauterine system and morethisterone for the treatment of idiopathic menorrhagia. Br J Obstet Gynaecol 105:592–598
29. Lahteenmaki P, Haukkamaa M, Puolakka J et al (1998) Open randomised study of use of levonorgestrel releasing intrauterine system as alternative to hysterectomy. BMJ 316:1122–1126
30. Mukherjee K, Jones K (2005) The treatment of dysfunctional uterine bleeding with the Mirena IUS: a survival analysis. Gynecol Surgery 2(4):251–254
31. Luukkainen T, Toivonen J (1995) Levonorgestrel–releasing IUD as a method of contraception with therapeutic properties. Contraception 52:269–276
32. Hurskainen R, Teperi J, Rissanen P et al (2001) Quality of life and cost-effectiveness of levonorgestrel-releasing intrauterine system versus hysterectomy for treatment of menorrhagia: a randomised trial. Lancet 357(9252):273–277
33. Haynes PJ, Hodgson H, Anderson AB, Turnbull AC (1977) Measurement of menstrual blood loss in patients complaining of menorrhagia. Br J Obstet Gynaecol 84:763–768
34. Ashermann JG (1948) Amenorrhea traumatica (atretica). Obstet Gynecol 55:23
35. Goldrath MH, Fuller TA, Segal S (1981) Laser photovaporization of the endometrium in the treatment of menorrhagia. Am J Obstet Gynecol 140:14–19
36. Garry R, Erian J, Grochmal SA (1991) A multi-centre collaborative study into the treatment of menorrhagia by Nd-YAG laser ablation of the endometrium. Br J Obstet Gynaecol 98:357–362
37. Erian J (1994) Endometrial ablation in the treatment of menorrhagia. Br J Obstet Gynaecol 101:19–22
38. Garry R, Shelley-Jones D, Mooney P, Phillips G (1995) Six hundred endometrial laser ablations. Obstet Gynecol 85:24–29
39. Shankar M, Naftalin N, Taub N et al (2003) The long-term effectiveness of endometrial laser ablation: a survival analysis. Eur Gynecol Reprod Biol 108:75–79
40. Philips G, Chien P, Garry R (1998) Risk of hysterectomy after 1000 consecutive laser ablations. Br J Obstet Gynaecol 105:897–903
41. Bhattacharya S, Cameron IM, Parkin DE et al (1997) A pragmatic randomised comparison of transcervical resection of the endometrium with endometrial laser ablation for the treatment of menorrhagia. Br J Obstet Gynaecol 104:601–607
42. De Cherney A, Polan ML (1983) Hysteroscopic management of intrauterine lesions and intractable uterine bleeding. Obstet Gynecol 61:392–397
43. A. Lethaby, M. Hickey and R. Garry (2005) Endometrial destruction techniques for heavy menstrual bleeding. Cochrane Database Syst Rev (4):CD001501
44. O'Connor H, Magos A (1996) Endometrial resection for the treatment of menorrhagia. N Engl J Med 335:151–156
45. O'Connor H, Broadbent JA, Magos AL et al (1997) Medical Research Council randomised trial of endometrial resection versus hysterectomy in management of menorrhagia. Lancet 349:897–901
46. Papadopoulos NP, Magos A (2007) First-generation endometrial ablation: roller-ball vs loop vs laser. Best Pract Res Clin Obstet Gynaecol 21:915–929
47. Lethaby A, Hickey M, Garry R, Penninx J (2009) Endometrial resection/ablation techniques for heavy menstrual bleeding. Cochrane Database Syst Rev (4):CD001501
48. Vancaillie TG (1989) Electrocoagulation of the endometrium with the ball-end resectoscope. Obstet Gynecol 74:425–427
49. Paskowitz RA (1995) Rollerball ablation of the endometrium. J Reprod Med 40:333–336
50. Overton C, Hargreaves J, Maresh M (1997) A national survey of the complications of endometrial destruction for menstrual disorders the MISTLETOE study. Br J Obstet Gynaecol 104:1351–1359
51. Jansen FW, Vredevoogd CB, van Ulzen K et al (2000) Complications of hysteroscopy: a prospective, multicenter study. Obstet Gynecol 96:266–270
52. Vilos GA, Brown S, Graham G et al (2000) Genital tract electrical burns during hysteroscopic endometrial ablation: report of 13 cases in the United States and Canada. J Am Assoc Gynecol Laparosc 7:141–147
53. Practice Committee of American Society for Reproductive Medicine (2008) Indications and options for endometrial ablation. Fertil Steril 90(5 Suppl):S236–S240
54. Sowter MC, Lethaby A, Singla AA (2002) Pre-operative endometrial thinning agents before endometrial destruction for heavy menstrual bleeding. Cochrane Database Syst Rev (3): CD001124
55. Vilos G, Edris F (2007) Second-generation endometrial ablation technologies: the hot liquid ballons. Best Pract Res Clin Obstet Gynaecol 21(6):947–967
56. Garza-Leal J, Pena A, Donovan A et al (2010) Clinical evaluation of a third-generation thermal uterine balloon therapy system for menorrhagia coupled with curettage. J Min Inv Gynecol 17(1):82–90
57. Gurtcheff SE, Sharp HT (2003) Complications associated with global endometrial ablation: the utility of the MAUDE database. Obstet Gynecol 102:1278–1282
58. Weisberg M (2004) Complications associated with global endometrial ablations: the utility of the MAUDE database. Obstet Gynecol 103:995
59. Ulmsten U, Carstensen H, Falconer C et al (2001) The safety and efficacy of MenoTreat, a new balloon device for thermal endometrial ablation. Acta Obstet Gynecol Scand 80:52–57
60. Vihko KK, Raitala R, Taina E (2003) Endometrial thermoablation for treatment of menorrhagia: comparison of two methods in outpatients setting. Acta Obstet Gynecol Scand 82:269–274
61. Ciantar E, Jones K (2007) Preventing hysterectomies for dysfunctional uterine bleeding with the HTA™: a survival analysis. Gynecol Surgery 4(1):39–43
62. Sharp NC, Cronin N, Feldberg I et al (1995) Microwaves for menorrhagia: a new fast technique for endometrial abllation. Lancet 346:1003–1004

63. Jameel JK, Ahmed T, Noble W, Philips K, Tised J (2005) Microwave endometrial ablation (MEA) and bowel injury. Gynecol Surgery 2(2):131–133
64. Sambrook AM, Cooper KG, Campell MK et al (2009) Clinical outcomes from a randomized comparison of microwave endometrial ablation with thermal balloon endometrial ablation for the treatment of heavy menstrual bleeding. BJOG 116(8):1038–1045
65. Donnez J, Polet R, Mathieu PE et al (1996) Endometrial laser interstitial hyperthermy: a potential modality for endometrial ablation. Obstet Gynecol 87:459–464
66. Donnez J, Polet R, Rabinivitz R et al (2000) Endometrial laser intrauterine thermotherapy: the first series of 100 patients observed for 1 year. Fertil Steril 74:791–796
67. Perino A, Castelli A, Cucinella G et al (2004) A randomized comparison of endometrial laser intrauterine thermotherapy and hysteroscopic endometrial resection. Fertil Steril 82(3):731–734
68. Marlies B (2007) Second generation endometrial ablation treatment: Novasure. Best Pract Res Clin Obstet Gynaecol 21(6):989–994
69. Cooper J, Gimpelson R, Laberge P et al (2002) A randomized, multicenter trial of safety and efficacy of the Novasure system in the treatment of menorrhagia. L Am Assoc Gynecol Laparoc 9 (4):418–428, o
70. Abbott J, Hawe J, Hunter D, Garry R (2003) A double blind randomized trial comparing the Cavatherm and the NovaSure endometrial ablation systems for the treatment of dysfunctional uterine bleeding. Fertl Steril 80:223–232
71. Bongers MY, Bourdrez P, Mol BW et al (2004) Randomized controlled trial of bipolar radio frequency endometrial ablation and balloon endometrial ablation. Br J Obstet Gynaecol 111:1095–1102
72. Bongers MY, Bourdez P, Van Der Steeg JW, Heintz AP, Brolmann HA (2005) Thermal endometrial ablation in dysfunctional uterine bleeding: an economic comparison of bipolar ablation and balloon ablation. Gynecol Surgery 2(4):271–277
73. Della Badia C, Nyirjesy P, Ata A (2007) Endometrial ablation devices: review of a manufacturer and user facility device experience database. Jmig 14:436–441
74. Pados G (2005) Laparoscopic hysterectomy: why is it not popular. In controversies in obstetrics-gynecology and infertility. Ben-Rafaeln T, Creatsas G, Shoham T (eds) Oren Publisher Ltd, International Proceedings Division, pp 518–522
75. Lethaby A, Shepperd S, Farquhar C, Cooke I (1999) Endometrial resection and ablation versus hysterectomy for heavy menstrual bleeding. Cochrane Database Syst Rev (2):CD000329
76. Lumsden MA, Twaddle S, Hawthorn R et al (2000) A randomized comparison and economic evaluation of laparoscopic-assisted hysterectomy and abdominal hysterectomy. Br J Obstet Gynaecol 107:1386–1391
77. Maresh MJA, Metcalfe MA, McPherson K et al (2002) The VALUE national hysterectomy study: description of the patients and their surgery. Br J Obstet Gynaecol 109:302–312
78. Marjoribanks J, Lethaby A, Farquhar C (2006) Surgery versus medical therapy for heavy menstrual bleeding. Cochrane Database Syst Rev (2):CD003855
79. Coulter A, Peto V, Doll H (1994) Patient's preferences and general practitioners' decisions in the treatment of menstrual disorders. Fam Pract 11:67–74
80. Cooper KG, Grant AM, Garratt AM (1997) The impact of using a partially randomized patient preference design when evaluating alternative managements for heavy menstual bleeding. Br J Obstet Gynaecol 104:1367–1373
81. Coulter A (1997) Partnerships with patients: the pros and cons of shared clinical discision making. J Health Serv Res Policy 2:112–121
82. Gambone JC, Reiter RC (1997) Hysterectomy: improving the patient's decision-making process. Clin Obstet Gynecol 40:868–877
83. Nagele F, Rubinger T, Magos A (1998) Why do women choose endometrial ablation rather than hysterectomy? Fertil Steril 69:1063–1066
84. Vercelleni P, Oldani S, Yaylayan L et al (1999) Randomised comparison of vaporising electrode and cutting loop for endometrial ablation. Obstet Gynecol 94:521–527
85. Pellicano M, Guida M, Acunzo G et al (2002) Hysteroscopic transcervical endometrial resection versus thermal destruction for menorrhagia: a prospective randomized trial on satisfaction rate. Am J Obstet Gynecol 187:545–550
86. Corson S (2001) A multicenter evaluation of endometrial ablation by hydrothermablator and rollerball for treatment of menorrhagia. J Am Assoc Gynecol Laparosc 8:359–367
87. Cooper J, Gimpelson R, Laberge P et al (2002) A randomized, multicenter trial of safety and efficacy of the NovaSure in the treatment of menorrhagia. J Am Assoc Gynecol Laparosc 9:418–428

Permissions

All chapters in this book were first published in GS, by Springer; hereby published with permission under the Creative Commons Attribution License or equivalent. Every chapter published in this book has been scrutinized by our experts. Their significance has been extensively debated. The topics covered herein carry significant findings which will fuel the growth of the discipline. They may even be implemented as practical applications or may be referred to as a beginning point for another development.

The contributors of this book come from diverse backgrounds, making this book a truly international effort. This book will bring forth new frontiers with its revolutionizing research information and detailed analysis of the nascent developments around the world.

We would like to thank all the contributing authors for lending their expertise to make the book truly unique. They have played a crucial role in the development of this book. Without their invaluable contributions this book wouldn't have been possible. They have made vital efforts to compile up to date information on the varied aspects of this subject to make this book a valuable addition to the collection of many professionals and students.

This book was conceptualized with the vision of imparting up-to-date information and advanced data in this field. To ensure the same, a matchless editorial board was set up. Every individual on the board went through rigorous rounds of assessment to prove their worth. After which they invested a large part of their time researching and compiling the most relevant data for our readers.

The editorial board has been involved in producing this book since its inception. They have spent rigorous hours researching and exploring the diverse topics which have resulted in the successful publishing of this book. They have passed on their knowledge of decades through this book. To expedite this challenging task, the publisher supported the team at every step. A small team of assistant editors was also appointed to further simplify the editing procedure and attain best results for the readers.

Apart from the editorial board, the designing team has also invested a significant amount of their time in understanding the subject and creating the most relevant covers. They scrutinized every image to scout for the most suitable representation of the subject and create an appropriate cover for the book.

The publishing team has been an ardent support to the editorial, designing and production team. Their endless efforts to recruit the best for this project, has resulted in the accomplishment of this book. They are a veteran in the field of academics and their pool of knowledge is as vast as their experience in printing. Their expertise and guidance has proved useful at every step. Their uncompromising quality standards have made this book an exceptional effort. Their encouragement from time to time has been an inspiration for everyone.

The publisher and the editorial board hope that this book will prove to be a valuable piece of knowledge for researchers, students, practitioners and scholars across the globe.

List of Contributors

R. J. Detollenaere and H. W. F. van Eijndhoven
Isala klinieken, GK Zwolle, The Netherlands

M. P. H. Vleugels
Rivierenland hospital, Tiel, The Netherlands

George H. Shade and Michael P. Diamond
Department of Obstetrics and Gynecology, Wayne State University/Detroit Medical Center 60 West Hancock Street, Detroit, MI 48201, USA

Mieke Lane
Cascadia Women's Clinic, Vancouver, WA, USA

Guri Baardstu Majak and Marit Lieng
Department of Gynecology, Oslo University Hospital—Ullevål, Kirkeveien 166, 0407 Oslo, Norway

Erik Qvigstad
University of Oslo, Norway, Oslo, Norway

Béla G. Molnár, Zsolt Kormányos and Virág Márton
Obstetrics and Gynaecology, University of Szeged, Szeged, Hungary

Luka Anðelic and Andor Góli
Obstetrics and Gynaecology, Opšta Bolnica Subotica, Subotica, Serbia

Francesco Paolo Giuseppe Leone, Stefania Calabrese, Carmelo Marciante and Irene Cetin
Department of Obstetrics and Gynecology, Clinical Sciences Institute L. Sacco, University of Milan, Via G.B. Grassi 74, 20157 Milan, Italy

Enrico Ferrazzi
Childrens' Hospital Buzzi, University of Milan, Milan, Italy

A. Hackethal, K. Eskef and H.-R. Tinneberg
Department of Obstetrics and Gynaecology, Justus-Liebig-University of Giessen
Klinikstr. 33, 35385 Giessen, Germany

M. Koppan
Department of Obstetrics and Gynecology, Health Science Center, University of Pécs, 17 Édesanyák Street, 7624 Pécs, Hungary

Henrik Skensved
Frederiksgade 2 A, 3400 Hillerod, Denmark

Mitsuru Shiota, Yasushi Kotani, Masahiko Umemoto, Takako Tobiume and Hiroshi Hoshiai
Department of Obstetrics and Gynecology, Kinki University Faculty of Medicine, 377-2 Ohno-higashi, Osaka-sayama Osaka 589-8511, Japan

Céline Castellier, Lucie Bresson, Michel Cosson and Jean-Philippe Lucot
Pôle de chirurgie gynécologique, Hôpital Jeanne de Flandre, Avenue Eugène Avinée, 59 037 Lille Cedex, France

Sharon P. Rodrigues, Moniek ter Kuile and Frank W. Jansen
Department of Gynecology, K6-76, Leiden University Medical Center, 2300 RC Leiden, The Netherlands

Jenny Dankelman and Frank W. Jansen
Department of BioMechanical Engineering, Delft University of Technology, Delft, The Netherlands

Ivo Brosens
Leuven Institute for Fertility and Embryology, Leuven, Belgium

Georg Kunz
Department of Obstetrics and Gynaecology, St-Johannes-Hospital, Dortmund, Germany

Giuseppe Benagiano
Department of Gynaecology, Obstetrics and Urology, University of Rome, Sapienza, Italy

Claire F. la Chapelle and Frank Willem Jansen
Department of Gynecology, Leiden University Medical Center, K6 room 76, 2300 RC Leiden, the Netherlands

Willem A. Bemelman
Department of Surgery, Academic Medical Center, Amsterdam, the Netherlands

Bart M. P. Rademaker
Department of Anesthesiology, Onze Lieve Vrouwe Gasthuis, Amsterdam, the Netherlands

Teus A. van Barneveld
Department of Quality in Healthcare, Dutch Association of Medical Specialists, Utrecht, the Netherlands

Midgley Gonzales, João Antônio Dias Junior, Sérgio Podgaec, Edmund Chada Baracat and Maurício Simões Abrão
Department of Obstetrics and Gynecology, University of São Paulo Medical School, Rua São Sebastião 550, 04708-001 São Paulo, São Paulo, Brazil

Leandro Accardo de Matos and Manoel Orlando da Costa Gonçalves
Digimagem Diagnósticos, São Paulo, Brazil

Roberto Blasbalg
Department of Radiology, University of São Paulo Medical School, São Paulo, Brazil

Maria-Laura Marotta, Nathalie Michaux and Olivier Donnez
Department of Gynecology, CHU Mont-Godinne, Université Catholique de Louvain, Av. G. Thérasse, 1, 5530 Yvoir, Belgium

Jacques Donnez
Pôle de Recherche en Gynécologie, Institut de Recherche Expérimentale et Clinique (IREC), Université Catholique de Louvain (UCL), 1200 Brussels, Belgium
Department of Gynecology, Cliniques Universitaires Saint-Luc, 1200 Brussels, Belgium

Michaël Dupont
Department of Radiology, CHU Mont-Godinne, Université Catholique de Louvain, 5530 Yvoir, Belgium

Monique Delos
Department of Anatomopathology, CHU Mont-Godinne, Université Catholique de Louvain, 5530 Yvoir, Belgium

Vinod Kumar
University Hospitals Birmingham NHS Foundation Trust, Birmingham, UK

Jonathan Chester
Good Hope Hospital, Birmingham, UK

Janesh Gupta and Manjeet Shehmar
Birmingham Women's NHS Foundation Trust, Birmingham, UK

Ayman Qatawneh, Fawaz Al-Kazaleh, Shawqi Saleh, Fida Thekrallah, Majed Bata and Issa Sumreen
Department of Obstetrics and Gynaecology, Faculty of Medicine, The University of Jordan, Amman 11942, Jordan

Mahmoud Al-Mustafa
Department of Anaesthesia, Faculty of Medicine, The University of Jordan, Amman, Jordan

Fiona L. Mackie
Education and Research Centre, Pennine Acute Trust, Royal Oldham Hospital, Rochdale Road, Oldham OL12JH, UK

Sofia Dias
School of Social and Community Medicine, University of Bristol, Canynge Hall, 39 Whatley Road, Bristol BS8 2PS, UK

Andrew Watson
FRCOG, Department of Obstetrics and Gynaecology, Tameside General Hospital, Fountain Street, Ashton Under Lyne, Lancashire OL6 9RW, UK

Gaity Ahmad
MRCOG, Department of Obstetrics and Gynaecology, Pennine Acute Trust, Royal Oldham Hospital, Rochdale Road, Oldham OL12JH, UK

Togas Tulandi
Department of Obstetrics and Gynecology, McGill University, 687 Pine Ave. West, Montreal, Quebec H3A 1A1, Canada

Deirdre J. Lyell
Department of Obstetrics and Gynecology, Stanford University, Stanford, CA, USA

Sylvie Gordts, Patrick Puttemans, Rudi Campo, Marion Valkenburg and Stephan Gordts
LIFE, Tiensevest 168, Leuven 3000, Belgium

O. E. O'Sullivan, M. O'Carroll, M. Hewitt and B. A. O'Reilly
Department of Obstetrics and Gynaecology, Cork University Maternity Hospital, Cork, Ireland

B. M. E. Adriaanse
Department of Obstetrics and Gynaecology, VU University Medical Centre, PK 6Z 170, De Boelelaan 1117, 1081 HV Amsterdam, The Netherlands

R. Natté
Department of Pathology, Haga Teaching Hospital, The Hague, The Netherlands

B. W. J. Hellebrekers
Department of Obstetrics and Gynaecology, Haga Teaching Hospital, The Hague, The Netherlands

Tania Dexter
49, Kennedy Road, Horsham, West Sussex RH13 5DB, England UK

Vincent Boama
Department of Obstetrics and Gynaecology, Hampshire Hospitals NHS Foundation Trust, Aldermaston Road, Basingstoke, Hampshire RG 24 9FT, UK

Vinod Kumar
Community Sexual and Reproductive Healthcare, University Hospitals Birmingham NHS Foundation Trust, Birmingham, UK

Janesh Kumar Gupta
Clinical and Experimental Medicine, University of Birmingham, Birmingham Women's NHS Foundation Trust, Edgbaston, B15 2TG Birmingham, UK

Anita J. Merritt, Ilze Zommere, Richard J. Slade and Brett Winter-Roach
Department of Gynaecology, Salford Royal Hospitals NHS Trust, Stott Lane, Salford M6 8HD, UK

J. Claeys, I. Hellendoorn, T. Hamerlynck and S. Weyers
Department of Obstetrics and Gynecology, Ghent University Hospital, Ghent, Belgium

J. Bosteels
Department of Obstetrics and Gynecology, Imelda Hospital, Bonheiden, Belgium

Arpita Ghosh, Daniel Borlase, Tosin Ajala and Anthony James Kelly
Brighton and Sussex University Hospitals NHS Trust, Brighton, UK

Zaky Ibrahim
Western Sussex Hospitals NHS Trust, West Sussex, UK

Patrick Campbell, Caitriona Monaghan and Michael Parker
Obstetrics & Gynaecology, Altnagelvin Area Hospital, Londonderry, Northern Ireland, UK

Vicente Payá, Juan José Hidalgo-Mora, Cesar Diaz-Garcia and Antonio Pellicer
Department of Gynecology and Human Reproduction, La Fe University Hospital, Bulevar Sur, 46026 Valencia, Spain

Fady Shehata, Einat Shalom-Paz and Togas Tulandi
Department of Obstetrics and Gynecology, McGill University Health Center, 687 Pine Avenue West, Montreal, QC, Canada H3A 1A1

Afsoon Zarei
Department of Obstetrics and Gynecology, Shiraz University of Medical Sciences Shiraz, Iran

Seumas Eckford
Department of Obstetrics and Gynaecology, North Devon District Hospital, Barnstaple, Devon, UK

Sharif I. M. F. Ismail
Department of Obstetrics and Gynaecology, North Devon District Hospital, Barnstaple Devon, UK
Department of Obstetrics and Gynaecology, Singleton Hospital, Swansea, South Wales, UK
Department of Obstetrics and Gynaecology, Wrexham Maelor Hospital, Wrexham, North Wales, UK
Department of Obstetrics and Gynaecology, Royal Bournemouth Hospital, Dorset, UK
Department of Obstetrics and Gynaecology, Yeovil District Hospital, Somerset, UK
Department of Obstetrics and Gynaecology, Royal Sussex County Hospital, Brighton BN2 5BE, UK

S. Eckford
Department of Obstetrics and Gynaecology, North Devon District Hospital, Barnstaple Devon, UK

Salih Taşkın, Tolga Taşcı, Murat Sönmezer and Cem Atabekoğlu
Department of Obstetrics and Gynecology, Ankara University Medical Faculty, Ankara, Turkey

Murat Gözüküçük
Ankara Universitesi Tip Fak, Kadin Dog, AD 06100 Cebeci, Ankara, Turkey

Santiago Domingo, Marta Gurrea and Antonio Pellicer
Gynecology Oncology Service, Department of Obstetrics and Gynecology, Hospital Universitario La Fe, Avda Campanar, 21, 46009 Valencia, Spain

M. Setälä
Department of Obstetrics and Gynecology, Päijät-Häme Central Hospital, Lahti, Finland

P. Suvitie, A. Perheentupa and J. Mäkinen
Turku University Hospital, Turku, Finland

J. Jalkanen and P. Härkki
Department of Obstetrics and Gynecology, Helsinki University Hospital, Helsinki, Finland

J. Fraser
Department of Obstetrics and Gynecology, North Karelian Central Hospital, Joensuu, Finland

J. Kössi
Department of Surgery, Päijät-Häme Central Hospital, Lahti, Finland

Boaz Sheizaf, Beniamin Almog, Kareemah Salamah, Fady Shehata, Janet Takefman and Togas Tulandi
Department of Obstetrics and Gynecology, McGill University, 687 Pine Avenue West, Montreal, QC, Canada H3A 1A1

George Pados, Dimitrios Athanatos, Dimitrios Tsolakidis, Panagiotis Stamatopoulos and Basil Tarlatzis
First Department OB-GYN, Aristotle University, Thessaloniki, Greece

Index

www.ingramcontent.com/pod-product-compliance
Lightning Source LLC
LaVergne TN
LVHW060941220926
848485LV00015B/1210